D1506802

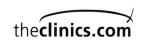

PHYSICAL MEDICINE AND REHABILITATION CLINICS

OF NORTH AMERICA

Gender Specific Medicine: The Physiatrist and Women's Health

GUEST EDITORS
Sheila A. Dugan, MD and
Heidi Prather, DO

CONSULTING EDITOR
George H. Kraft, MD, MS

August 2007 • Volume 18 • Number 3

SAUNDERS

An Imprint of Elsevier, Inc.
PHILADELPHIA   LONDON   TORONTO   MONTREAL   SYDNEY   TOKYO

W.B. SAUNDERS COMPANY
A Division of Elsevier Inc.

1600 John F. Kennedy Blvd. • Suite 1800 • Philadelphia, Pennsylvania 19103

http://www.theclinics.com

PHYSICAL MEDICINE AND REHABILITATION	**Volume 18, Number 3**
CLINICS OF NORTH AMERICA	**ISSN 1047-9651**
August 2007	**ISBN 1-4160-5113-9**
Editor: Debora Dellapena	**978-1-4160-5113-8**

The ideas and opinions expressed in *Physical Medicine and Rehabilitation Clinics of North America* do not necessarily reflect those of the Publisher. The Publisher does not assume any responsibility for any injury and/or damage to persons or property arising out of or related to any use of the material contained in this periodical. The reader is advised to check the appropriate medical literature and the product information currently provided by the manufacturer of each drug to be administered to verify the dosage, the method and duration of administration, or contraindications. It is the responsibility of the treating physician or other health care professional, relying on independent experience and knowledge of the patient, to determine drug dosages and the best treatment for the patient. Mention of any product in this issue should not be construed as endorsement by the contributors, editors, or the Publisher of the product or manufacturers' claims.

Physical Medicine and Rehabilitation Clinics of North America (ISSN 1047-9651) is published quarterly by Elsevier Inc., 360 Park Avenue South, New York, NY 10010-1710. Months of publication are February, May, August, and November. Business and Editorial Offices: 1600 John F. Kennedy Blvd., Suite 1800, Philadelphia, PA 19103-2899. Customer Service Office: 6277 Sea Harbor Drive, Orlando, FL 32887-4800. Periodicals postage paid at New York, NY and additional mailing offices. Subscription price per year is $179.00 (US individuals), $275.00 (US institutions), $90.00 (US students), $218.00 (Canadian individuals), $352.00 (Canadian institutions), $123.00 (Canadian students), $252.00 (foreign individuals), $352.00 (foreign institutions), and $123.00 (foreign students). Foreign air speed delivery is included in all *Clinics* subscription prices. All prices are subject to change without notice. POSTMASTER: Send address changes to *Physical Medicine and Rehabilitation Clinics of North America*, Elsevier Periodicals Customer Service, 6277 Sea Harbor Drive, Orlando, FL 32887-4800. **Customer Service: 1-800-654-2452 (US). From outside of the US, call 1-407-345-4000.**

Physical Medicine and Rehabilitation Clinics of North America is indexed in *Excerpta Medica, Index Medicus, Cinahl*, and *Cumulative Index to Nursing and Allied Health Literature*.

Printed in the United States of America.

CONSULTING EDITOR

GEORGE H. KRAFT, MD, MS, Alvord Professor of Multiple Sclerosis Research; Professor, Department of Rehabilitation Medicine; Adjunct Professor, Neurology; Director, Electrodiagnostic Medicine, Western Multiple Sclerosis Center; and Co-Director, Muscular Dystrophy Clinic, University of Washington, Seattle, Washington

GUEST EDITORS

SHEILA A. DUGAN, MD, Director, Women's Spine Program, Chicago Institute of Neurosurgery and Neuroresearch; Assistant Professor, Department of Physical Medicine and Rehabilitation; Assistant Professor, Department of Preventive Medicine, Rush Medical College, Rush University Medical Center, Chicago, Illinois

HEIDI PRATHER, DO, Associate Professor; Chief, Section of Physical Medicine and Rehabilitation, Department of Orthopaedic Surgery, Washington University School of Medicine, Washington University, St. Louis, Missouri

CONTRIBUTORS

JOANNE BORG-STEIN, MD, Assistant Professor, Physical Medicine and Rehabilitation, Harvard Medical School; Medical Director, Spaulding-Wellesley Rehabilitation Center, Wellesley, Massachusetts; and Medical Director, Newton Wellesley Hospital Spine Center, Newton, Massachusetts

ANDREA L. CHEVILLE, MD, MSCE, Senior Associate Consultant, Department of Physical Medicine and Rehabilitation, Mayo Clinic, Rochester, Minnesota

JOHN CLOHISY, MD, Associate Professor; Co-Chief, Adult Reconstructive Surgery; Director, Adolescent and Young Adult Hip Service, Department of Orthopaedic Surgery, Washington University School of Medicine, Washington University, St. Louis, Missouri

BARBARA J. DELATEUR, MD, MS, Professor, Department of Physical Medicine and Rehabilitation, Johns Hopkins University, Johns Hopkins Hospital; and Rehabilitation Services, Johns Hopkins Bayview Medical Center, Baltimore, Maryland

SHEILA A. DUGAN, MD, Director, Women's Spine Program, Chicago Institute of Neurosurgery and Neuroresearch; Assistant Professor, Department of Physical Medicine and Rehabilitation; Assistant Professor, Department of Preventive Medicine, Rush Medical College, Rush University Medical Center, Chicago, Illinois

JENNIFER E. EARL, PhD, ATC, Assistant Professor of Human Movement Sciences, University of Wisconsin, Milwaukee, Athletic Training Education Program; Clinical Assistant Professor, Medical College of Wisconsin, Department of Orthopaedic Surgery, Milwaukee, Wisconsin

LOUIS A. GILULA, MD, Professor, Mallinckrodt Institute of Radiology, Washington University School of Medicine, St. Louis, Missouri

DANICA N. GIUGLIANO, BA, Ludwig Research Fellow, Women's Sports Medicine Center, Hospital for Special Surgery, New York, New York

DAVID D. GUTTERMAN, MD, Professor, Cardiovascular Medicine, Cardiovascular Center, Medical College of Wisconsin, Milwaukee, Wisconsin

ANNE Z. HOCH, DO, FACSM, Associate Professor, Departments of Orthopaedic Surgery and Physical Medicine and Rehabilitation, Medical College of Wisconsin, Milwaukee; Director, Women's Sports Medicine Fellowship; Director, Women's Sports Medicine Program/Sports Medicine Center, Medical College of Wisconsin, Milwaukee, Wisconsin

DEVYANI HUNT, MD, Clinical Instructor; Co-Director Women's Health Service, Physical Medicine and Rehabilitation, Department of Orthopaedic Surgery, Washington University School of Medicine, Washington University, St. Louis, Missouri

JASON W. JURVA, MD, Assistant Professor, Cardiovascular Medicine, Cardiovascular Center, Medical College of Wisconsin, Milwaukee, Wisconsin

SOPHIA LAL, DO, Instructor; Fellow, Women's Sports Medicine Program/Sports Medicine Center, Department of Orthopaedic Surgery, Medical College of Wisconsin, Milwaukee, Wisconsin

HEIDI PRATHER, DO, Associate Professor; Chief, Section of Physical Medicine and Rehabilitation, Department of Orthopaedic Surgery, Washington University School of Medicine, Washington University, St. Louis, Missouri

WENDY S. SHORE, PhD, Department of Physical Medicine and Rehabilitation, Johns Hopkins University, Johns Hopkins Hospital, Baltimore, Maryland

JULIE K. SILVER, MD, Assistant Professor, Harvard Medical School, Department of Physical Medicine and Rehabilitation, Boston, Massachusetts

MEHRSHEED SINAKI, MD, MSc, Consultant, Department of Physical Medicine and Rehabilitation, Mayo Clinic; Professor of Physical Medicine and Rehabilitation, Mayo Clinic, Rochester, Minnesota

JENNIFER L. SOLOMON, MD, Assistant Attending Physiatrist, Women's Sports Medicine Center, Hospital for Special Surgery; and Clinical Instructor of Physical Medicine and Rehabilitation, Weill Medical College, Cornell University, New York, New York

THERESA MONACO SPITZNAGLE, PT, DPT, MHS, Clinical Instructor, Program In Physical Therapy, Washington University School of Medicine, St. Louis, Missouri

CAROLE S. VETTER, MD, ATC, Assistant Professor, Division Sports Medicine, Department of Orthopaedic Surgery, Medical College of Wisconsin, Milwaukee, Wisconsin

JOHN O. WATSON, MD, Instructor, Section of Physical Medicine and Rehabilitation, Washington University Orthopedics, St. Louis, Missouri

KATHLEEN M. WEBER, MD, Assistant Professor, Department of Internal Medicine; Assistant Professor, Department of Orthopedic Surgery, Rush Medical College, Midwest Orthopedics, Chicago, Illinois

CONTENTS

> The past 35 years have seen a tremendous increase in the number
> of female athletes at all ages and abilities. Recent research has
> shown a myriad of benefits for girls and women who participate
> in sports. Physical activity positively influences almost every as-
> pect of a young woman's health, from her physiology to her social
> interactions and mental health. As the level of girls participation in
> sports increases, it is important to examine their risk factors for
> sports-related injuries.

> In the past 35 years, a significant increase has occurred in sports
> participation by women. An estimated 3 million girls and young
> women compete in American high school sports. Women who par-
> ticipate in sports and fitness programs are generally healthier and
> have higher self-esteem. However, an increase has also been seen
> in gender-specific injuries and medical problems. The female ath-
> lete triad is a syndrome of separate but interrelated conditions of
> disordered eating, amenorrhea, and osteoporosis. Athletic ame-
> norrhea is known to have a hormonal profile similar to menopause

characterized by decreased circulating estrogens. Menopause is known to be associated with osteoporosis and accelerated cardiovascular disease. Although enhanced risk for cardiovascular disease is theoretically possible, it has not been explored in the young athletic population. Premature cardiovascular disease first manifests as endothelial dysfunction, which can be examined noninvasively with ultrasound. This article discusses disordered eating, amenorrhea, osteoporosis, and the potential for heightened cardiovascular risk in young athletic women.

The Child Bearing Years

Musculoskeletal Disorders of Pregnancy, Delivery and Postpartum

Joanne Borg-Stein and Sheila Dugan

Gender-specific care of musculoskeletal impairments is increasingly important in women's health. This is most relevant and of paramount importance as it relates to identification and management of musculoskeletal and peripheral neurologic disorders of pregnancy, delivery, and postpartum. The specific anatomic and physiologic changes of pregnancy predispose to a specific set of diagnoses. Virtually all women experience some degree of musculoskeletal discomfort during pregnancy. This article provides an overview of the more common pregnancy-related musculoskeletal conditions and includes a discussion of epidemiology, risk factors, diagnosis, prognosis, and management.

Recognizing and Treating Pelvic Pain and Pelvic Floor Dysfunction

Heidi Prather, Theresa Monaco Spitznagle, and Sheila A. Dugan

The reported prevalence rates of pain within the pelvis range from 3.8% to 24% in women aged 15 to 73 years. Despite the significant number of women affected, pelvic floor pain and dysfunction are commonly overlooked in women seeking medical care. Physiatrists are uniquely qualified to manage these patients because of their knowledge of the musculoskeletal and nervous systems and their awareness of the relationships among pain, physiology, and function. When evaluating women who have pelvic pain, practitioners must ask questions about history of urinary or fecal incontinence, dyspareunia, or pelvic pain with certain activities or associated with menses, surgery, or trauma. If left unidentified, pelvic floor dysfunction can deter individuals from normal bowel and bladder function, intimacy, and even engagement in work and social functions. This article introduces pelvic floor anatomy, neurophysiology, and function and provides an overview of pelvic pain and pelvic floor dysfunctions and their recognition and treatment.

Acetabular Labral Tears of the Hip in Women

Devyani Hunt, John Clohisy, and Heidi Prather

Acetabular labral tears are a major cause of hip dysfunction in young patients and a primary precursor to hip osteoarthritis. In addition, labral disease more commonly occurs in women and can present with nonspecific symptoms. It is possible to diagnose, quantify, and treat labral tears before the onset of secondary joint deterioration. However, the diagnosis requires a high index of suspicion, special attention to subtle patterns of presentation, and timely consideration for imaging studies. Treatment options are still evolving and include a wide array of nonsurgical and surgical techniques. Treatment should also address secondary dysfunction that can be associated with hip pathology. An initial trial of conservative management is recommended and failure to progress is an indication for surgical consultation.

Rehabilitation in Women with Breast Cancer 521
Julie K. Silver

The diagnosis and treatment of breast cancer in women has undergone profound changes in the past century. Although much research and clinical attention has been focused on saving the lives of women with this condition, less focus has been on rehabilitation aspects. This postacute care should be a distinct phase of treatment. The field of physical medicine and rehabilitation has much to offer women who undergo extremely toxic although life-prolonging therapies for breast cancer. The focus of rehabilitation should include improving strength and cardiovascular conditioning, alleviating pain and improving fatigue. With respect to exercise, this can help women to physically recover from treatment and potentially prevent cancer recurrence. Many exciting opportunities will be available for rehabilitation specialists to improve the care of women with breast cancer and to participate in research in the field of oncology rehabilitation.

Current and Future Trends in Lymphedema Management: Implications for Women's Health 539
Andrea L. Cheville

Breast cancer has served as a catalyst for improvements in lymphedema care and research for the last 20 years. Awareness must be extended to other instigating factors in light of shifting epidemiology. The aging population, obesity epidemic, and higher 5-year cancer survival rates are changing the face of lymphedema. Lymphedema patients are now older, heavier, and more medically complex. A higher proportion have nonbreast malignancies and advanced cancer. This article describes the current standard of care, as well as recent concessions for patient comfort, convenience, and economic reality. Primary prevention remains underemphasized. Patient education, timely diagnosis, and the early initiation of treatment represent important targets for improvement. Hopefully, new diagnostic tools for detecting subclinical lymphedema, identifying modifiable risk factors, and better understanding lymphedema pathogenesis will improve primary prevention and care.

Midlife Women

As noted in research on frailty in women, regular exercise can limit age-related functional decline. However, physical activity has been implicated in the etiology of such musculoskeletal disorders as osteoarthritis. Proper exercise plans must strike a balance between promoting health and limiting the risk of injury. This article discusses age-related musculoskeletal changes and gender-specific conditions that may predispose midlife and older women to musculoskeletal injuries. The controversy about how physical activity may relate to osteoarthritis is discussed, along with common osteoarthritic-related spinal and appendicular conditions. Exercise prescription for women is briefly presented. The consistent message in the literature is that exercise is a safe and powerful tool to prevent and treat many medical, psychological, and musculoskeletal conditions in females at midlife and beyond.

Post-Menopause

As the aging population grows, vertebral compression fractures are becoming an important source of pain and dysfunction. Management can be complex, because care may require multiple treatment modalities and the treatment plan must be tailored to the individual's pain, functional limitations, and goals. Treatment options usually involve a combination of medications, bracing, and physical therapy. This article reviews current recommendations for managing vertebral compression fractures. Indications, complications, and treatment options, including vertebral augmentation, are discussed.

Locomotion has always been a major criterion for human survival. Thus, it is no surprise that science supports the dependence of bone health on weight-bearing physical activities. The effect of physical activity on bone is site-specific. Determining how to perform osteogenic exercises, especially in individuals who have osteopenia or osteoporosis, without exceeding the biomechanical competence of bone always poses a dilemma and must occur under medical advice. This article presents the hypothesis that back exercises performed in a prone position, rather than a vertical position, may have a greater effect on decreasing the risk for vertebral fractures without resulting in compression fracture. The risk for vertebral fractures can be reduced through improvement in the horizontal trabecular connection of vertebral bodies.

Frailty is a complex subject, and all aspects of frailty are intertwined. This article identifies and discusses the individual aspects of frailty. These aspects, including sarcopenia, nutrition, obesity, relative strength, inflammatory markers, osteopenia and osteoporosis, aerobic capacity, absolute strength, balance, and prevention of frailty, must be reunited, albeit in varying combinations, if the effects of frailty on women are to be understood and treated. This article does not exhaust the topic, but covers what the authors consider to be the major issues.

FORTHCOMING ISSUES

RECENT ISSUES

VISIT OUR WEB SITE

The Clinics are now available online!
Access your subscription at www.theclinics.com

ELSEVIER
SAUNDERS

Phys Med Rehabil Clin N Am
18 (2007) xv–xvi

PHYSICAL MEDICINE
AND REHABILITATION
CLINICS OF
NORTH AMERICA

Foreword

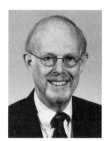

George H. Kraft, MD, MS
Consulting Editor

Dr. Heidi Prather is a star. She is an associate professor and director of Physical Medicine and Rehabilitation at the Washington University School of Medicine in St.Louis. Her Spine Fellowship and musculoskeletal medicine teaching programs are popular and highly sought after by graduating Physical Medicine and Rehabilitation residents. Dr. Prather is active in the American Academy of Physical Medicine and Rehabilitation (AAPM&R) and the Physiatric Association of Spine, Sports, and Occupational Medicine.

In 2005, Dr. Heidi Prather was honored by the AAPM&R at its annual meeting in Philadelphia, where she gave the Richard and Hinda Rosenthal Foundation lecture. After hearing that lecture, I understood why my residents were raving about her teaching, and asked her to be the Guest Editor of an issue on women's health and musculoskeletal medicine.

Dr. Prather accepted, and recruited Dr. Sheila A. Dugan, a physiatrist at the Chicago Institute for Neurosurgery and Neuroresearch in Elmhurst, Illinois, to assist with the issue as her Co-Guest Editor. This August 2007 issue is the outstanding result.

Gender Specific Medicine: The Physiatrist and Women's Health focuses on the rehabilitative treatment of sports-related injuries in women. But it covers much more than that. This issue also delves into activity-associated problems of females, both in active stages of youth as well as in aging.

Topics covered include the role of physical activity in bone health—and reduction of spinal fractures—as well as in cardiovascular health. Stress fractures, patellofemoral pain, ACL tears, and acetabular labral tears are specifically discussed. Frequent problems of women such as breast cancer,

1047-9651/07/$ - see front matter © 2007 Elsevier Inc. All rights reserved.
doi:10.1016/j.pmr.2007.06.003   *pmr.theclinics.com*

lymphedema, problems of pregnancy (pre partum, delivery, and post partum), and pelvic pain are also examined. The discussions range from diseases of the young female athlete to the postmenopausal and geriatric woman.

This is a comprehensive *Clinics* issue that will appeal to all physicians who treat women—especially those women engaged in sports or other forms of physical activity. I hope that the practicing physician will keep this issue handy. It will be used frequently.

George H. Kraft, MD, MS
University of Washington
Box 356490, 1959 NE Pacific Street
Seattle, WA 98195-6490, USA

E-mail address: ghkraft@u.washington.edu

ELSEVIER
SAUNDERS

Phys Med Rehabil Clin N Am
18 (2007) xvii–xviii

PHYSICAL MEDICINE
AND REHABILITATION
CLINICS OF
NORTH AMERICA

Preface

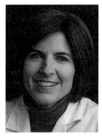 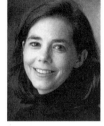

Sheila A. Dugan, MD   Heidi Prather, DO
Guest Editors

Historically, women's health services have been relegated to reproductive concerns. Physiatrists consider women's health in a much broader context, as we have been trained to do for all patients. This larger context inspired us to bring together this issue of the *Physical Medicine and Rehabilitation Clinics*. Because of their knowledge of the musculoskeletal system, the nervous system, and awareness of the relationship between pain, physiology, and function, physiatrists are uniquely qualified to manage girls and women who have painful and debilitating conditions.

One key factor in providing appropriate care is matching the patient's problem with the patient's place in her lifespan. Health behaviors in childhood set the stage for bone development, skill acquisition, weight management, body image, and self-esteem. The childbearing years bring unique experiences to women's lives with associated biomechanical, hormonal, and psychosocial changes that set the tone for her future mind and body. Cancers specific to the reproductive system and their sequelae, such as lymphedema, bring medical and functional challenges to women and health care providers. For women who have cancer, physiatrists can provide care that focuses on function during and after treatment that goes beyond the focus of the oncology health care providers. Midlife and the hormonal changes and changes in body composition bring a host of associated medical problems. Exercise and physical activity can mediate these problems and maintain and improve failing physical function, especially in the setting of chronic health conditions such as osteoarthritis and heart disease. Aging women have expectations for health, quality of life, and independence.

doi:10.1016/j.pmr.2007.06.002

Physiatrists can partner with older women for conservative management of osteoporosis, with the focus, again, being on function. Physiatrists are leading the way in research and education about osteoporosis and prevention and treatment of frailty.

We are delighted to present this issue of *Physical Medicine and Rehabilitation Clinics*. We hope you will benefit from the expertise of your colleagues. These authors have dedicated their clinical and research careers to making a difference in the lives of girls and women by tackling challenging health concerns such as the female athlete triad, hip and knee disorders, and pregnancy-related musculoskeletal issues, to name only a few. We truly appreciate their affirmative responses when we asked each of them to share their unique perspective on girls' and women's health issues.

We would like to dedicate this edition to those women who have inspired us personally and professionally. We embrace and celebrate your mentorship and strength of purpose.

Sheila A. Dugan, MD
University Physical Medicine and Rehabilitation
Rush University Medical Center
1725 W. Harrison Street, Suite 970
Chicago, IL 60612, USA

E-mail address: Sheila_Dugan@rush.edu

Heidi Prather, DO
Washington University Orthopedics
Suite 11300, One Barnes Jewish Hospital Plaza
St. Louis, MO 63110

E-mail address: pratherh@wudosis.wustl.edu

ELSEVIER
SAUNDERS

Phys Med Rehabil Clin N Am
18 (2007) 361–383

PHYSICAL MEDICINE
AND REHABILITATION
CLINICS OF
NORTH AMERICA

Factors That Affect the Young Female Athlete

Sophia Lal, DO*, Anne Z. Hoch, DO, FACSM

Sports Medicine Center, Medical College of Wisconsin, Milwaukee, WI 53226, USA

History of women in sports

The past 35 years have seen a tremendous increase in the number of female athletes at all ages and abilities. The civil rights federal law Title IX of 1972 [1] prohibits sex discrimination at any educational institutions that receive federal funds, including school-sponsored sports. The number of high school girls playing competitive sports increased from fewer than 300,000 before Title IX to almost 3 million in 2005–2006, an increase of 1004% (Fig. 1) [2].

Historically, women were excluded from most sports. In 1896, the first modern Olympics did not let women compete because of a concern that they could injure their reproductive organs. Women were introduced gradually into the Olympic arena; in 1904 archery was added, in 1908 lawn tennis and figure skating were included, and then women's diving and swimming were added to the 1912 Stockholm Olympics. The 1920s saw a trend toward the elimination of interscholastic competition for girls because of its "undue stress" and "morbid social influences." During these times, Babe Didrikson Zaharias, who is considered the female athletic phenomenon of the 20th century, found very limited opportunities to compete in sports [3]. Throughout her athletic career, she endlessly challenged the public's stereotype while excelling in multiple sports, including those dominated by men. The Associated Press ultimately named Zaharias the Woman Athlete of the Half Century in 1950 [4].

Sport has been one of the most important sociocultural learning experiences for boys and men, and those same benefits were becoming available to girls and women especially in the last 35 years. ABC televised the 1968 Winter Games live and in color for the first time, and the enduring image is of

---

* Corresponding author.

E-mail address: sophialal@hotmail.com (S. Lal).

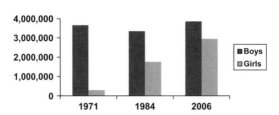

Fig. 1. Participation by boys and girls in interscholastic high school athletics from 1971–2006.

Peggy Fleming's free-skating program. She won the Gold Medal, the only Gold Medal the United States brought home from Grenoble [5]. During the 1968 Summer Olympics, Georgia's Wyomia Tyus set a world record running the 100 meter in 11.08 seconds [6]. By the end of her career, Tyus held world records at both 100 yards and 100 meters, won eight National AAU titles, five of them outdoors, and was elected to the U.S. Olympic Hall of Fame in 1985. At those same Summer Games, Debbie Meyer won a gold medal in the 200, 400, and 800-meter freestyles, making her the first woman swimmer to win three individual gold medals at one Olympic Games. Over the course of her career, Meyer broke 20 world and 24 American records. She was named Swimming World magazine's Swimmer of the Year from 1967 to 1969. She won the 1968 Sullivan Award as the top amateur athlete in the country. She was inducted into the International Swimming Hall of Fame in 1977 and into the U.S. Olympic Hall of Fame in 1987 [7].

In 1973, just 1 year after Title IX was passed and during the infancy of the Equal Rights Movement, Billie Jean King brought women's tennis and women's sports into prime time as she defeated Bobby Riggs in the internationally televised "Battle of the Sexes." In 1974, she helped establish a player's union and professional women's tour and fought for equal pay [8]. She then founded the Women's Sports Foundation, a charitable educational organization dedicated to advancing the lives of girls and women through sports and physical activity [9]. By 1996, Women's Team Events dominated the Atlanta Olympics in soccer, basketball, softball, and gymnastics, witnessing a 27% increase in participation compared with the previous 1992 Olympic Games in Los Angeles [10]. Mia Hamm and the United States women's national soccer team won the gold medal in front of 80,000 spectators, an all-time record for any women's sporting event [11]. In 1999, Women's Soccer USA became the World Cup Champions, and by 2001, the Women's United Soccer Association held its first game [12]. The Women's National Basketball Association (WNBA) began play in June 1997. In 2001, WNBA games were broadcast to nearly 60 million fans in 23 different languages and 167 countries [13].

Obvious financial differences exist between compensation for the professional male and female athlete. So far the WNBA's monetary success has not mirrored that of the NBA's. The maximum salary for a WNBA player in 2007 was $100,000. Many WNBA players choose to supplement their salaries by playing in Australian women's basketball leagues during the WNBA off-season [14]. 2006 WNBA hard salary cap was $700,000 and the minimum for a four-year veteran was about $47,000 [15]. In comparison, the 2006-07 NBA salary cap was $53.135 million and the average salary was $5.215 million [16,17]. At the top of Forbes list of highest-paid athletes, Tiger Woods is recognized as the world's best-paid athlete. According to David Carter, professor of sports business at the University of Southern California, Woods has what it takes to be marketable. He is not only artic-ulate but also attractive, clean-cut, and scandal-free. "Ultimately, it boils down to whether an athlete has charisma, believability and the ability to communicate. Tiger Woods has all of these things." Another solid Nike in-vestment like Woods, tennis player Maria Sharapova is the world's best-compensated female athlete [18]. She is safe and likable, and beautiful. In comparison to Woods who earned $87 million in 2005, Sharapova earned $18+ million in the same year. Annika Sorenstam, the world's top-ranked female golfer, made $7.3 million that year [18]. The number of women on the Forbes list is less than a handful.

Women athletes have been successful at increasing their earnings. When the Ladies Professional Golf Association (LPGA) first began in 1950, the top purse was $15,000 and grew to $30.3 million by 1997 (43 events). Michelle Wei won the U.S. Women's Amateur Public Links Championship at age 13. At age 14, Wie narrowly missed becoming the first woman to make a cut on the men's United States tour since 1945. Now at 17 years old, according to Golf World magazine, Wie will be the most recognized female athlete in the world, because not only is she capable of rewriting female golf's record books but she also has an almost perfect profile for advertisers. With a Ko-rean background and born in Hawaii, Wie is the ideal sponsorship vehicle for both golf's biggest current market, the United States, and its biggest new market, the Far East. "Once the apparel line gets rolling and you have a cou-ple of other major endorsements her earnings could reach $30–40 million a year," said Brandon Steiner of Steiner Sports Marketing [19]. The women's winner of the 2005 New York City Marathon took home $130,000. The women's purse was the largest purse in marathon history and was $30,000 larger than the 2005 men's purse [20]. Although female athletes are making strides financially, they still have a large monetary gap to close.

Recent research has shown a myriad of benefits for girls and women who participate in sports. Physical activity positively influences almost every as-pect of a young woman's health, from her physiology to her social interac-tions and mental health. High school girls who are active in sports have higher graduation rates, fewer unwanted pregnancies, and greater self-esteem than those who are not active [21]. Regular exercise has been shown to decrease the risk for multiple diseases, including obesity and type II dia-betes, and has shown modest protection against breast cancer [22], coronary heart disease, hypertension, osteoporosis, depression [23], and some cancers of the reproductive system [24]. The U.S. Preventive Services Task Force

and the Office of Disease Prevention and Health Promotion have emphasized that physical activity and fitness must be viewed as a health priority
among the older population (with women as the majority). Clearly, encouraging an active lifestyle among women is critical to the long-term health of
the United States [25]. With these benefits, health care providers should become aware of the unique issues these women face as athletes.

Body image

For at least the past 40 years, Western cultures have valued and idealized
youthfulness and slimness in women. For the past 44 years, men have
swooned over James Bond's women. The Bond Girls have become an
icon of film history and broken fashion boundaries with their sexy, mesmer-
izing style. The Bond films always show a strong appreciation for the silhouette of a woman's body (such a silhouette is featured in the classic opening
of the films). As Playboy founder Hugh Hefner states,

> As much as I think of Sean Connery as the first and the best of the Bonds, I
> think Ursula Andress, the first of the Bond Girls, was the most memorable.
> The Bond Girl had that very contemporary good girl / bad girl quality that
> defined the nature of sexuality, particularly in the '60s and '70s, and it was
> timed to the arrival of the sexual revolution. These were independent
> women, always beautifully attired and coifed — and a lot of fun [26].

Perhaps not surprisingly, Hefner said the Bond Girl's style is "exactly"
the same as that of a Playboy girl. In fact, the magazine launched in
1953, the same year Ian Fleming published "Casino Royale." Playboy
also published advance excerpts of several Bond books, and the Playboy
Club was featured in several of the films. With each film, the look, shape,
and personality of the Bond Girls have changed. "They're not as voluptuous
as they used to be back in the '60s," said swimsuit designer Melissa Oda-
bash. "Now they're more athletic" [27].

Young girls in today's American society deal with daily media that potentially changes the way they think about their own developing body. Numerous articles have been written about the children's toys, books, and
television shows, among other things, that teach children that only skinny
is beautiful, including many Disney movies such as Beauty and the Beast,
Cinderella, and Snow White. Barbie dolls also have this effect on children.
A study by Davidson and colleagues [28] examining the body-shape preferences of young children in the United States, Mainland China, and Turkey
determined that all children did not necessarily prefer the slim body image,
but preferred what the people from their area preferred. For example, the
young girls from the Middle East favored larger-sized women, whereas
the young children from China didn't even believe that extremely overweight people existed [28]. The children from the United States ranked being
slim as their top choice [28]. However, children of the Middle East do not

necessarily have the same amount of freedom as to which foods they can eat, and in fact don't always have enough food, which is perhaps why they prefer the bigger model compared with a slim one. Maybe they think that the more obese model has enough food and doesn't have to worry about where their next meal comes from.

One study of Saturday morning toy commercials found that 50% of commercials aimed at girls spoke about physical attractiveness, whereas none of the commercials aimed at boys referred to appearance [29]. Another study found 50% of advertisements in teen girl magazines and 56% of television commercials aimed at female viewers used beauty as a product appeal [30]. Toys such as the famous Barbie Doll make girls and women feel as if they have to try to somehow attain her certain body type. Not only would she be 7-feet 2-inches tall, but also she'd have an impressive 40-inch bust line, a tiny 22-inch waist, and 36-inch hips. In addition to these absurd and physiologically impossible statistics, her neck would be twice the length of a normal human being [31]. Barbie would not have enough room in her tiny waistline to have full-sized organs, nor would she be able to menstruate. Because of her proportions, she would have to walk on all fours because her body would not be able to adequately support her [31]. Regardless, Barbie's figure and other media-driven advertisements can make some girls feel unhappy with their bodies, even though Barbie's body type is impossible to attain. However, when Mattell, the company that markets and produces the Barbie Doll, tried to change Barbie's body because of pressure from today's society, the doll they introduced with the regular body type failed in the market [32].

Studies have shown that both women and men, young women and girls in particular, are highly influenced by sociocultural factors concerning body image and eating habits, the latter of which is closely correlated with self-image [33]. Researchers are concerned that, at such a young age, individuals have an unhealthy need to be skinny. Although the incidence of obesity is increasing among teenagers, adolescent girls of average weight are almost as likely to be dieting as their overweight peers [34]. The desire to be thin not only affects girls who are considered medically overweight but also girls who are at a healthy weight. Reasons given by children for wanting to lose weight are rather varied and include "teasing by peers, pressure from family, feeling uncomfortable or embarrassed, wanting to feel better or look better, changing sports ability, not liking [current] weight, and wanting to be healthier" [35].

In a survey of 12-year-olds performed to determine which adults influence children the most about dieting and related eating behaviors, 77% responded that they first heard about the concept of dieting from a family member, usually a parent [35]. Friends and peers also play an integral role in shaping attitudes concerning body image and weight loss behaviors. For younger girls aged 8 to 13 years, the strongest influences concerning the pressure to lose weight were found to be mothers and best female friends [33]. Peers and close friends are often considered credible sources on the subject of dieting, particularly if they seem knowledgeable in controlling weight-related behaviors

[36]. In fact, adolescent girls reported their peers as one of the primary sources of information on weight control and dieting [34].

Girls' attitudes and behaviors about weight stem from three main sociocultural influences: parents, peers, and the media. Experts have found that most young children discover the concept of dieting from their parents, either through parental attitudes or modeling. The role that peers have in terms of girls' body image is very similar to that of parents. Peers are often a primary source of weight-control information and can influence other girls by pressuring them to lose weight through comments and teasing, and also by performing dieting behavior themselves.

These interactions between individuals, paired with the ever-present media, serve to perpetuate the thinness ideal. After examining each of these factors in turn, the overall process of socialization for young girls clearly contributes to the perpetuation of the thinness ideal, which for many girls increases body dissatisfaction and subsequent weight-control behaviors [47]. The current American weight loss culture can include childhood preoccupation with a thin body and social pressure about weight. This obsession can be associated with the development of binge eating disorders in adolescence [37]. In bulimia nervosa (BN), individuals may be slightly underweight, of normal weight, overweight, or obese. The primary diagnostic criteria for BN are behavioral; individuals binge and then engage in compensatory methods to prevent weight gain at least twice a week for an average 3-month period. Other criteria include excessive influence of body weight and shape on self-evaluation, and binging and purging that does not occur only during episodes of anorexia nervosa (AN). Two BN subtypes identified are purging type, in which laxative use, vomiting, diuretics, or enemas are used to prevent weight gain; and nonpurging type, which includes excessive exercise as the regular method of preventing weight gain [38]. According to the 2003 Youth Risk Behavior Survey, 36% of adolescent girls believed that they were overweight and 59% were attempting to lose weight. In the 30 days before questioning, 8% of adolescent girls reported they had either attempted vomiting or had taken laxatives to help control their weight [39]. The American Psychiatric Association identifies two subtypes of AN: restricting type and binge-eating/purging type. In the former, a low body mass index (BMI) is attained or maintained through dieting, fasting, or excessive exercise; in the latter, binge eating or purging is present [38]. Eating disorder not otherwise specified (EDNOS) is used for diagnostic purposes when the disorder does not meet the all of the criteria for AN or BN [38].

An estimated 1 to 2 million American women meet the criteria for BN as defined by the Diagnostic and Statistical Manual of Mental Disorders, Fourth Edition (DSM-IV) [40]. BN most often begins in late adolescence through young adulthood with a course that may be chronic or intermittent and lead to various physiologic problems [38]. Half a million women meet the diagnostic criteria for AN [40]. The onset of AN is often identified as occurring in mid- to late adolescence, ages 14 to 18 years. Although rare, onset can occur in the mid-adult years. The course of this disorder can be chronic, especially if untreated, and can result in numerous medical complications, including death [38].

EDNOS occurs in approximately 3% to 5% of women between ages 15 and 30 years in Western countries. Questions have been raised about the femininity and appearance of highly successful female athletes. Society has produced a stereotype of how a female should look. Today's "healthy" look is thin, according to society's current definition. Unfortunately, unhealthy behaviors are associated with this very slender appearance, and athletic performance diminishes as a result [41].

No consensus has been reached regarding the precise causes of eating disorders. An individual can experience a decreased sense of self-esteem or self-control because of predisposing factors (eg, biology, family history, traumatic events) and may then use dieting behavior or weight loss to provide a sense of stability or control [42]. Our culture's obsession with achieving lower weight conveys an almost unavoidable message to maturing adolescents. Several factors have been noted to be associated with the development of eating disorders. In a 3-year study of 44 secondary schools in Australia, students, initially aged 14 to 15 years, dieting was the most important predictor of a new eating disorder. High rates of earlier dieting and psychiatric morbidity in female subjects accounted for differences in eating disorder incidence between sexes. In adolescents, controlling weight through exercise rather than diet restriction seems to carry less risk for the development of eating disorders [43]. Researchers believe that numerous low-calorie diets, weight loss programs, and the increase in articles and advertisements on dieting in women's magazines and the media are associated with the increase in eating disorders [44]. They have studied television as a purveyor of cultural standards of beauty and have found that the female characters are thinner and younger than the male characters [45]. By 1990, researchers had concluded that Western culture's emphasis on slimness in women was related to the development of eating disorders [46].

Epidemiology of sports- and activity-related injuries

As the level of girls' participation in sports increases, it is important to examine their risk factors for sports-related injuries. The risk factors for lower extremity injuries have been divided into both extrinsic (ie, from factors outside the body) and intrinsic (ie, from factors within the body). Extrinsic risk factors include level of competition, skill level, shoes and orthotic equipment, and playing surface. Intrinsic risk factors include age, sex, phase of the menstrual cycle, ligamentous laxity, previous injury, aerobic fitness, body size, limb girth, limb dominance, flexibility, muscle strength and imbalance, reaction time, postural stability, anatomic alignment, and foot morphology [48]. Table 1 [49–83] reviews intrinsic and extrinsic risk factors for knee injury in female athletes.

Table 1
Risk factor for knee injury in female athletes

Risk factor for knee injury	Reference
Female gender	
NCAA injury rates differ, female > male	Arendt and Dick [49]
High school injury rates differ, female > male	Chandy and Grana [50]
	Powell and Barber-Foss [51]
	Zilmer et al [52]
Professional Basketball Injury Rates Differ, Female > Male	Zelisko et al [53]
Sex hormones	
Injury rate differs by menstrual cycle phase	Myklebust et al [54]
	Wojtys et al [55]
	Slauterbeck et al [56]
No variation in ligament laxity in different phases	Belanger et al [57]
Oral contraceptive use offered no injury protection	Arendt et al [58]
Anatomic considerations	
Q angle higher in injured female athletes	Shambaugh et al [59]
Static postural faults correlated with higher injury rate	Loudon et al [60]
Femoral notch parameters associated with injury (consensus paper)	Griffin et al [61]
Notch size associated with increased injury risk	Shelbourne et al [62]
Notch size not associated with increased injury risk	Schickendantz and Weiker [63]
	Teitz et al [64]
Notch shape associated with increased injury risk	Ireland [65]
Neuromuscular imbalances	
Proprioception deficits in anterior cruciate ligament deficient or anterior cruciate ligament injured	Barrack et al [66]
	Wojtys and Huston [67]
	Barrett [68]
	Corrigan et al [69]
Single leg stance deficits, females > males	Hewett et al [70,71]
Jumping and landing strategies differ, female versus male	Schultz and Perrin [72]
	Rozzi et al [73]
Jump landing did not differ, female versus male	Fagenbaum and Darling [74]
Females with greater valgus dominant knee	Ford et al [75]
Females with highly dominant leg	Hewett et al [76]
Preseason strength and conditioning deficits associated with injury	Knapik et al [77]
Preseason conditioning program associated with reduced injury	Hewett et al [78]
	Caraffa et al [79]
Quadriceps dominant pattern in female athletes	Huston and Wojtys [80]
Quadriceps dominant pattern in elite athletes	Baratta et al [81]
Eccentric muscle fatigue in female athletes	Nyland et al [82]
Stiffness/elasticity differences, female versus males	Winter and Brookes [83]

Dugan SA. Sports-related knee injuries in female athletes: what gives? Am J Phys Med Rehabil 2005;84(2):125; with permission.

Since 1975, women soldiers have been integrated with their male counterparts in training and barracks living. Shaffer and colleagues [84] collected data from 2962 women undergoing basic training in South Carolina. Variables collected included baseline performance on a timed run (a measure of aerobic fitness), anthropometric measurements, and a baseline questionnaire highlighting exercise and menstrual status. One hundred fifty-two recruits (5%) experienced 181 confirmed lower extremity stress fractures, with the most common sites being the tibia (25%), metatarsals (22%), pelvis (22%), and femur (20%). Logistic regression models showed that having low aerobic fitness (a slower time on the timed run) and no menses during the past year were significantly associated with the occurrence of any stress fracture and with pelvic or femoral stress fracture during boot camp.

Tracking injury rates at the high school and collegiate levels is also important. Injuries must be defined and reported rates must clarify the numerator and denominator. The National Collegiate Athletic Association (NCAA) [85] has injury surveillance systems that follow the types and body parts of athletes sustaining injuries in 16 sports. Data are compiled from injury reports completed by athletic trainers from participating institutions. The reports indicate the number of injuries per 1000 exposure hours. Gender-based differences exist in the college lacrosse rules and apparatus used in gymnastics. Comparison of injuries in different sports and between genders is an important aspect of planning coverage of events and prevention strategies [86]. The National Center for Catastrophic Sports Injury Research in Chapel Hill, NC, has been recording fatalities and catastrophic and serious injuries in United States high schools and colleges. Cheerleading incidents resulted in the highest number of catastrophic injuries in female athletes [87]. Computerized reporting packages are now available for better documentation of injury types and severity.

Epidemiology of participation

According to the National Federation of State High School Associations, participation of female high school athletes in interscholastic sports has gained momentum since the passage of Title IX and has risen annually since 1983, with almost 3 million female athletes (7.16 million total high school athletes) competing in sports in the United States during the 2005–2006 school year (see Fig. 1) [88]. Based on competition at the high school level in the 2005–2006 school year, the National Federation of State High School Associations lists the top sports in which girls participated (Table 2) [89]. Table 3 [90] shows the gender gap in high schools across the nation, broken down by state. Overall, the national average of high school sports participation is 49.1% girls compared with 50.9% boys, a difference of −1.8% (range: −1.9 to −19.4, with a national average of −7.7%). These statistics further exemplify the disparity between girls and boys sports participation in different regions of the United States.

Table 2
2005–06 High school athletics participation survey

Ten most popular programs			
Number of female participants		Number of male participants	
Basketball	452,929	Football: 11-player	1,071,775
Track and field: outdoor	439,200	Basketball	546,335
Volleyball	390,034	Track and field: outdoor	533,985
Softball: fast pitch	369,094	Baseball	470,671
Soccer	321,555	Soccer	358,935
Cross country	175,954	Wrestling	251,534
Tennis	173,753	Cross country	208,303
Swimming and diving	147,413	Golf	161,284
Competitive spirit squad	98,570	Tennis	153,006
Golf	64,195	Swimming and diving	107,468
TOTAL:	2,632,697		3,863,296

From 2005–06 High school athletics participation survey, p. 2. The national federation of state high school associations; 2006. *Data from* the National Federation of State High School Associations. 2005–2006 high school athletics participation survey; 2006. Available at: http://www.nfhs.org/core/contentmanager/uploads/2005_06NFHSparticipationsurvey.pdf. Accessed on January 10, 2007.

Gender differences (anatomic and physiologic) that may affect performance

Adult females, compared with their male counterparts, tend to have shorter stature and limbs, weigh less, and have smaller articular surfaces. These differences result in less power for striking, kicking, and throwing [91,92]. Women have wider pelves but also narrower shoulders and smaller thoraces than men [93,94]. Their leg length per total height is less than men's and most of their subcutaneous fat is in their hips and lower body, resulting in a lower center of gravity and, hence, better balance [91,93].

Comparing equally trained and conditioned women and men, men have more muscle mass per total body weight [93,95] and therefore can run faster, jump higher, and lift more weight. Female athletes are more buoyant and better insulated because they have a greater percentage of body fat per body weight [93,95–97] and therefore may have an advantage in cold water sports.

Women have a smaller stroke volume because they have a smaller heart size and heart volume. This means that they have an increased heart rate for a given submaximal cardiac output (cardiac output = stroke volume × heart rate) [93,95,98]. Because a woman's stroke volume is less, even with an increased heart rate, her cardiac output is approximately 30% lower than an equally trained man's cardiac output [95]. Her systolic blood pressure is also lower than a man's [93]. Because men have approximately 6% more red blood cells and 10% to 15% more hemoglobin per 100 mL of blood than women, the blood of men has a greater oxygen-carrying capacity [99,100].

Compared with women, adult men, because of their chest size, have a greater vital capacity [91], which is the maximal volume of air that can be moved through the lungs from a maximal inspiration to a maximal expiration. A man's residual volume, the volume of air that remains in the lungs after maximal expiration, is also greater. Women have less total lung capacity because their smaller vital capacity and residual volume. Finally, an adult woman's breathing capacity is approximately 10% less than her age-matched male counterpart [95].

Women have a smaller tidal volume but a faster respiratory rate than men at the same submaximal minute volume (tidal volume × respiratory rate) [95]. Oxygen pulse (ie, the quantity of oxygen used by the body per heartbeat), which is a measure of the efficiency of the cardiovascular and respiratory systems, is approximately three times higher in adult men [91]. These differences give men a greater maximum oxygen uptake (VO_{2max}) [95,98]. VO_{2max} assesses cardiovascular fitness or aerobic ability by measuring the lung's ability to extract oxygen from the air and deliver it to the blood, the blood's ability to circulate that oxygen to muscle tissue, and the muscle's ability to use oxygen effectively in energy pathways. Before puberty, VO_{2max} is about the same for both sexes. By the late teens, both sexes reach their peak VO_{2max}; however, postpubertal men have an average 28% greater VO_{2max} than women when expressed per total body weight [95] and 15% to 25% more than that of a woman when expressed per fat-free weight (Tables 4 and 5) [95].

Lactate threshold values are similar in male and female endurance athletes [101]. At distances greater than 42.2 km (26.2 miles, the distance of a marathon), sex differences in running speeds are negligible, with females potentially outperforming men at distances greater than 70 km (43.5 miles). One of the potential reasons given for enhanced performance of women in long-distance running events (>42.2 km) is the fatigue resistance of their muscles [102,103]. Through conditioning in warm weather, both men and women can increase the amount of sweat and the rate of sweating [104–106].

Women mature physiologically earlier than men. The adolescent growth spurt, which precedes sexual maturation, occurs in girls at about 11 years of age; the adolescent growth spurt in boys does not begin until approximately 1 to 3 years later. Bone growth in girls ceases at about age 20 years, but in boys growth continues until the early 20s [107].

A study in 2000 by Bailey and colleagues [108] investigated calcium retention and accretion rates over the short-term, using dual-energy X-ray absorptiometry (DXA), which allows the precise and accurate determination of whole-body bone mineral content (BMC) with minimal (approximately 1 mrem) radiation exposure. A series of these scans in one individual over the adolescent growth spurt shows the change in BMC accrual rates. These can be converted into calcium accretion rates, because the calcium fraction of bone mineral has been determined. In this study, six whole-body DXA scans for each of 60 boys and 53 girls were measured annually. Boys had a 26% higher mean peak bone mineral accrual rate (407 g/y; SD = 93 g/y)

Table 3
Athletic gender gap: rank order 2005–2006

	High school enrollment[a]		% High school enrollment		Athletic participation[a]		% Athletic participation[b]		Enrollment versus % female athletic	States for female participation
	Female	Male	Female	Male	Female	Male	Female	Male		
NH-New Hampshire	32,571	33,964	49.0%	51.1%	20,780	23,399	47.0%	53.0%	−1.9%	1
PA-Pennsylvania	288,680	301,652	48.9%	51.1%	124,715	142,432	46.7%	53.3%	−2.2%	2
ME-Maine	30,304	32,241	48.5%	51.6%	26,110	30,578	46.1%	53.9%	−2.4%	3
NM-New Mexico	48,153	50,049	49.0%	51.0%	22,586	25,918	46.6%	53.4%	−2.5%	4
VT-Vermont	15,554	16,575	48.4%	51.6%	10,361	12,351	45.6%	54.4%	−2.8%	5
KY-Kentucky	91,054	95,613	48.8%	51.2%	43,327	53,130	44.9%	55.1%	−3.9%	6
MN-Minnesota	136,335	143,721	48.7%	51.3%	95,359	118,117	44.7%	55.3%	−4.0%	7
CO-Colorado	110,176	115,105	48.9%	51.1%	55,055	67,740	44.8%	55.2%	−4.1%	8
CT-Connecticut	84,705	88,516	48.9%	51.1%	46,070	57,075	44.7%	55.3%	−4.2%	9
AK - Alaska	19,906	21,083	48.6%	51.4%	10,038	12,615	44.3%	55.7%	−4.3%	10
MT-Montana	23,207	24,699	48.4%	51.6%	14,594	19,120	43.3%	56.7%	−5.2%	11
WY-Wyoming	13,185	14,263	48.0%	52.0%	7,543	10,142	42.7%	57.3%	−5.4%	12
VA-Virginia	178,220	184,254	49.2%	50.8%	73,974	95,035	43.8%	56.2%	−5.4%	13
DE-Delaware	17,362	18,130	48.9%	51.1%	10,269	13,413	43.4%	56.6%	−5.6%	14
WV-West Virginia	40,409	42,165	48.9%	51.1%	15,137	19,820	43.3%	56.7%	−5.6%	15
HI-Hawaii	26,162	28,130	48.2%	51.8%	14,394	19,562	42.4%	57.6%	−5.8%	16
WA-Washington	157,176	166,483	48.6%	51.4%	68,380	91,909	42.7%	57.3%	−5.9%	17
MA-Massachusetts	144,908	148,491	49.4%	50.6%	91,248	119,268	43.3%	56.7%	−6.1%	18
NC-North Carolina	198,033	201,981	49.5%	50.5%	76,133	99,449	43.4%	56.6%	−6.2%	19
OK-Oklahoma	85,908	89,291	49.0%	51.0%	31,825	42,465	42.8%	57.2%	−6.2%	20
NY-New York	418,297	422,652	49.7%	50.3%	151,813	198,536	43.3%	56.7%	−6.4%	21
IA-Iowa	74,771	78,541	48.8%	51.2%	61,783	84,322	42.3%	57.7%	−6.5%	22
ID-Idaho	37,918	39,784	48.8%	51.2%	19,021	25,983	42.3%	57.7%	−6.5%	23
DC-District of Columbia	9,203	8,522	51.9%	48.1%	1,747	2,120	45.2%	54.8%	−6.7%	24
MI-Michigan	255,400	265,638	49.0%	51.0%	135,377	185,873	42.1%	57.9%	−6.9%	25
MO-Missouri	134,685	140,773	48.9%	51.1%	71,168	98,581	41.9%	58.1%	−7.0%	26

State	Female enrollment[a]	Male enrollment[a]	Female %	Male %	Female athletes[b]	Male athletes[b]	Female %	Male %	% Difference	Rank
OR-Oregon	78,981	83,673	48.6%	51.4%	39,198	56,136	41.1%	58.9%	−7.4%	27
MD-Maryland	132,614	135,530	49.5%	50.5%	43,830	60,518	42.0%	58.0%	−7.5%	28
SD-South Dakota	19,067	19,840	49.0%	51.0%	11,826	16,766	41.4%	58.6%	−7.7%	29
CA-California	921,050	963,269	48.9%	51.1%	278,716	399,303	41.1%	58.9%	−7.8%	30
AZ-Arizona	155,954	164,736	48.6%	51.4%	42,988	62,809	40.6%	59.4%	−8.0%	31
IN-Indiana	147,407	153,802	48.9%	51.1%	65,377	94,421	40.9%	59.1%	−8.0%	32
NE-Nebraska	44,037	46,908	48.4%	51.6%	32,435	48,233	40.2%	59.8%	−8.2%	33
ND-North Dakota	16,203	17,188	48.5%	51.5%	10,631	15,833	40.2%	59.8%	−8.4%	34
NJ-New Jersey	198,361	201,575	49.6%	50.4%	102,137	145,772	41.2%	58.8%	−8.4%	35
FL-Florida	385,654	395,884	49.3%	50.7%	87,426	126,597	40.8%	59.2%	−8.5%	36
WI-Wisconsin	139,116	147,590	48.5%	51.5%	77,655	118,280	39.6%	60.4%	−8.9%	37
OH-Ohio	276,694	288,264	49.0%	51.0%	126,746	189,783	40.0%	60.0%	−8.9%	38
IL-Illinois	300,420	311,157	49.1%	50.9%	129,946	193,757	40.1%	59.9%	−9.0%	39
KS-Kansas	68,636	72,228	48.7%	51.3%	38,936	59,786	39.4%	60.6%	−9.3%	40
RI-Rhode Island	24,064	24,707	49.3%	50.7%	10,239	15,518	39.8%	60.2%	−9.6%	41
NV-Nevada	0	0	49.1%	50.9%	15,148	23,911	38.8%	61.2%	−10.3%	42
TX-Texas	594,522	626,426	48.7%	51.3%	283,775	458,566	38.2%	61.8%	−10.5%	43
AR-Arkansas	66,066	68,575	49.1%	50.9%	19,961	32,289	38.2%	61.8%	−10.9%	44
UT-Utah	71,606	76,554	48.3%	51.7%	17,866	29,845	37.4%	62.6%	−10.9%	45
GA-Georgia	213,351	215,624	49.7%	50.3%	61,138	101,999	37.5%	62.5%	−12.3%	46
SC-South Carolina	98,732	98,580	50.0%	50.0%	30,955	52,760	37.0%	63.0%	−13.1%	47
MS-Mississippi	66,251	63,002	51.3%	48.7%	31,099	55,152	36.1%	63.9%	−15.2%	48
LA-Louisiana	96,699	93,713	50.8%	49.2%	31,429	58,728	34.9%	65.1%	−15.9%	49
AL-Alabama	102,452	105,931	49.2%	50.8%	28,028	58,859	32.3%	67.7%	−16.9%	50
TN-Tennessee	0	0	49.1%	50.9%	30,813	72,874	29.7%	70.3%	−19.4%	51
TOTALS[c]			49.1%	50.9%	2,947,105	4,217,448	41.4%	58.6%	−7.7%	

Girls receive 1.3 million less participation opportunities than boys at the high school level.

[a] Based on most recent available data: 2004–2005 National Center for Educational Statistics (NCES) (http://nces.ed.gov/) high school enrollment data for grades 9–12.

[b] Based on most recent available data: 2005–2006 National Federation High School Athletic Association (www.nfhs.org) athlete data.

[c] In the case of two states with no gender breakdown of high school enrollment (Nevada and Tennessee), national average high school enrollment was used (49.1% female and 50.9% male).

Courtesy of the Women's Sports Foundation, East Meadow, NY; with permission.

Table 4
Men and women athletes: impact on performance of anatomic differences[a]

Anatomic differences

Factor	Women	Men	Impact
Height	64.5 in	68.5 in	
Weight	56.8 kg	70.0 kg	
Limb length	Shorter	Longer	Men can achieve a greater force for hitting or kicking
Articular surface	Smaller	Larger	May provide men with greater joint stability; men have greater surface area to dissipate impact force
Body shape	Narrower shoulders	Wider shoulders	Women have lower center of gravity and therefore greater balance ability; women have an increased valgus angle at the knee which increases knee injuries; women and men have different running gaits
	Wider hips	Narrower hips	
	Legs 51.2% of height	Legs 52% of height	
	More fat in lower body	More fat in upper body	
% Muscle/TBW[a]	Approximately 36%	Approximately 44.8%	Men have greater strength and greater speed
% Fat/TBW[b]	Approximately 22%–26%	Approximately 13%–16%	Women are more buoyant and better insulated; they may be able to convert to fatty acid metabolism more rapidly

Abbreviation: TBW, total body weight.
[a] Comparisons are made for average postpubertal male and female.
[b] Varies somewhat with age, sport, and level of conditioning.
From Yurko-Griffin L, Harris SS. Female athletes. In: Sullivan JA, Anderson SJ, editors. Care of the young athlete. Rosemont (IL): American Academy of Orthopaedic Surgeons; 1999. p. 137–48; with permission.

than girls (322 g/y; SD = 66 g/y). The results showed that a bone mineral growth spurt continues after height velocity has peaked. The mean ages of peak calcium accretion rates were 14.0 years for the boys (1.0 years; 12.0–15.9 years) and 12.5 years for the girls (0.9 years; 10.5–14.6 years). The ages at peak height velocity were 13.4 years (SD = 1.0) in boys and 11.8 years (SD = 0.9) in girls, which lagged behind peak BMC by 0.6 years (boys) and 0.7 years (girls) (Table 6). This time lag could have important implications; if linear growth in stature represents the growth of skeletal volume (ie, bone breadths follow the same growth pattern as stature), the lag suggests that

Table 5
Men and women athletes: impact on performance of physiologic differences[a]

System/Factor	Women	Men	Impact
Physiologic differences			
Cardiovascular			
Heart size	Smaller	Larger	Women's stoke volume is less, necessitating an increased heart rate for a given submaximal cardiac output; cardiac output in women is approximately 30% less than men; women may be less at risk of developing hypertension
Heart volume	Smaller	Larger	
Systolic blood pressure	Lower	Higher	
Hemopoietic			
Hemoglobin		10%–15% per 100 mL blood	Men's blood has a greater oxygen-carrying capacity
Pulmonary			
Chest size	Smaller	Larger	Total lung capacity in men is greater than in women
Lung size	Smaller	Larger	
Vital capacity	Smaller	Larger	
Residual volume	Smaller	Larger	
Efficiency of cardiorespiratory system			
Oxygen pulse	Lower	Higher	Higher oxygen pulse provides men an advantage in aerobic activity
Level of aerobic fitness (reflects performance of cardiorespiratory and muscular systems)			
VO_{2max}	Lower	Higher	Men have greater aerobic ability
Metabolism (BMR)	Approximately 6%–10% lower (when related to body surface area)	Approximately 6%–10% higher (when related to body surface area)	Women need fewer calories to sustain same activity level as men
Thermoregulation	Female = Male	Female = Male	Both sexes can adequately sweat in hot weather to decrease core body temperature

Abbreviation: BMR, basal metabolic rate.

[a] Comparisons are made for average postpubertal male and female.

From Yurko-Griffin L, Harris SS. Female athletes. In: Sullivan JA, Anderson SJ, editors. Care of the young athlete. Rosemont (IL): American Academy of Orthopaedic Surgeons; 1999. p. 137–48; with permission.

Table 6
Peak values and ages at which they occurred

Variable	Boys (SD)	Girls (SD)
Age at PHV (y)	13.4 (1.0)	11.8 (0.9)
Age at peak BMC velocity (y)	14.0 (1.0)	12.5 (0.9)
Peak BMC velocity (g/y)	407 (93)	322 (66)
Peak Ca accretion rate (mg/d)	359 (82)	284 (59)
Mean Ca intake (mg/d)	1140 (392)	1113 (378)
Apparent retention efficiency (%)	36.5 (12.3)	29.6 (8.5)

Abbreviations: BMC, bone mineral content; Ca, calcium; PHV, peak height velocity.
Data from Bailey DA, Martin AD, McKay HA, et al. Calcium accretion in girls and boys during puberty: a longitudinal analysis. J Bone Miner Res 2000;15(11):2245–50.

bone mineralization does not keep up with the rapidly expanding skeletal volume [109].

Strength training has several benefits for women. Because women tend be at higher risk for osteoporosis, strength training provides enhanced bone modeling to increase bone strength and reduce the risk for osteoporosis. Strength training increases functional strength for sports and daily activities, decreases nonfunctional body fat, and increases lean body mass. It creates a higher metabolic rate because of an increase in muscle and decrease in fat. From a psychological aspect, it improves self-esteem and confidence [110].

Women, on average, have roughly two thirds the absolute strength and power output of men. A greater difference is typically found between men and women in absolute upper body strength compared with lower body strength. Women possess approximately 40% to 60% of the upper body strength and 70% to 75% of the lower body strength of men. When measuring strength, factoring in lean body mass is important. Based on a strength-to-lean-body-mass ratio, women are almost equal in strength to men, and when strength is calculated per cross-sectional area of muscle, significant gender difference does not exist [110]. For this reason, women should train in the same ways as men.

Hormones also play a role in the development of absolute strength in men and women. The androgens from the adrenal glands and ovaries are the hormones that influence strength. The most important androgens for strength development are testosterone and androstenedione. Average women have approximately one tenth the testosterone of men. Women who have higher testosterone levels may have a greater potential for strength and power development. Although hormones help in strength development, whether they are the reason for the differences in absolute strength is uncertain [110].

Despite the research and its known benefits, strength training is a persistent medical issue for women. A lack of accurate information persists and feeds misconceptions, keeping women away from strength training or preventing them from training in optimal ways. Some myths include the ideas that strength training causes women to become larger and heavier, women should use different training methods than men, and women should avoid high-intensity or high-load training. In fact, women should strength train in the same ways as men, using the same program design, exercises, intensities, and volumes relative to their body size and level of strength so they can achieve the maximum physiologic and psychological benefits [110]. The number of elite female athletes participating in strength and conditioning programs is increasing. This type of training is important in improving their athletic performance and preventing injury.

Awareness of the anatomic differences between men and women is important because they may help explain the different observed injury rates and patterns. For example, women have a higher rate of anterior cruciate ligament injuries than men. In 2004, Hewett and colleagues [111] established that, before maturation, male and female athletes have similar forces and motions about the knee when they land from a jump, and girls have decreased neuromuscular control of the knee from early to late puberty. Boys, on the other hand, show better neuromuscular control of the knee in late puberty than early puberty. Hewett studied 181 middle-school and high-school soccer and basketball players (100 girls and 81 boys), measuring their dynamic knee joint control, knee joint torques, and lower-extremity bone length, and compared results according to maturational stage. They documented changes in how girls and boys land from a jump after the onset of maturation, showing that female athletes had greater total medial motion of the knees and a greater maximum lower-extremity valgus angle with landing than the male athletes. The girls also showed decreased knee flexor torques compared with the boys, and a significant difference between the maximum valgus angles of their dominant and nondominant lower extremities after maturation. Boys regained neuromuscular control after their so-called "neuromuscular spurt," whereas girls did not seem to make a similar neuromuscular adaptation [111], potentially leading to decreased dynamic knee stability in female athletes. The study remarked that future controlled prospective longitudinal research is needed and should focus on defined populations of female athletes followed up through multiple sports seasons to correlate neuromuscular profiles with injury risk. Only then can the relative injury risk be predicted with high sensitivity [111].

Summary

Great strides have been made in the world of female athletics, especially in the past 35 years. Continued efforts to thwart discrimination are still required for many reasons. "Keeping Score: Girls' Participation in High School Athletics in Massachusetts," undertaken by the National Women's Law Center and Harvard Prevention Research Center on Nutrition and Physical Activity, used public health data to assess gender disparities in physical activity among high school students in Massachusetts, and then interviewed girls and their coaches about access to team sports and treatment of their teams. These girls were less likely than boys to participate in organized sports, physical education classes, or informal forms of exercise. The report suggested that persistent discrimination in the state's high school athletics programs may be one reason for the disparities and provides recommendations for improving gender equity in youth physical activity [112].

If researchers and clinicians continue to heighten awareness and knowledge of the differences young female athletes have in areas such as body image, epidemiology, and gender, they can make a difference in the future of youth and humanity. "Sports and physical activity participation can help girls avoid the dangerous minefields of adolescence and reach their full potential," said past Health and Human Services Secretary Shalala. "We've come a long way in breaking down barriers for girls, but now we need to work together to help get girls off the sidelines and onto the fields" [113].

References

[1] Title IX of the Education Amendments of 1972. In: 20 U.S.C. § 1681; 1972.
[2] 2005–06 High school athletics participation survey. Based on Competition at the High School Level in the 2005-06 School Year. National Federation of State High Schools. The National Federation of State High Schools Association Handbook. Kansas City (MO): NFSHSA; 2005–2006.
[3] Available at: http://womenshistory.about.com/gi/dynamic/offsite.htm?zi=1/XJ/Ya&;sdn=womenshistory&cdn=education&tm=14&f=10&tt=14&bt=1&bts=1&zu=http%3A//www.greatwomen.org/women.php%3Faction%3Dviewone%26id%3D177. Accessed January 10, 2007.
[4] Available at: http://www.gale.com/free_resources/whm/bio/didriksonzaharias_b.htm. Accessed January 10, 2007.
[5] Available at: http://www.peggyfleming.net/story.html. Accessed January 10, 2007.
[6] Available at: http://kclibrary.nhmccd.edu/decade60.html#sports. Accessed January 10, 2007.
[7] Available at: http://www.usaswimming.org/USASWeb/ViewMiscArticle.aspx?TabId=472&;Alias=Rainbow&Lang=en&mid=791&Itemid=775. Accessed January 10, 2007.
[8] Available at: http://www.yogiberramuseum.org/prog_womeninsports.html#top. Accessed January 10, 2007.
[9] Available at: http://www.womenssportsfoundation.org/cgi-bin/iowa/about/more.html. Accessed January 10, 2007.
[10] Wiggins DL, Wiggins ME. The female athlete. Clin Sports Med 1997;16:593–612.
[11] Available at: http://en.wikipedia.org/wiki/Mia_Hamm. Accessed January 10, 2007.
[12] Available at: http://www.womenssportsfoundation.org/cgi-bin/iowa/issues/history/article.html?record=51. Accessed January 10, 2007.
[13] Available at: http://www.wnba.com/about_us/historyof_wnba.html. Accessed January 10, 2007.
[14] Available at: http://en.wikipedia.org/wiki/Europe or http://en.wikipedia.org/wiki/Women%27s_National_Basketball_League/oWomen's National Basketball League. Accessed June 17, 2007.
[15] Available at: http://www.usatoday.com/sports/basketball/wnba/draft/2006-04-04-lynx_x.htm. Accessed June 17, 2007.

[16] Available at: http://sports.espn.go.com/nba/news/story?id=2516704, Article by By Chad Ford, ESPN Insider, http://x.go.com/cgi/x.pl?goto=http://search.espn.go.com/keyword/search?searchString=chad_ford&name=SEARCH_m_archive&srvc=sz. Accessed June 17, 2007.

[17] WNBA, 2005; Wikipidia; NBA; 2005.

[18] Available at: http://www.forbes.com/business/2006/03/22/woods-sharapova-nike_cx_lr_0322athletes_2.html. Accessed January 10, 2007.

[19] Available at: http://news.bbc.co.uk/sport1/hi/golf/4309396.stm. Accessed January 10, 2007.

[20] New York Times, June 16; 2005.

[21] The Women's Sports Foundation. Sport and teen pregnancy. East Meadow (NY): The Women's Sports Foundation; 1998.

[22] Bernstein L, Patel AV, Ursin G, et al. Lifetime recreational exercise activity and breast cancer risk among black women and white women. Journal of the National Cancer Institute 2005;97(22):1671–9.

[23] Shakib S, Spruijt-Metz D, Figueroa-Colon RF, et al. Aerobic fitness and depressive symptoms in children. Presented at the North American association for the study of obesity (NAASO) annual meeting, 2000. Long Beach, CA, 2000.

[24] Kolonel LN. Nutrition and prostate cancer. Cancer Causes & Control 1996;7(1):44–83.

[25] Callahan LR, Hannafin JA, Sheridan M. The female athlete. In: Paget S, Gibofsky A, Beary A, et al, editors. Hospital for special surgery manual of rheumatology and outpatient orthopedic disorders: diagnosis and therapy. 5th edition. Philadelphia, PA: Lippincott Williams & Wilkins; 2006. p. 198–202.

[26] Available at: http://www.mtv.com/movies/news/articles/1545872/20061115/story.jhtml. Accessed on January 10, 2007.

[27] Available at: http://www.vh1.com/movies/news/articles/1545872/story.jhtml. Accessed on January 10, 2007.

[28] Davidson D, Welborn T, Azure D, et al. Male and female body shape preferences of young children in the United States, Mainland China, and Turkey. Child Study Journal 2002; 32(3):131–3.

[29] Dittrich L. About-Face facts on the MEDIA. About-Face web site. Online: Available at: http://aboutface.org/resources/facts/media.html. 2000. Accessed on January 10, 2007.

[30] Woznicki K., Pop culture hurts body image. On Health web site. Online: Available at: http://www.onhealth.com/ch1/briefs/item,55572.asp. 1999. Accessed on January 10, 2007.

[31] Fein GG. Toys and stories. In: Pellegrini AD, editor. The future of play theory. Albany (NY): State University of New York Press; 1995. p. 151–65.

[32] J Oakes. Young girls: body image & well being—where do they learn harmful habits? Ecclectica: April 2006. Available at: http://www.ecclectica.ca/issues/2006/1/index.asp? Article=25. Accessed on January 10, 2007.

[33] McCabe MP, Ricciardelli LA. A prospective study of pressures from parents, peers, and the media on extreme weight change behaviours among adolescent boys and girls. Behaviour Research and Therapy 2005;43:653–68.

[34] Phares V, Steinberg AR, Thompson JK, et al. Gender differences in peer and parental influences: body image disturbance, self-worth, and psychological functioning in preadolescent children. Journal of Youth and Adolescence 2004;33(5):421–9.

[35] Schur EA, Sanders M, Steiner H, et al. Body dissatisfaction and dieting in young children. International Journal of Eating Disorders 2000;27:74–82.

[36] Balaam BJ, Haslam SA. A closer look at the role of social influence in the development of attitudes to eating. Journal of Community and Applied Social Psychology 1998;8: 195–212.

[37] The McKnight Investigators. Risk factors for the onset of eating disorders in adolescent girls: results of the McKnight longitudinal risk factor study. Am J Psychiatry 2003;160(2): 248–54.

[38] American Psychiatric Association. Diagnostic and statistical manual of mental disorders. 4th edition. Washington (DC): American Psychiatric Association; 2000.

[39] Grunbaum JA, Kann L, Kinchen S. Youth risk behavior surveillance–United States, 2003. MMWR Surveill Summ 2004;53(2):1–96.

[40] Abstract for Reference 10 of 'Eating disorders: Epidemiology, pathogenesis, and clinical features'. International academy of eating disorders. Position statement on equity in insurance coverage for eating disorders. Available at: www.aedweb.org/disorders.html. Accessed on January 10, 2007.

[41] Smith A. The female athlete triad: causes, diagnosis, and treatment [electronic version]. The Physician and Sportsmedicine 1996;24.

[42] Garner DM, Garfinkel PE. Handbook of treatment for eating disorders. 2nd edition. New York: Guilford Press; 1997.

[43] Patton GC, Selzer R, Coffey C, et al. Onset of adolescent eating disorders: population based cohort study over 3 years. BMJ 1999;318(7186):765–8.

[44] Nasser M. Culture and weight consciousness. J Psychosom Res 1988;32:573–7.

[45] Perdue L, Silverstein B. A comparison of the weights and ages of women and men on television. Presented at the annual Meeting of the Eastern Psychological Association. Boston, MA, March 21–24, 1985.

[46] Anderson AE, DiDomenico L. Diet vs. shape content of popular male and female magazines: a dose response relationship to the incidence of eating disorders? Int J Eating Dis 1992;11:283–7.

[47] Available at: http://www.ecclectica.ca/issues/2006/1/index.asp?Article=26#sdfootnote16anc. Accessed January 10, 2007.

[48] Dugan SA. Sports-related knee injuries in female athletes: what gives? American Journal of Physical Medicine and Rehabilitation 2005;84(2):122–30.

[49] Arendt E, Dick R. Knee injury patterns among men and women in collegiate basketball and soccer. NCAA data and review of the literature. Am J Sports Med 1995;23:694–701.

[50] Chandy TA, Grana WA. Secondary school athletic injury in boys and girls. A three year comparison. Physician Sports Med 1985;13:106–11.

[51] Powell JW, Barber-Foss KD. Sex-related injury patterns among selected high school sports. Am J Sports Med 2000;28:385–91.

[52] Zillmer DA, Powell JW, Albright JP. Gender specific injury patterns in high school varsity basketball. J Women's Health 1992;1:69–76.

[53] Zelisko JA, Noble HB, Porter M. A comparison of men's and women's professional basketball injuries. Am J Sports Med 1982;10:297–9.

[54] Myklebust G, Haehlum S, Holm I, et al. A prospective cohort study of anterior cruciate ligament injuries in elite Norwegian team handball. Scand J Med Sci Sports 1998; 8:149–53.

[55] Wojtys EM, Huston LJ, Boynton MD, et al. The effects of the menstrual cycle on anterior cruciate ligament injuries in women as determined by hormone levels. Am J Sports Med 2002;30:182–8.

[56] Slauterbeck JR, Fuzie SF, Smith MP, et al. The menstrual cycle, sex hormones, and anterior cruciate ligament injury. J Athlet Training 2002;37:275–80.

[57] Belanger MJ, Moore DC, Crisco JJ, et al. Knee laxity does not vary with the menstrual cycle, before or after exercise. Am J Sports Med 2004;32:1150–7.

[58] Arendt EA, Bershadsky B, Agel J. Periodicity of noncontact anterior cruciate ligament injuries during the menstrual cycle. J Gend Specif Med 2002;5:19–26.

[59] Shambaugh JP, Klein A, Herbert JH, et al. Structural measures as predictors of injury in basketball players. Med Sci Sports Exerc 1991;23:522–7.

[60] Loudon JK, Jenkins W, Loudon KL. The relationship between static posture and ACL injury in female athletes. J Orthop Sports Phys Ther 1996;24:91–7.

[61] Griffin LY, Agel J, Albohm MJ, et al. Noncontact anterior cruciate ligament injuries: risk factors and prevention strategies. J Am Acad Orthop Surg 2000;8:141–50.

[62] Shelbourne KD, Thorp TJ, Klootwyk TE. The relationship between intercondylar notch width of the femur and the incidence of anterior cruciate ligament tears: a prospective study. Am J Sports Med 1998;26:402–7.

[63] Schickendantz MS, Weiker GG. The predictive value of radiographs in the evaluation of unilateral and bilateral anterior cruciate ligament injuries. Am J Sports Med 1993;21:110–3.

[64] Teitz CC, Lind BC, Sacks BM. Symmetry of the femoral notch width index. Am J Sports Med 1997;25:687–90.

[65] Ireland ML. Special concerns of the female athlete. In: Fu FH, Stone DA, editors. Sports injuries: mechanism, prevention, and treatment. edition 2. Baltimore (MA): Williams and Wilkins; 1994. 1. p. 153–62.

[66] Barrack RL, Skinner HB, Buckley SL. Proprioception in the anterior cruciate deficient knee. Am J Sports Med 1989;17:1–16.

[67] Wojtys EM, Huston LJ. Neuromuscular performance in normal and anterior cruciate ligament-deficient lower extremities. Am J Sports Med 1994;22:89–104.

[68] Barrett DS. Proprioception and function after anterior cruciate ligament reconstruction. J Bone Joint Surg 1994;76B:654–9.

[69] Corrigan JP, Cashman WF, Brady MP. Proprioception in the cruciate deficient knee. J Bone Joint Surg 1992;74B:247–50.

[70] Hewett, TE, Paterno, MV, Noyes, FR. Differences in single leg balance on an unstable platform between female and male normal, ACL-deficient and ACL-reconstructed knees. Presented at the Twenty-fifth Annual Meeting of the American Orthopedic Society for Sports Medicine. Traverse City, Michigan, 1999.

[71] Hewett TE, Paterno MV, Myer GD. Strategies for enhancing proprioceptive and neuromuscular control of the knee. Clin Ortho Rel Research 2002;402:76–94.

[72] Schultz SJ, Perrin DH. Using surface electromyography to assess sex differences in neuromuscular response characteristics. J Athletic Training 1999;34:165–76.

[73] Rozzi SL, Lephart SM, Gear WS, et al. Knee joint laxity and neuromuscular characteristics of male and female soccer and basketball players. Am J Sports Med 1999;27:312–9.

[74] Fagenbaum R, Darling WG. Jump landing strategies in male and female college athletes and the implications of such strategies for anterior cruciate ligament injury. Am J Sports Med 2003;31:233–40.

[75] Ford KR, Myer GD, Hewett TE. Valgus knee motion during landing in high school female and male basketball players. Med Sci Sports Exerc 2003;25:1745–50.

[76] Hewett TE, Stroupe AL, Nance TA, et al. Plyometric training in female athletes. Decreased impact forces and increased hamstring torques. Am J Sports Med 1996;24:765–73.

[77] Knapik JJ, Bauman CL, Jones BH, et al. Preseason strength and flexibility imbalances associated with athletic injuries in female collegiate athletes. Am J Sports Med 1991;19:76–81.

[78] Hewett TE, Riccobene JV, Lindenfeld TN. The effect of neuromuscular training on the incidence of knee injury in female athletes. A prospective study. Am J Sports Med 1999;27: 699–706.

[79] Caraffa A, Cerulli G, Projetti M, et al. Prevention of anterior cruciate ligament injuries in soccer: a prospective controlled study of proprioceptive training. Knee Surg Sports Traumatol Arthroscopy 1996;4:19–21.

[80] Huston LJ, Wojtys EM. Neuromuscular performance characteristics in elite female athletes. Am J Sports Med 1996;24:427–36.

[81] Baratta R, Solomonow M, Zhou BH, et al. Muscular coactivation: the role of the antagonist musculature in maintaining knee stability. Am J Sports Med 1988;16:113–22.

[82] Nyland JA, Caborn DN, Shapiro R, et al. Fatigue after eccentric quadriceps femoris work produces earlier gastrocnemius and delayed quadriceps femoris activation during crossover cutting among normal athletic women. Knee Surg Sports Traumatol Arthrosc 1999;5: 162–7.

[83] Winter EM, Brookes FBC. Electromechanical response times and muscle elasticity in men and women. Eur J Appl Physiol 1991;63:124–8.

[84] Shaffer RA, Rauh MJ, Brodine SK, et al. Predictors of stress fracture susceptibility in young female recruits. American Journal of Sports Medicine 2006;34(1):108–15.

[85] Available at: www.ncaa.org. Accessed January 10, 2007.

[86] Ryan JB, Ireland ML. Epidemiology of injuries. In: Ireland ML, Nattiv A, editors. The female athlete. Philadelphia: Saunders; 2002. p. 15–26.

[87] Cantu RC, Mueller FO. Fatalities and catastrophic injuries in high school and college sports, 1982–1997: lessons in improving safety. Physician Sportsmed 1999;27(8):35–49.

[88] Athletic Participation Survey Totals, p. 2. The national federation of state high school associations, 2006. Available at: http://www.reference.com/browse/wiki/National_Federation_of_State_High_School_Associations. Accessed January 10, 2007.

[89] 2005–06 High school athletics participation survey, p 2. The national federation of state high school associations. 2006. Available at: http://www.reference.com/browse/wiki/National_Federation_of_State_High_School_Associations. Accessed January 10, 2007.

[90] Women's Sports Foundation. 1/11/2007.

[91] Arnheim D. Modern principles of athletic training. 7th edition. St. Louis (MO): Mosby; 1989. p. 64–111.

[92] Thomas C. Factors important to women participants in vigorous athletics. In: Strauss R, editor. Sports medicine and physiology. Philadelphia: WB Saunders; 1979. p. 304–19.

[93] Hale RW. Factors important to women engaged in regular physical activity. In: Strauss R, editor. Sports medicine and physiology. Philadelphia: WB Saunders; 1984. p. 250–69.

[94] Klafs C, Lyon J. The female athlete. 2nd edition. St. Louis (MO): Mosby; 1978. p. 15–46.

[95] Wells CL. Women, sport and performance. 2nd edition. Champaign (IL): Human Kinetics; 1991. p. 3–34.

[96] Wilmore JH. Alterations in strength, body composition and anthropometric measurements consequent to a 10-week weight training program. Med Sci Sports Exerc 1974;6:133–8.

[97] Wilmore J, Brown C. Body physic and composition of the female distance runner. In: Milvy P, editor. The marathon: physiological, medical, epidemiologic, and psychological studies. New York: New York Academy of Sciences; 1977. p. 764–76.

[98] Marshall JL. Myths about women's sports. In: Marshall JL, editor. The sports doctor's fitness book for women. New York: Delacorte; 1981. p. 6–13.

[99] Astrand P, Rodahl K. Textbook of work physiology. 2nd edition. New York: McGraw Hill; 1977.

[100] DeVries H. Physiology of exercise for physical education and athletics. 3rd edition. Dubuque (IA): William C. Brown; 1980.

[101] Weyand PG, Cureton KJ, Conley DS, et al. Peak oxygen deficit predicts sprint and middle-distance track performance. Med Sci Sports Exerc 1994;26:1174–80.

[102] Clarke DH. Sex differences in strength and fatigability. Res Q Exerc Sport 1986;57: 144–9.

[103] Misner JE, Massey BH, Going SB, et al. Sex differences in static strength and fatigability in three different muscle groups. Res Q Exerc Sport 1990;61:238–42.

[104] Ferstle J, Wells C. Asking the right questions. Physician Sportsmed 1982;14:157–60.

[105] Haymes E. Physiologic responses of female athletes to heat stress, a review. Physician Sportsmed 1984;12:45–59.

[106] Wells CL. Response of physically active and acclimatized men and women to exercise in a desert environment. Med Sci Sports Exerc 1980;12:9–13.

[107] Tanner J. Growth at adolescence. 2nd edition. Oxford: Blackwell; 1962.

[108] Bailey DA, Martin AD, McKay HA, et al. Calcium accretion in girls and boys during puberty: a longitudinal analysis. Journal of Bone & Mineral Research 2000;15(11):2245–50.

[109] Yurko-Griffin L, Harris SS. Female athletes. In: Sullivan JA, Anderson SJ, editors. Care of the young athlete. Rosemont (IL): American Academy of Orthopaedic Surgeons; 1999. p. 137–48.

[110] Ebben W, Jensen R. Strength training for women: debunking myths that block opportunity. The Physician and Sportsmedicine 1998;26:86–97.

[111] Hewett TE, Myer GD, Ford KR. Decrease in neuromuscular control about the knee with maturation in female athletes. Journal of Bone & Joint Surgery [Am] 2004;86(8): 1601–8.

[112] Available at: http://www.hsph.harvard.edu/now/feb6/obesity.html. Accessed January 10, 2007.

[113] Available at: http://www.girlpower.gov/press/research/sports.htm. Accessed January 10, 2007.

ELSEVIER
SAUNDERS

Phys Med Rehabil Clin N Am
18 (2007) 385–400

PHYSICAL MEDICINE
AND REHABILITATION
CLINICS OF
NORTH AMERICA

The Female Athlete Triad and Cardiovascular Dysfunction

Anne Z. Hoch, DO, FACSM*, Sophia Lal, DO,
Jason W. Jurva, MD, David D. Gutterman, MD

*Medical College of Wisconsin, 9200 West Wisconsin Avenue,
Milwaukee, WI 53226, USA*

In the past 35 years, a significant increase has occurred in sports participation by women. An estimated 3 million girls and young women compete in American high school sports. Women who participate in sports and fitness programs are generally healthier and have higher self-esteem. However, an increase has also been seen in gender-specific injuries and medical problems. The female athlete triad (Triad) is a syndrome of separate but interrelated conditions of disordered eating, amenorrhea, and osteoporosis. Athletic amenorrhea is known to have a hormonal profile similar to menopause characterized by decreased circulating estrogens. Menopause is known to be associated with osteoporosis and accelerated cardiovascular disease. Although enhanced risk for cardiovascular disease is theoretically possible, it has not been explored in the young athletic population. Premature cardiovascular disease first manifests as endothelial dysfunction, which can be examined noninvasively with ultrasound. This article discusses disordered eating, amenorrhea, osteoporosis, and the potential for heightened cardiovascular risk in young athletic women.

In the early 1900s women were excluded from the Olympic Games. Athletic competition was believed to be too stressful for women and that their reproductive organs were at risk for injury. Fortunately, the past 35 years have seen an explosion in sports participation by women, largely because of Title IX, the Educational Amendment Act of 1972, which mandated equal access to sports participation in public schools and universities for men and women. In 1972, 1 in 27 high school girls played a varsity high

* Corresponding author. Women's Sports Medicine Program/Sports Medicine Center, Departments of Orthopaedic Surgery/PM&R, Medical College of Wisconsin, 9200 West Wisconsin Avenue, Milwaukee, WI 53226.
E-mail address: azeni@mcw.edu (A.Z. Hoch).

1047-9651/07/$ - see front matter © 2007 Elsevier Inc. All rights reserved.
doi:10.1016/j.pmr.2007.05.001

pmr.theclinics.com

school sport. In 2007, 1 in 2 girls played a varsity sport, an increase of more than 1000%.

From this explosion in sports participation, we have learned that exercise and competitive sports are beneficial to women in many ways. Premenopausal women younger than 45 years who exercise aerobically at least 4 hours per week have a 37% reduction in breast cancer risk [1]. Lopiano [2] reports that high school girls involved in sports are less likely to experience unwanted pregnancies and become involved with drugs. Furthermore, women who play sports have higher self-esteem and lower levels of depression [2]. Experts have also found that sports traditionally teach values that carry over into the competitive workplace [2]. Several studies have shown that exercise increases bone mineral density (BMD) [3,4]. Teegarden and colleagues [5] found that active girls who participate in high school sports have significantly greater BMD, which may help prevent osteoporosis in the future. Lastly, vigorous physical activity and aerobic exercises are known to lessen symptoms of the menstrual cycle, such as cramping, low back pain, headache, and depression [6].

However, an increasing prevalence of exercise-associated medical problems, including the Triad, has also been found. The Triad was initially defined in 1992 by a special American College of Sports Medicine (ACSM) task force on women's issues, and a position stand was published in 1997 defining the condition in detail [7]. Since then, a significant amount of research on the Triad has been performed, and in 2003 the ACSM established a special writing team of researchers and clinicians to publish a revised position stand, which will be published soon.

In a study by Nichols and colleagues [8], the prevalence of the Triad was examined in 170 high school athletes from eight different sports in southern California. Disordered eating was assessed with the Eating Disorder Examination Questionnaire (EDE-Q) [9]. Menstrual status was also examined with a questionnaire, and BMD was tested with dual energy x-ray absorptiometry (DXA) using Lunar model DPX-NT (Lunar/GE Corp, Madison, Wisconsin).

Of the 170 athletes in the sample, 18.2% met criteria for disordered eating, with vomiting (7%) as the most common pathogenic behavior for controlling weight, and 24% had oligomenorrhea/amenorrhea, with oligomenorrhea (17.1%) the most common menstrual irregularity. Twenty two percent had low BMD for their age based on World Health Organization (WHO) criteria (Z-score < -1.0), whereas 4.1% met the International Society for Clinical Densitometry criteria (Z-score < -2.0) for low bone mass. Ten athletes (5.9%) met criteria for any two Triad components, and two athletes (1.2%) had all three components. Oligomenorrheic/amenorrheic athletes, after adjusting for body mass index (BMI), reported significantly higher dietary restraint and EDE-Q global scores when compared with eumenorrheic athletes. They were also significantly older in menarcheal age and had significantly lower trochanter BMD after adjusting for chronologic age, ethnicity, BMI, and percentage of body fat. These data help alert health care professionals, coaches, and parents that several components of the Triad are present in high school age athletes, which is a critical time for bone mineral accrual [8].

In another study looking at prevalence of the Triad, the authors [10] studied 80 varsity high school athletes from a competitive all-girls' school in the Midwest. Results showed that 55% of the girls had low energy availability, with an average deficit of 575 kcal; 33% had amenorrhea; 16% had a Z-score less than −1.0; 1% had a Z-score less than −2.0; and 19% had a history of stress fractures.

Disordered eating

Women, including female athletes, are under intense pressure to be thin and have a low percentage of body fat, not only for aesthetic purposes but also because of the misperception that a thin physique will increase athletic performance. Hence, eating disorders are much more common in female athletes compared with nonathletes. *Disordered eating* refers to a spectrum of abnormal eating patterns ranging from a mild preoccupation with calories and body image to frank anorexia nervosa and bulimia nervosa, which is a strict Diagnostic and Statistical Manual of Mental Disorders, Fourth Edition (DSM–IV) diagnosis [18]. By definition, hypothalamic amenorrhea is one of the criteria for anorexia nervosa. Bulimia nervosa can further be divided into purging and nonpurging type. The latest edition of DSM–IV has included a third classification of eating disorders, "eating disorder not otherwise specified (NOS)." This diagnosis covers a wider variety of abnormal eating patterns with different, less-stringent criteria than anorexia nervosa and bulimia nervosa. Box 1 lists the diagnostic criteria for these conditions.

However, DSM–IV criteria for eating disorders are based on nonathletic women. Therefore, some authors believe that disordered eating in athletes should have its own criteria that are more athlete-specific, such as those listed for anorexia in Table 1 [11]. Pathologic eating patterns used by athletes commonly include consumption of diets low in fat and calories, and use of diet pills, laxatives, diuretics, fasting, self-induced vomiting, and excessive exercise to control weight. In a survey of female athletes, Rosen and colleagues [12] found that 25% reported routine use of diet pills, 16% reported laxative abuse, and 14% reported self-induced vomiting. Ultimately, these practices may lead to excessive weight loss, dehydration, loss of fat free mass, and subsequent decreased athletic performance [13].

The specific etiology and pathophysiology of eating disorders remains largely unknown. Most experts agree that they are multifactorial and complex regarding genetics, environment, biology, cultural influences, and behavior factors [14]. In addition, clinical eating disorders are often

Box 1. Diagnostic criteria for anorexia nervosa, bulimia nervosa, and eating disorder not otherwise specified.

Anorexia nervosa

Refusal to maintain body weight at or above 85% of normal weight for age and height

Intense fear of gaining weight or becoming fat, although underweight

Disturbance in the way one's body weight or shape is experienced, undue influence of body weight or shape on self-evaluation, or denial of the seriousness of the current low body weight

Amenorrhea in postmenarchal women

Bulimia nervosa

Recurrent episodes of binge eating. An episode of binge eating is characterized by:

    Eating, within a discrete period (eg, any 2-hour period), an amount of food that is definitely larger than most people would eat during a similar period under similar circumstances

    A sense of lack of control over eating during the episode (eg, a feeling that one cannot stop eating or control what or how much one is eating)

Recurrent inappropriate compensatory behavior to prevent weight gain, such as self-induced vomiting, misuse of laxatives, diuretics, enemas, or other medications; fasting; or excessive exercise

Binge eating and inappropriate compensatory behaviors occur, on average, at least twice a week for 3 months

Self-evaluation is unduly influenced by body shape and weight

The disturbance does not occur exclusively during episodes of anorexia nervosa

Eating disorder not otherwise specified

For women, all criteria for anorexia nervosa are met except that the individual has regular menses

All criteria for anorexia nervosa are met except that, despite significant weight loss, the person's current weight is in the normal range

All criteria for bulimia nervosa are met except that the binge eating and inappropriate compensatory mechanisms occur at a frequency of less than twice a week for a duration of less than 3 months

The regular use of inappropriate compensatory behavior by an individual of normal body weight after eating small amounts of food (eg, self-induced vomiting after the consumption of two cookies)

Repeatedly chewing and spitting out, but not swallowing, large amounts of food

Binge-eating disorder: recurrent episodes of binge eating in the absence of the regular use of inappropriate compensatory behavior characteristics of bulimia nervosa

---

From American Psychiatric Association. Eating disorders. In: First M, editor. Diagnostic and statistical manual of mental disorders. 4th edition. Washington, DC: American Psychiatric Publishing, Inc.; 1994. p. 549–50; with permission.

accompanied by comorbid psychological conditions, such as obsessive–compulsive disorder, depression, and anxiety disorder [15]. However, several factors are associated with the development of abnormal eating patterns, including extreme pressures from coaches, parents, society, and the athletes themselves to be thin or achieve an "ideal body weight" or "optimal" body fat. Women who participate in sports such as ballet, gymnastics, and figure skating, which emphasize a lean physique or low body weight, are at greater risk [11,16,17]. Women participating in endurance sports, such as long distance running, cross country skiing, and Iron Man triathletes, are also at higher risk. Many of these athletes have the misperception that weight loss will increase their performance. Finally, sports with a weight category, such as lightweight crewing, rowing, and martial arts, have a higher risk.

In the nonathletic female population, 1% have anorexia nervosa and between 1% and 4% have bulimia nervosa as defined by DSM-IV [18]. The true prevalence of disordered eating in athletes is unknown. Obtaining prevalence data in female athletes is difficult because athletes are typically in denial or secretive about their eating disorders. Underreporting is also a large problem because of the fear of being discovered and potential consequence to their athletic careers [19]. The prevalence of eating disorders among female collegiate athletes, including low energy availability, disordered eating, pathogenic weight control, subclinical eating disorders, and frank anorexia and bulimia, range from 1% to 62% [7,8,10,12,19–22].

Eating disorders are chronic conditions with significant health consequences, including dehydration, malnutrition, cardiac arrhythmia, menstrual dysfunction, osteoporosis, psychologic disorders, and death. Treatment requires a multidisciplinary team approach with physicians, psychologists, dietitians, family members, coaches, and athletic trainers participating in the healing process. Most importantly, the athletes must be part of the treatment team; for the treatment to be successful, they must want to

Table 1
Anorexia athletica

Common features	Sundgot-Borgen[a]
Weight loss[b]	+
Delayed puberty[c]	(+)
Menstrual dysfunction[d]	(+)
Gastrointestinal complaints	+
Absence of medical illness or affective disorder explaining the weight reduction	+
Distorted body image[b]	(+)
Excessive fear of becoming obese	+
Restriction of food (<1200 kcal/d)	+
Use of purging methods[e]	(+)
Binging[b]	(+)
Compulsive exercise[b]	(+)

[a] +, absolute criteria; (+), relative criteria.
[b] >5% of expected body weight.
[c] No menstrual bleeding at age 18 (primary amenorrhea).
[d] Primary amenorrhea, secondary amenorrhea, or oligomenorrhea.
[e] Self-induced vomiting, laxatives, and diuretics.
From Sundgot-Borgen J. Prevalence of eating disorders in elite female athletes. Int J Sport Nutr 1993;3(1):29–40; with permission.

change behaviors and break disordered eating habits. Behavior contracts may have to be used with some more challenging athletes.

The sports physician must have a high index of suspicion for all female athletes, regardless of the sport, and play an active role in prevention and early detection. Tools that can be used for screening include the "Eat-26" questionnaire [23,24]. This survey includes 26 questions related to eating attitude and the potential for an eating disorder. Each question is scored 1 to 6 points. A score of 20 or greater suggests an eating disorder [24]. Validated body image forms are also available and helpful [25]. The Harris Benedict basal metabolic energy expenditure equation is useful for determining basal energy requirements:

$$BEE = 655.1 + (9.563 \times W) + (1.850 \times H) - (4.676 \times A)$$

where W is weight in kg, H is height in cm, and A is age in years

However, this tool becomes inaccurate when subjects are in a low energy deficit. Used in combination with a 3-day food diary to determine caloric input and an exercise log to determine caloric expenditure, whether an athlete is in a positive or negative energy balance can be determined. The dietitian will then create a meal plan with specific recommendations to promote healthy eating. Continued follow-up sessions are often needed to promote and support a behavior change. Treatment and recovery from an eating disorder is notoriously difficult. According to Lebrun [26], 40% of patients who have an eating disorder will recover, 30% will recover but have relapses, and the remaining 30% will be chronically affected.

Menstrual dysfunction in athletes

Menarche refers to the age menses begins, which on average occurs at 12.5 years of age for nonathletic Caucasian American girls. Athletic females experience menarche at a later age, with retrospective studies varying between 14 and 15.4 years [27]. Warren and Perlroth [27] followed up pubertal progression for 4 years in 15 ballet dancers. The average age of menarche in 13 of the ballet dancers was 15.4 years; however, 2 still had primary amenorrhea at age 18. *Primary amenorrhea* has recently been redefined by the American Society of Reproductive Medicine as the absence of menstruation by 15 years of age in girls with secondary sex characteristics [28]. This age was lowered from 16 years because the age of menarche has become younger in developed countries. Secondary amenorrhea is diagnosed when menstrual cycles stop for at least three consecutive months in women who were previously menstruating normally. Oligomenorrhea is characterized by menstrual cycles at intervals greater than 35 days. Eumenorrhea refers to normal ovulatory menstrual cycles repeating every 28 to 30 days. Luteal phase dysfunction is described as a shortened secretory phase of the menstrual cycle, typically less than 10 days. It is associated with low progesterone levels and may be an adaptive response to exercise.

The prevalence of secondary amenorrhea in the general nonathletic population is between 2% and 5% [7]. Reports in the athletic population vary significantly mainly because of methodologic differences and have been reported to range from 6% to 79% [7,27]. Health consequences of amenorrhea can be potentially devastating. Hypothalamic athletic amenorrhea is a significant risk factor for osteoporosis and osteopenia. Drinkwater and colleagues [29] landmark study showed that young amenorrheic runners had lower vertebral body BMD (1.12 g/cm^2) compared with eumenorrheic runners (1.30 g/cm^2). In 1999, Gibson and colleagues [30] prospectively studied 34 middle and long distance runners aged 18 to 35 years diagnosed with athletic amenorrhea or oligomenorrhea. The runners were placed into one of three treatment arms: estrogen replacement therapy plus 1000 mg of calcium, 1000 mg of calcium alone, and no treatment. No overall change was seen in BMD at 12 months, although a trend toward an increase (1.5%) in spinal BMD occurred at 12 months in the hormone replacement group [30]. This study controlled for calcium intake, but not total caloric intake. However, in a randomized, controlled clinical trial by Hergenroeder [31], ethinyl estradiol (0.035 mg) was found to increase BMD in young women who had hypothalamic amenorrhea. The numbers were small in this study and the beneficial effect was only noted in the lumbar spine and total body, not in the femur [32].

Infertility, another health consequence of athletic amenorrhea, is usually considered reversible if normal menses returns. However, athletes who have regular menstrual cycles every 28 days may have hidden menstrual irregularities, such as chronic anovulatory cycles or inadequate luteal phase [27,33]. Shangold and colleagues [34] has found that only 50% of eumenorrheic runners ovulated during a test month compared with 83% of controls. Chronic anovulation and unopposed estrogen secretion promotes endometrial proliferation, which could increase the risk for hyperplasia and adenocarcinoma of the uterus.

Treatment of athletic amenorrhea is a challenge to all involved. Based on Louck's and colleagues [35] low energy availability theory, the ultimate goal is to return these athletes to a positive energy balance. This result can be difficult to achieve and requires a comprehensive team approach that is dedicated to the female athlete. A skilled sports dietitian can assist by determining the exact caloric deficit and devising a meal plan with suggestions for small diet changes to increase caloric consumption at 50 to 100 kcal intervals. Adequate calcium intake is important, because athletic amenorrhea is associated with low BMD and risk for osteoporosis. NIH recommends between 1200 and 1500 mg of calcium and 400 and 800 IU of vitamin D for all girls between ages 11 and 24 years [36]. Sports psychologists and psychiatrists are important in assisting with stress reduction and in-depth treatment of eating disorders. Hormone replacement can be used if menses does not resume in 10 to 12 months. However, many female athletes are reluctant to take hormones because of fear of weight gain and subsequent decreased athletic performance. Moreover, the return of menses secondary to hormone replacement does not necessarily mean that a positive energy balance has been restored. To confuse the picture even further, a recent study by Weaver and colleagues [37] showed that women taking oral contraceptive pills who underwent a program of resistive exercise and jumping rope for 24 months had a lower BMD than controls who were not taking oral contraceptive pills. Calcium intake but not total caloric intake was taken into account.

Osteoporosis

The U.S. Department of Agriculture recently reported that only 13.5% of girls and 36.3% of boys aged 12 to 19 years in the United States get the recommended daily amount of calcium, placing them at serious risk for osteoporosis and other bone diseases. Furthermore, peak bone mineral acquisition seems to occur earlier in girls (aged 11–14) than boys (aged 13–17). The National Institute of Child Health and Human Development has stated that the nation's youth are in the midst of a calcium crisis [38].

The third component of the Triad defined by the initial position stand is osteoporosis. *Osteoporosis* is defined as decreased bone mass and density and an increased risk or incidence of fracture in postmenopausal women by an NIH Consensus Group in 2000. Osteoporosis is diagnosed by DXA, which is the most accurate technique in pre- and postmenopausal women [7,39–41]. BMD is normally distributed and expressed in standard deviation units relative to its T or Z distribution [40]. The T-score compares BMD of the test subject with that of "normals" based on a 20-year-old woman divided by the standard deviation of the population. Therefore, this definition does not apply to female athletes younger than 20 years. Z-scores compare BMD to age-matched controls, which may be more meaningful in the young athletic population. The WHO defines osteoporosis in postmenopausal women based on T-scores, which also predict fracture risk [40]. A T-score less than −1.0 is considered a criterion for osteopenia, and one less than −2.5 is consistent with osteoporosis. However, these criteria were not established for use in, nor do they apply to, premenopausal women. Presently, few data are available describing normal BMD in women, and more specifically female athletes, younger than 20 years. Furthermore, because of variable rates of puberty, quantifying BMD is difficult for this age. Lunar recently published manufacturers' normal values for women aged 6 to 20 years; however, the subjects were nonathletes. Future research should be directed at establishing ranges of BMD for the athletic and sedentary adolescent population.

The International Society for Clinical Densitometry (ISCD) recently proposed using Z-scores in premenopausal women, which is relative to chronologic age [41]. They also suggest using the term "low bone mass for chronologic age" and reserve the diagnosis of osteoporosis for women with risk factors [39]. Only a few studies have examined the prevalence of low bone mass/osteoporosis in young athletes. The largest study, conducted by Torstveit and Sundgot-Borgen [42], assessed 186 elite Norwegian athletes and showed that 10.2% had a Z-score less than −1.0 and 2% had one less than −2.0. In contrast, Nichols and colleagues [8] studied 170 high school athletes and found that 21.8% had a Z-score less than −1.0 and 4.1% had one less than −2.0. In 80 varsity high school athletes this article's authors [10] showed that 16% had a Z-score less than −1.0 and 1% had one less than −2.0.

The female athlete triad and cardiovascular disease

Cardiovascular disease is the number one cause of death in women in the United States. Cardiovascular disease risk increases significantly after menopause, with one in four women ultimately dying of a cardiac event [43]. The key pathophysiologic event of menopause is suppression of hypothalamic pituitary reproductive axis and ultimately ovarian failure and decreased circulating estrogens. Epidemiologic observations suggest that estrogen may have a significant cardioprotective influence. This hypothesis is supported by Walsh and colleagues [44], who showed that estrogen can reduce low-density lipoprotein (LDL) cholesterol levels and increase high-density lipoprotein (HDL) cholesterol levels. However, based on a regression analysis that showed that only 50% of the reduction in cardiovascular events is caused by the lipid-lowering effect of estrogen, Bush and colleagues [45] suggests that additional mechanisms contribute to the cardioprotective effect of estrogen.

Coronary and peripheral vessels contain estrogen receptors on the vascular endothelium, and estrogens stimulate the production of nitric oxide (NO). NO is also released in response to increased blood flow and shear stress, causing vasodilation or flow-mediated vasodilation (FMD). Chemical stimuli, including acetylcholine, serotonin, thrombin, and substance P, are also known to increase the release of NO. NO not only is a potent vasodilator but also prevents platelet aggregation, leukocyte adhesion, and vascular smooth muscle proliferation and migration, which are each key components of the atherosclerotic process [46,47]. The importance of endothelial function in cardiovascular health is evident by the finding that individuals who have risk factors for coronary artery disease, such as diabetes, hypertension, hyperlipidemia, tobacco use, and even a family history of coronary disease, experience reduced endothelial-dependent vasodilation before developing atherosclerotic plagues. Reduced endothelium-dependent vasodilation seems to be one of the earliest signs of cardiovascular disease [48]. Brachial artery and coronary artery endothelial dysfunction are strongly correlated, making this a valid marker for cardiovascular disease risk [49]. Furthermore, vascular endothelial dysfunction has been shown to predict long-term atherosclerotic disease progression and cardiovascular event rates [50].

Menopause was recently shown to be associated with reduced endothelium-dependent dilation, presumably secondary to reduced estrogen levels [51]. Lieberman and colleagues [52] also showed that estrogen replacement therapy improves endothelium-dependent vasodilation in postmenopausal women. In addition, both short-term and long-term estrogen administration improves endothelium-dependent vasodilation in the coronary arteries of atherosclerotic monkeys after oophorectomy [52]. Collectively, these studies support the hypothesis that estrogen exerts a cardioprotective effect through its interaction with the vascular endothelium. However, this hypothesis must be tempered by the results of a recent large prospective randomized trial of estrogen replacement that showed an increase in cardiovascular events in postmenopausal women treated with estrogens, which markedly reduced the use of postmenopausal estrogen therapy [53].

Exercise-induced amenorrhea is a complex physiologic condition. Because the exact cause of hypothalamic athletic amenorrhea remains unclear, it continues to be a diagnosis of exclusion. However, the pathophysiology is very similar to menopause in terms of reduced circulating estrogens. In theory, young premenopausal amenorrheic athletes, similar to postmenopausal women, most likely have reduced endothelium-dependent dilation, a precursor to cardiovascular disease. The clinical implications of this dysfunction are twofold. First, loss of FMD in conduit arteries (an endothelium-dependent process) will restrict exercise-induced dilation of these vessels and limit the maximum perfusion available to the tissue supplied, which could reduce exercise capacity through restricting flow to critical muscles involved in exercise. Second, chronic impairment of endothelial function leads to accelerated development of atherosclerosis in animal models and increased cardiovascular events in humans. Loss of endothelial function in athletes may hasten the development of cardiovascular disease and events by years or decades.

Celermajer and colleagues [54,55] recently described a noninvasive technique for assessing endothelial function that has revolutionized the way investigators study important vascular parameters. In 1992, he published the first study in which he used noninvasive, high-resolution external vascular ultrasound to examine the brachial artery. Celermajer and colleagues [55] initially described the technique by measuring the diameter of the brachial artery under three different conditions. Baseline measurements were made after a 4-hour fast and at least 10 minutes in the supine position. Fasting is required because many substances can alter endothelial dilation, such as caffeine, fatty meals, vitamin C, and cigarette smoking. Brachial artery diameter was recorded again during reactive hyperemia, induced by inflating a blood pressure cuff on the forearm to 40 mmHg above systolic pressure for 5 minutes. Deflating the blood pressure cuff induces increased flow (reactive hyperemia) that, in turn, stimulates an endothelium-dependent vasodilation of the brachial artery (FMD) visualized with the overlying transducer. Finally, brachial artery diameter is measured after administration of sublingual nitroglycerin (0.4 mg), which causes endothelium-independent vasodilation and assesses the reactivity of the underlying vascular smooth muscle [55]. Brachial artery diameter can be measured accurately with computer analysis using automated vascular edge detection. This measurement is accurate to within 0.1 mm and has low intraobserver and interobserver variability.

The mechanisms of FMD have been well-studied. Shear stress acting on the endothelium stimulates calcium flux into the endothelial cell, activating the constitutively expressed dimerized enzyme NO synthase. NO synthase uses tetrahydrobiopterin, rac, HSP90, and NADPH as cofactors and arginine as a substrate to produce NO and citrulline. NO, as a nonpolar molecule, diffuses from the endothelium to the smooth muscle, binding to the heme domain of guanylyl cyclase and activating the conversion of GTP to cGMP. The attendant increased in cGMP activates a signaling cascade that results in smooth muscle relaxation. FMD of the brachial artery is almost exclusively caused by the release of NO from the endothelium, and treatment with nonmetabolized congeners of l-arginine, such as l-arginine mononmethyl ester, inhibit the enzyme and block FMD. Thus, FMD is essentially a bioassay for NO from the endothelium. NO, in addition to its vasodilator properties, is a potent inhibitor of platelet aggregation, smooth muscle proliferation, leukocyte adhesion, LDL oxidation, and other proatherosclerotic processes [46,47]. Therefore, reduced FMD increases the propensity for atherosclerotic cardiovascular disease.

Several factors can influence FMD. For example, FMD can vary up to 50% during different phases of the menstrual cycle. Hashimoto and colleagues [56] examined 17 male and female medical students to determine if FMD was affected by changes in ovarian hormone levels and if a difference occurred between men and women. His study showed that during menstruation, when estrogen levels are at their lowest level, FMD was 11%. However, during the follicular phase when estradiol levels increase, FMD increased to 18%. In the luteal phase, when estradiol levels remain high and progesterone levels increase by way of production from the corpus luteum, FMD remained at 18%. This study further exemplifies the complex interactions of the menstrual cycle and cardiovascular function.

The authors [57] tested 10 amenorrheic, 11 oligomenorrheic, and 11 control/eumenorrheic college runners for endothelial dysfunction using the brachial artery technique described by Celermajer and colleagues [54,55]. No differences were seen in estradiol, estrone, total estrogen, progesterone, or carbohydrate, fat, or protein intake among the groups. Levels of prolactin, thyroid stimulating hormone (TSH), cholesterol (Chol), and hemoglobin, or the total caloric, calcium, and phosphate intake, showed little difference among groups. All the women consumed less than the daily recommended 1500 mg of calcium. The baseline brachial artery diameters and the endothelium-independent dilation to nitroglycerin were similar. However, the vasodilator response to reactive hyperemia was significantly less in the amenorrheic group (1.1%) compared with the control/eumenorrheic group (5.6%). This study was the first to show that endothelial function was reduced in women runners who have amenorrhea.

Rickenlund and colleagues [58] similarly explored this question and, in addition to reduced FMD, also showed an unfavorable lipid profile in amenorrheic athletes. This study compared young endurance athletes who had amenorrhea, oligomenorrhea, and regular cycles (eumenorrhea) with sedentary controls. Results confirmed that FMD was significantly impaired in the amenorrheic group compared with the others. Additionally, the amenorrheic athletes had a significantly higher level of Chol and LDL compared with the other athletes. The amenorrheic group also had the highest levels of serum lipid apolipoprotein B (Apo B) and the lowest cytokine interleukin 6 levels, which may be caused by estrogen deficiency.

Another study conducted by Rickenlund and colleagues [59] investigated the effects of oral contraceptives (OC) on endothelial function, lipid profile, and markers of inflammation. Subjects included Swedish female athletes participating in endurance sports from universities, high schools, and public sports events. Three groups, amenorrheic athletes, regularly menstruating athletes, and regularly menstruating sedentary controls, were examined before and after 9 months of low-dose, monophasic, combined OC treatment (30 μg ethinyl estradiol and 150 μg levonorgestrel on days 1–21, followed by a hormone and tablet-free interval days 22–28). The amenorrheic athletes showed decreased FMD at baseline, significantly increased FMD during

OC treatment, but no significant differences after treatment. No significant differences were seen in lipid levels (triglyceride, Chol, HDL, Apo A, and Apo B) and inflammatory markers among the groups at baseline. However, the amenorrheic group had the highest levels of Chol, LDL, and Apo B before treatment. During OC treatment, HDL decreased and Apo B, high-sensitivity C-reactive protein, and tumor necrosis factor-alpha increased in all groups. This study provides supportive evidence that OC treatment restores endothelial function in amenorrheic athletes through the protective action of estrogen, noting that some associated changes occur in the lipid profile and inflammatory markers [59].

Other interventions may be available that can improve endothelial function. Recent studies have shown that folic acid supplementation improves endothelial-dependent FMD in patients who have hypercholesterolemia [60,61]. The authors have also shown that folic acid improved FMD in eumenorrheic runners [62].

Summary

The female athlete triad position stand was published by the ACSM in 1997 [7]. It described in detail three distinct, yet interrelated, medical conditions. In the past 10 years, a tremendous effort has focused on prevention, education, and treatment of this condition. Understanding the pathophysiology of athletic amenorrhea raises the additional question of whether these athletes also at risk for premature vascular dysfunction. If current ongoing studies prove that they are, a better name for the condition may be the *Female Athlete Tetrad*, referring to the interrelatedness of disordered eating, amenorrhea, osteoporosis, and augmented cardiovascular risk.

References

[1] Thune I, Brenn T, Lund E, et al. Physical activity and the risk of breast cancer. N Engl J Med 1997;336(18):1269–75.

[2] Lopiano D. Gender equity in sports. In: Agostini R, editor. Medical and orthopedic issues of active and athletic women. Philadelphia: Hanley & Belfus; 1994. p. 13–22.

[3] Prince RL, Smith M, Dick IM, et al. Prevention of postmenopausal osteoporosis. A comparative study of exercise, calcium supplementation, and hormone-replacement therapy. N Engl J Med 1991;325(17):1189–95.

[4] Nichols DL, Bonnick SL, Sanborn CF. Bone health and osteoporosis. Clin Sports Med 2000; 19(2):233–49.

[5] Teegarden D, Proulx WR, Kern M, et al. Previous physical activity relates to bone mineral measures in young women. Med Sci Sports Exerc 1996;28:105–13.

[6] Lebrun CM. Effects of the menstrual cycle and birth control pills on athletic performance. In: Agostini R, editor. Medical and orthopaedic issues of active and athletic women. Philadelphia: Hanely & Belfus; 1994. p. 78–91.

[7] Otis CL, Drinkwater B, Johnson M, et al. American College of Sports Medicine position stand. The female athlete triad. Med Sci Sports Exerc 1997;29(5):1669–71.

 [8] Nichols JF, Rauh MJ, Lawson MJ, et al. Prevalence of the female athlete triad syndrome among high school athletes. Arch Pediatr Adolesc Med 2006;160(2):137–42.
 [9] Fairburn CG, Beglin SJ. Assessment of eating disorders: interview or self-report questionnaire? Int J Eat Disord 1994;16(4):363–70.
[10] Hoch AZ, Stavrakos JE, Bobb VL, et al. Prevalence of components of the Female Athlete Triad in high school athletes. Med Sci Sports Exerc 2006;38(5):S345.
[11] Sundgot-Borgen J. Prevalence of eating disorders in elite female athletes. Int J Sport Nutr 1993;3(1):29–40.
[12] Rosen LW, McKeag DB, Hough DO, et al. Pathogenic weight-control behavior in female athletes. The Physician and Sportsmedicine 1986;14(1):79–86.
[13] Nattiv A. The female athlete triad. In: Garrett WE, Lester GE, McGowan J, et al, editors. Women's health in sports and exercise. Rosemont (IL): American Academy of Orthopaedic Surgeons; 2001. p. 451–65.
[14] Brownell K, Foryet J, editors. Handbook of eating disorders: physiology, psychology and treatment of obesity, anorexia nervosa and bulimia nervosa. New York: Basic Books; 1986.
[15] Fairburn CG, Brownell K, editors. Eating disorders and obesity: a comprehensive handbook. 2nd edition. New York: Gilford Press; 2001.
[16] Sundgot-Borgen J, Torstveit MK. Prevalence of eating disorders in elite athletes is higher than in the general population. Clin J Sport Med 2004;14(1):25–32.
[17] Fogelholm M, Hiilloskorpi H. Weight and diet concerns in Finnish female and male athletes. Med Sci Sports Exerc 1999;31(2):229–35.
[18] American Psychiatric Association. Eating Disorders. In: First M, editor. Diagnostic and statistical manual of mental disorders. 4th edition. Washington, DC: American Psychiatric Publishing, Inc.; 1994. p. 539–50.
[19] Sanborn CF, Horea M, Siemers BJ, et al. Disordered eating and the female athlete triad. Clin Sports Med 2000;19(2):199–213.
[20] Burckes-Miller ME, Black DR. Male and female college athletes: prevalence of anorexia nervosa and bulimia nervosa. Athletic Training 1988;23:137–40.
[21] Brownell K, Rodin J. Prevalence of eating disorders in athletes. In: Brownell K, Rodin J, Wilmore J, editors. Eating, body weight and performance in athletes: disorders of modern society. Philadelphia: Lea & Febiger; 1992. p. 128–45.
[22] Byrne S, McLean N. Eating disorders in athletes: a review of the literature. J Sci Med Sport 2001;4(2):145–59.
[23] Garner DM, Olmstead MP, Polivy J. Development and validation of a multidimensional eating disorder inventory for anorexia nervosa and bulimia. International Journal of Eating Disorders 1983;2(2):15–34.
[24] Garner DM, Olmsted MP, Bohr Y, et al. The eating attitudes test: psychometric features and clinical correlates. Psychol Med 1982;12(4):871–8.
[25] Stunkard AJ, Sorensen T, Schulsinger F. Use of the Danish Adoption Register for the study of obesity and thinness. Res Publ Assoc Res Nerv Ment Dis 1983;60:115–20.
[26] Lebrun CM. Special issues of the female athlete. In: Johnson R, editor. Sports medicine in primary care. Philadelphia: W.B. Saunders; 2000. p. 243–55.
[27] Warren MP, Perlroth NE. The effects of intense exercise on the female reproductive system. J Endocrinol 2001;170(1):3–11.
[28] Practice Committee of the American Society for Reproductive Medicine. Current evaluation of amenorrhea. Fertil Steril 2004;82(1):266–72.
[29] Drinkwater BL, Nilson K, Chesnut CH, et al. Bone mineral content of amenorrheic and eumenorrheic athletes. N Engl J Med 1984;311(5):277–81.
[30] Gibson JH, Mitchell A, Reeve J, et al. Treatment of reduced bone mineral density in athletic amenorrhea: a pilot study. Osteoporos Int 1999;10(4):284–9.
[31] Hergenroeder AC. Bone mineralization, hypothalamic amenorrhea, and sex steroid therapy in female adolescents and young adults. J Pediatr 1995;126(5 Pt 1):683–9.

[32] Nattiv A, Armsey TD Jr. Stress injury to bone in the female athlete. Clin Sports Med 1997; 16(2):197–224.
[33] De Souza MJ, Miller BE, Loucks AB, et al. High frequency of luteal phase deficiency and anovulation in recreational women runners: blunted elevation in follicle-stimulating hormone observed during luteal-follicular transition. J Clin Endocrinol Metab 1998;83(12): 4220–32.
[34] Shangold M, Freeman R, Thysen B, et al. The relationship between long-distance running, plasma progesterone, and luteal phase length. Fertil Steril 1979;31(2):130–3.
[35] Loucks AB, Verdun M, Heath EM. Low energy availability, not stress of exercise, alters LH pulsatility in exercising women. J Appl Physiol 1998;84(1):37–46.
[36] NIH Consensus conference. Optimal calcium intake. NIH Consensus Development Panel on optimal calcium intake. JAMA 1994;272(24):1942–8.
[37] Weaver CM, Teegarden D, Lyle RM, et al. Impact of exercise on bone health and contraindication of oral contraceptive use in young women. Med Sci Sports Exerc 2001;33(6): 873–80.
[38] NIH News Release. "Calcium crisis" affects. American youth. expanded web site seeks to inform children of dangers of low calcium intake. 2001. Available at: http://www.nih.gov/ news/pr/dec2001/nichd-10.htm. Accessed June 25, 2006.
[39] IOC Medical Commission Working Group Women in Sport. Position stand on the female athlete triad. Available at: www.olympic.org/common/asp/download_report.asp?file=en_report_ 917.pdf&;id=917. Accessed December 2, 2006.
[40] World Health Organization. Assessment of risk fracture and its application to screening for postmenopausal osteoporosis. World Health Organ Tech Rep Ser 1994;843:1–129.
[41] Leib ES, Lewiecki EM, Binkley N, et al. Official positions of the International Society for Clinical Densitometry. J Clin Densitom 2004;7(1):1–6.
[42] Torstveit MK, Sundgot-Borgen J. Low bone mineral density is two to three times more prevalent in non-athletic premenopausal women than in elite athletes: a comprehensive controlled study. Br J Sports Med 2005;39(5):282–7.
[43] Barrett-Connor E, Bush TL. Estrogen and coronary heart disease in women. JAMA 1991; 265(14):1861–7.
[44] Walsh BW, Schiff I, Rosner B, et al. Effects of postmenopausal estrogen replacement on the concentrations and metabolism of plasma lipoproteins. N Engl J Med 1991;325(17): 1196–204.
[45] Bush TL, Barrett-Connor E, Cowan LD, et al. Cardiovascular mortality and noncontraceptive use of estrogen in women: results from the Lipid Research Clinics Program Follow-up Study. Circulation 1987;75(6):1102–9.
[46] Dusting GJ, Fennessy P, Yin ZL, et al. Nitric oxide in atherosclerosis: vascular protector or villain? Clin Exp Pharmacol Physiol Suppl 1998;25:S34–41.
[47] Moncada S, Higgs A. The L-arginine-nitric oxide pathway. N Engl J Med 1993;329:2002–12.
[48] Celermajer DS. Endothelial dysfunction: does it matter? Is it reversible? J Am Coll Cardiol 1997;30:325–33.
[49] Anderson TJ, Uehata A, Gerhard MD, et al. Close relation of endothelial function in the human coronary and peripheral circulations. J Am Coll Cardiol 1995;26:1235–41.
[50] Schachinger V, Britten MB, Zeiher AM. Prognostic impact of coronary vasodilator dysfunction on adverse long- term outcome of coronary heart disease. Circulation 2000;101(16): 1899–906.
[51] Perregaux D, Chaudhuri A, Mohanty P, et al. Effect of gender differences and estrogen replacement therapy on vascular reactivity. Metabolism 1999;48(2):227–32.
[52] Lieberman EH, Gerhard MD, Uehata A, et al. Estrogen improves endothelium-dependent, flow-mediated vasodilation in postmenopausal women. Ann Intern Med 1994;121:936–41.
[53] Rossouw JE, Anderson GL, Prentice RL, et al. Risks and benefits of estrogen plus progestin in healthy postmenopausal women: principal results From the Women's Health Initiative randomized controlled trial. JAMA 2002;288(3):321–33.

[54] Celermajer DS. Testing endothelial function using ultrasound. J Cardiovasc Pharmacol 1998;32(Suppl 3):S29–32.

[55] Celermajer DS, Sorensen KE, Gooch VM, et al. Non-invasive detection of endothelial dysfunction in children and adults at risk of atherosclerosis. Lancet 1992;340(8828): 1111–5.

[56] Hashimoto M, Akishita M, Eto M, et al. Modulation of endothelium-dependent flow-mediated dilatation of the brachial artery by sex and menstrual cycle. Circulation 1995; 92(12):3431–5.

[57] Hoch AZ, Dempsey RL, Carrera GF, et al. Is there an association between athletic amenorrhea and endothelial cell dysfunction? Med Sci Sports Exerc 2003;35(3):377–83.

[58] Rickenlund A, Eriksson MJ, Schenck-Gustafsson K, et al. Amenorrhea in female athletes is associated with endothelial dysfunction and unfavorable lipid profile. J Clin Endocrinol Metab 2005;90(3):1354–9.

[59] Rickenlund A, Eriksson MJ, Schenck-Gustafsson K, et al. Oral contraceptives improve endothelial function in amenorrheic athletes. J Clin Endocrinol Metab 2005;90(6):3162–7.

[60] Verhaar MC, Wever RM, Kastelein JJ, et al. Effects of oral folic acid supplementation on endothelial function in familial hypercholesterolemia: a randomized placebo-controlled trial [in process citation]. Circulation 1999;100:335–8.

[61] Stroes ES, van Faassen EE, Yo M, et al. Folic acid reverts dysfunction of endothelial nitric oxide synthase. Circ Res 2000;86:1129–34.

[62] Hoch AZ, Adams B, Syed AQ, et al. Folic acid supplementation improves endothelial function in eumenorrheic runners. Med Sci Sports Exerc 2005;37(5):S52.

ELSEVIER
SAUNDERS

Phys Med Rehabil Clin N Am
18 (2007) 401–416

PHYSICAL MEDICINE
AND REHABILITATION
CLINICS OF
NORTH AMERICA

Stress Fractures and Rehabilitation

Sheila A. Dugan, MD[a],*, Kathleen M. Weber, MD[b]

[a]Rush Medical College, Rush University Medical Center, 1725 West Harrison Street,
#970, Chicago, IL 60612, USA
[b]Rush Medical College, Midwest Orthopedics, 800 S. Wells, Suite M3,
Chicago, IL 60607, USA

Stress fractures are common sports injuries accounting for approximately 10% of all overuse injuries [1]. Studies have shown a 1.5 to 3.5 times increased risk for stress fractures in female athletes compared with male athletes [2–4]. Women military recruits are 1.2 to 10 times more likely to sustain stress fractures compared with male recruits [5–7]. A plethora of medical literature has been published discussing the demographics, risk factors, anatomic distribution, diagnostic evaluation, and treatment of stress fractures [8–12]. However, the literature contains a void regarding the rehabilitation and preventive aspects of this frequent injury. This article briefly reviews the risk factors, common sites, and sport-specific and gender-specific stress fractures. In addition, the common clinical presentation, physical examination findings, and diagnostic evaluation are discussed, including high-risk stress fractures. Highlighted is an in-depth review of the treatment and prevention of stress fractures in women.

Defining stress fracture

Stress fractures are partial bone fractures resulting from repetitive microtrauma. They are classified as fatigue or insufficiency fractures. A fatigue fracture occurs when an abnormal amount of stress is placed on a normal bone. Insufficiency fractures develop when normal stress is applied to an abnormal bone, such as an osteoporotic bone. A third type of fractures occurs when abnormal stress is applied to abnormal bone such as occurs with some female athletes in training who have osteopenia [13].

* Corresponding author. Department of Physical Medicine & Rehabilitation, Rush Medical College, Rush University Medical Center, 1725 West Harrison Street, #970, Chicago, IL 60612.
   E-mail address: sheila_dugan@rush.edu (S.A. Dugan).

1047-9651/07/$ - see front matter
doi:10.1016/j.pmr.2007.04.003

Normal bone has ongoing remodeling allowing accommodation to loading. Stress reaction (microfractures) can result if this remodeling system does not keep pace with the applied force. A stress fracture, and most likely a complete fracture, will result if the inciting event continues. The literature debates whether the bone's failure to adapt has been related to excessive load-bearing forces or inadequate contractile muscular forces [3,14,15]. Whichever the cause, early intervention is associated with more rapid healing [16].

Risk factors

Both intrinsic and extrinsic risk factors have been implicated in the cause of stress fractures (Table 1) [17]. Intrinsic factors include those that are biomechanical (eg, limb malalignment, gait abnormality, muscle imbalance, and small tibia diameter) or biochemical (eg, hormonal imbalance, low bone mass density, bone disease, and nutritional deficits). Extrinsic factors include training errors (eg, overuse, lack of cross training, lack of conditioning, increases in training intensity and duration without an adequate buildup phase, poor technique), environment (eg, nonabsorbent training surface, banked track), and equipment (eg, inappropriate foot wear, prolonged use of foot wear, non–gender specific training equipment).

Although they have been studied individually, the interplay between intrinsic and extrinsic factors likely leads to increased risks for stress fractures. Specifically, the amount, intensity, and timing of training plays a significant role in the bone's ability to adapt to increasing demands. Overtraining and inadequate training surfaces in combination with poor muscular

Table 1
Risk factors for stress fractures

Extrinsic Factors	
Training errors	Overuse
	Lack of cross training (eg, cycling, elliptical trainer, weight training)
	Lack of conditioning
	Increasing intensity and duration too quickly
	Poor technique
Environment	Training surface (nonabsorbent, banked, same direction track or street running)
Equipment	Footwear (inappropriate or prolonged use)
Intrinsic Factors	
Biomechanical	Malalignment
	Gait abnormality
	Muscle imbalance
	Narrow tibia width
Biochemical	Hormonal imbalance
	Low bone mass density
	Bone disease
	Nutritional deficits

conditioning may overload the bone, resulting in a stress fracture [15]. Some evidence shows that muscle mass is inversely related to stress fracture incidence. Individuals who have less muscle mass may be predisposed to develop a stress fracture, because studies have shown that one of the major roles of muscles is energy absorption [18]. As muscles become fatigued, the nearby bone is exposed to greater forces. Experts have proposed that bone injury may be a secondary event after a primary failure of muscle function. Further studies are needed to define the role of conditioning and strengthening programs in the incidence and treatment of stress fractures in females.

Common sites for stress fractures

Stress fractures are seen most commonly in the lower extremities. The most common site for both males and females is the tibia [16]. Sport-specific sites include the tibia, metatarsals and fibula in runners and dancers, the humerus in overhead throwing athletes and the rib and clavicle in rowers [18–20]. Gender specific stress fracture patterns in women include femoral, pelvic, and metatarsal stress fractures (Table 2) [21].

Gender-specific issues

The incidence of stress fractures is higher in women than men. A proposed mechanism in young athletic women relates higher stress fracture

Table 2
Site- and sport-specific stress fractures

Site	Sport or activity
Lower extremity	
Pelvis	Running, race walking
Femur	Running
Patella	Jumping sports, soccer, basketball, baseball (catcher)
Tibia	Running, soccer, aerobics, ballet
Fibula	Running, skating
Metatarsals	Running (2nd and 3rd), ballet dancing (base of 2nd)
Axial skeleton	
Lumbar spine (pars intra-articularis)	Gymnastics, football (lineman), water-skiing
Ribs (1st)	Throwing sports
Ribs (other)	Rowing and swinging sports (tennis, golf, baseball batting)
Upper extremity	
Coracoid process of scapula	Trap shooting
Humerus	Throwing, racket sports
Olecranon	Throwing sports
Ulna	Tennis, javelin
Metacarpal	Tennis, handball

rates to premenopausal osteopenia or osteoporosis caused by a hypoestrogenic state resulting from hypothalamic amenorrhea. A positive correlation exists between menstrual dysfunction and low bone density [22,23]. Likewise, menstrual dysfunction and stress fractures are also positively correlated [23,24]. Cortical bone mass seems to be preserved in amenorrheic women [22]. One study correlated osteopenic dual energy x-ray absorptiometry (DEXA) scan results with cancellous (ie, femoral neck) more strongly than with cortical bone (ie, tibial) stress fractures [25]. This study helps support the use of DEXA scan screening in the active amenorrheic woman who has a stress fracture [8]. Other factors such as inadequate nutrition, inappropriate conditioning, and anatomic differences have been implicated in the increased incidence of stress fractures in female athletes [26].

Studies have shown a higher risk for stress fractures in female track and field athletes that had more restrictive eating habits [17]. Nutrition's role in stress fracture development is not fully understood. Matched by age and body mass index (BMI), ballet dancers who have stress fractures tend to show more restrictive eating habits compared with both nondancers and dancers who have no stress fractures [27].

Common clinical presentation

History

Stress fractures are characterized by the insidious onset of localized pain and swelling over the involved bone. Patients may report increased activity or change in training regimen before the onset of symptoms. Initially, the pain occurs with activity and responds to rest. The athlete may note a decline in performance secondary to pain. Pain may progress, occurring during activities of daily living such as walking. If the inciting activity continues, the patient will notice pain at rest and nocturnal symptoms may develop. Many patients have vague complaints, and without a high level of suspicion the stress fracture may be missed, especially in the hip region. When evaluating a female patient, practitioners must inquire about a history of menstrual abnormalities (eg, delayed menarche, amenorrhea, oligomenorrhea), stress fractures, disordered or restrictive eating habits, a family history of osteoporosis, or any other potential secondary causes of osteopenia/osteoporosis.

Examination

A comprehensive musculoskeletal and functional examination is important for diagnosing stress fractures. The key findings of this examination are listed in Box 1. Patients who have lower extremity stress fractures may present with antalgic gait. The lumbar spine and lower extremity alignment must be observed while patients are standing and, if feasible, while

---

Box 1. Physical examination key findings

Observation
Gait abnormality
    Antalgic on involved side
    Excessive pronation
Reduced muscle mass
Lower extremity biomechanical assessment
    Pes Cavus
    Pes Planus
    Rear foot or forefoot pronation
Poor functional strength
    Unable to maintain hip in neutral position during unilateral
      squat

Palpation
Localized tenderness
Edema

Strength
Weakness of supporting musculature, including adjacent joints

Flexibility
Tightness of musculature of involved extremity, especially
  muscles spanning two joints

Provocative maneuvers
Pain with application of tuning fork caused by vibratory stress
Pain with load applied in lever across fracture site (use caution;
  risk for completing fracture)

---

performing their sports-specific activity. This observation provides insight into patterns of load-bearing and may identify a biomechanical reason for the development of the stress fracture. For example, biomechanical foot abnormalities, including pes cavus or hyperpronation, may be observed in standing, gait, or sport-specific assessments.

Palpation over the affected region of the bone may reveal pain, sometimes exquisite and well-localized tenderness. Tibial stress fractures usually present along the medial border of the tibia in the lower or upper one third. Stress fracture is differentiated from medial tibial stress syndrome (previously known as shin splints), which present with more diffuse tenderness along the middle to distal third of the posteromedial border of the tibia at the origin of the medial ankle musculature. In fibular stress fractures, seen more commonly in men, the location is usually 6 to 8 cm proximal to the lateral malleolus. Tarsal or metatarsal stress fractures present with localized foot tenderness; in runners the distal 2nd and 3rd metatarsal shaft is involved, whereas the base of the 2nd metatarsal is most common in dancers.

Manual muscle testing and range-of-motion testing can identify strength and flexibility deficits that can be addressed during the rehabilitation program but should be performed with caution in the involved extremity (see "Rehabilitation" section). Beyond the usual seated myotomal strength testing, testing hip abduction strength against gravity in side-lying is important. Functional strength testing such as unilateral squatting may reveal common patterns of weakness in women, such as increased knee valgus, indicative of hip abduction weakness. Provoking pain over the suspected fracture site with a vibrating tuning fork or ultrasound should increase clinical suspicion of a stress fracture. Another clinical test used in the setting of clinical or radiographic uncertainty is a lever mechanism. For example, the examiner can evaluate for a femoral stress fracture by applying a force across the distal femur bone in the seated position using the edge of the examination table as a fulcrum while fixing the patient's proximal femur. Pain provocation is a positive finding. However, the load must be applied gradually and cautiously while monitoring the patient's reaction to avoid completing the fracture.

Diagnostic testing

Stress fractures are typically diagnosed clinically. Plain radiographs can be normal at presentation. If a stress fracture is strongly suspected, treatment should be initiated and radiographs repeated later. If the diagnosis is uncertain or early diagnosis is necessary, such as with an elite athlete or in the setting of a possible high-risk stress fracture, an MRI or triple-phase bone scan (technetium-99m diphosphonate) can be positive at an early stage. Radionuclide scanning is a more sensitive but less specific method for imaging bone stress injuries [28]. MRI identifies the bone stress injury with more specific anatomic localization and provides additional soft tissue information, which can be useful in differentiating a bone stress injury from a soft tissue injury. For example, MRI can be useful in specifying the exact location of a femoral neck stress fracture (tension versus compression side) (Fig. 1). This information can be helpful in clinical management. MRI grading systems have been developed that use the short T1 inversion recovery (STIR) sequences. Four grades of abnormality have been described, from grade 1 (positive for periosteal edema on STIR or T2-weighted images) through grade 4 (positive injury line on T1 or T2-weighted images) [29,30].

The use of DEXA scan in the active woman who has a stress fracture is useful in diagnosing concurrent osteopenia or osteoporosis but is not used routinely. Research is ongoing in the use of bone density testing in premenopausal female athletes who present with stress fractures with the goal of making evidence-based recommendations on bone density testing in this population.

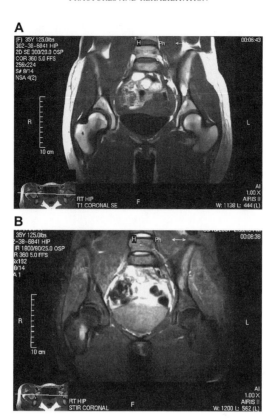

Fig. 1. MRI of femoral neck stress fracture with T1 coronal (*A*) and short T1 inversion recovery coronal (*B*) images showing compression side lesion.

Treatment

Acute-phase

RICE (rest, ice, compression, and elevation) and oral pain medications are used initially to manage pain. However, caution should be exercised in using pain medicine, because the reduction of pain may result in activity overuse and worsen the clinical situation. Activity modification is mandatory with discontinuation of activities that provoke pain. Alternative forms of nonimpact activities (eg, swimming, cycling, water running) may be substituted for the inciting activity until symptoms have abated. Educating the patient about their injury, the importance of activity restriction, and potential complications with noncompliance will enhance their understanding of the imposed exercise limitations. Immobilization may be required depending on the site of the stress fracture. For example, a metatarsal stress fracture can be treated with a removable boot cast for use with weight-bearing activity. If a removable boot cast is chosen, it is important to instruct the individual to wear a shoe with an equally elevated contralateral

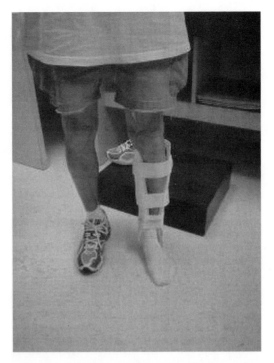

Fig. 2. Pneumatic leg brace used to treat a tibial stress fracture.

heel height. Immobilization with a pneumatic leg brace may be used for tibial stress fracture management to promote healing and limit the forces across the fracture site (Fig. 2). Studies have shown that subjects returned to activity sooner when a short leg pneumatic brace was used [31]. When acute treatment requires immobilization, postimmobilization muscle atrophy and loss of flexibility must be addressed in the subsequent rehabilitation program (see "Rehabilitation" section).

Bone stimulators have been shown to positively influence healing in nonunion tibial fractures [32]. Theoretically, these electromagnetic stimulation units have the potential to enhance healing in stress fractures. Their use has not been well studied in stress fractures, however, and remains controversial.

High-risk stress fractures

Stress fractures such as femoral neck, tarsal navicular, and anterior cortex tibial are considered high risk because of the possible complications, including progression to complete fracture, delayed union, nonunion, or avascular necrosis. A sports medicine specialist should be consulted in high-risk stress fractures and when diagnostic uncertainty exists [33].

Femoral neck fractures, seen more frequently in women, require a high index of clinical suspicion, because the clinical presentation may be vague. Typical complaints include groin, thigh, or even knee pain. Fractures occurring on the tension side (superior aspect) are high-risk stress fractures and can become displaced. They require strict non–weight bearing status with axillary crutches initially and require referral to orthopedic surgery for consideration of surgical intervention. Compression side (inferior aspect) femoral neck stress fractures also require strict non–weight bearing status initially but tend to be more stable and less likely to require surgical intervention.

Fractures with the propensity to progress to nonunion, such as stress fracture of the mid-shaft, anterior cortex of the tibia, require immobilization and symptom-driven weight bearing restrictions. Radiographs may reveal lucency in the cortex, referred to as the *dreaded black line* (Fig. 3). This finding heralds a defect that requires significant healing time and may eventually require surgical intervention [33]. Bone stimulators have been used to promote healing in this fracture type [32].

Tarsal navicular stress fractures may present with a paucity of physical findings. They are often missed initially. A high index of suspicion is needed to make the diagnosis. Bone scan is sensitive in detecting the fracture, although not specific. MRI and CT are more sensitive and specific [33]. Once confirmed, a CT scan is needed to define the extent of fracture [34]. These fractures require non–weight bearing, casting, and possibly surgical intervention. Custom orthotics are recommended during rehabilitation and return to play.

Rehabilitation

As with other musculoskeletal injuries, the principles of rehabilitation for stress fractures, listed in Box 2, are based on a gradual progression of activity with frequent re-evaluation of patient tolerance.

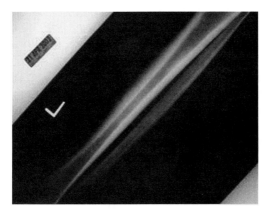

Fig. 3. Lucency at the anterior cortex of the tibial described as a "dreaded black line" heralding a bone defect.

Box 2. Principles of rehabilitation

Acute Phase
Minimize symptoms
Activity modification
    Consider weight-bearing restriction
Pain management
Reduce swelling
Deep-tissue massage to muscle trigger points, avoid fracture site
Maximize healing potential
Modality use (therapeutic electrical stimulation)
Minimize cardiovascular deconditioning
Cross-training (eg, cycling, swimming)
Maintain or restore normal joint range of motion and flexibility
Manual therapy
Stretching techniques
    Non–weight bearing stretching initially
Maintain or increase overall muscular strength and endurance
Continue noninvolved limb strengthening
Nonpainful isometric of involved limb initially

Subacute or recovery phase
Increase flexibility/restore lost flexibility from weight-bearing
    restriction
Weight-bearing and multiplane stretching
Increase local muscle strength
Progress to concentric and eccentric strengthening
Improve neuromuscular control and remediate maladaptive
    movement patterns
Non–weight bearing proprioceptive neuromuscular facilitation
    patterns initially
Progress to weight-bearing proprioceptive training
Gradual progression of activity
Pain indicates progressing too quickly

Functional phase
Maximize entire kinetic chain weight bearing neuromuscular control
Multiplane and plyometric training
Dynamic balance activities (ie, wobble board)
Restore functional activity, including sports, vocational, and other
    avocational pursuits
Agility drills
Sports specific activity patterns before return to play
Return to normal volume of training
Pain indicates progressing too quickly

Acute phase of rehabilitation

Ice is an effective local analgesic and anti-inflammatory agent. Physical therapy modalities (eg, heat, interferential electrical stimulation) are used to increase local blood flow and promote healing. No controlled studies have proven their efficacy, but these modalities are clinically useful in symptom control. Therapeutic ultrasound can reduce pain in muscles surrounding the fracture site but can aggravate bone pain at the fracture site. Ultrasound over the fracture site is contraindicated. Deep-tissue massage, including transverse friction massage, may be indicated to treat trigger points in muscles close to the stress fracture but not directly over the fracture site. This massage not only reduces pain but also enhances restoration of normal muscular flexibility, especially in patients who were immobilized for acute management.

Pain-free cardiovascular activities are encouraged because they not only prevent loss of cardiovascular conditioning but also allow patients to continue to be active and therefore more likely to comply with imposed activity restrictions. Examples of alternative activities for a metatarsal stress fracture in a runner would include pain-free aqua jogging, swimming, and upper-body ergometry. Pain during or after the activity is a clinical indication that the stress fracture is not healed; pain indicates that participation at that level is premature.

Stretching the muscles more proximal or distal to the fracture site may be initiated early if necessary. Loss of flexibility is acutely related to protective muscle guarding. Subsequent loss of adjacent joint range of motion occurs in patients who require restricted weight bearing or immobilization. Patients who have premorbid flexibility deficits, most commonly seen in muscles that span two joints (eg, the gastrocnemius) require a more rigorous stretching program. Occasionally, this program includes restoration of normal joint accessory movements. Non–weight bearing stretching can begin in the involved extremity only if it can be performed without pain provocation. Patients may continue a complete strengthening program in the uninvolved limbs and trunk as long as it can be performed in symptom-free positions. Isometric strengthening of the involved extremity is included as tolerated.

Subacute or recovery phase of rehabilitation

Modalities should no longer be required in the recovery phase. Persistent or recurrent swelling and pain indicates bone overload. Gradual progression of weight-bearing activity and stretching in weight-bearing positions is incorporated as tolerated.

Strength deficits have been implicated in the development of stress fractures [15]. In addition, deficits in local muscle strength can result from immobilization or activity limitations. As with stretching, strengthening of the involved limb is progressed from non–weight bearing isometric (static) exercises to concentric and finally eccentric training. Proprioceptive

neuromuscular facilitation can be used initially in retraining normal movement patterns, and the position can be modified to avoid strain on the fracture site.

Functional phase of rehabilitation

The athlete must go beyond the resolution of pain and improving flexibility and strength to a functional phase of rehabilitation where conditioning
and sports-specific activity meet or exceed returning-to-play criteria. In
many sports, plyometric (weight-bearing eccentric) training should precede
return to play. Neuromuscular re-education is a crucial part of a successful
return to activity. Weight-bearing proprioceptive training (balance board,
wobble board, mini-trampoline) is incorporated as appropriate (Fig. 4).
Sports-specific training must be addressed before return to play especially
when the patient has undergone a prolonged period of immobilization.
An athlete should be able to perform cutting and running drills pain-free
before returning to competition. Distance runners must be symptom-free

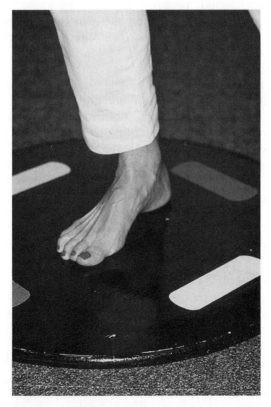

Fig. 4. Wobble board for weight-bearing proprioceptive training in the functional phase of
stress fracture rehabilitation.

with mileage progression. Practice and game time should be increased gradually as conditioning permits.

Prevention

Stress fractures are preventable injuries. The athlete and athletic program should be assessed to identify modifiable extrinsic and intrinsic risk factors for stress fractures. Extrinsic risk factors can be reduced through education on the proper progression of activity duration and intensity, which allows bone-appropriate adaptation to the imposed demands of the sport. Rest periods are mandatory to healthy training regiments. In addition, technique errors should be corrected. Videotaping and gait analysis are additional tools in evaluating an athlete's technique and providing education to coach and athlete. Cross training, including weight training, should be an essential part of any training regimen. It can facilitate both muscle strengthening and further aerobic conditioning while lowering the risk for harmful repetitive loading. Eccentric training is crucial to combat fatigue, which has been implicated in stress fracture development [15]. Absorbent training surface and properly fitted equipment can also reduce the risk for stress fractures. Shock-absorbing insoles, although controversial, may decrease the ground reaction forces and play a role in preventing stress fractures [35].

In addition, newer research looking at bone geometry shows that multidirectional loading, as seen in soccer players, leads to more symmetric bone geometry compared with single-plane runners' motion which leads to asymmetric bone geometry [36]. Symmetric bone geometry may be associated with less injury-prone bone. Incorporating multidirectional cross training may prove to be beneficial in injury prevention. Further studies are ongoing in this area.

Intrinsic risk factors also play a significant role in the development of stress fractures. Although some factors are non-modifiable, those that are modifiable should be identified and treated. In individuals who have significant forefoot or rearfoot biomechanical abnormalities, custom foot orthotics may be indicated [35]. The gait can be observed in the office or while the patient is running on a treadmill. If necessary, formal video gait analysis can be performed. Identified abnormalities should be corrected.

Patients who have known menstrual abnormalities should undergo a more detailed menstrual and nutritional history, physical examination, and workup to detect potential treatable conditions. Oral contraceptive pills (OCPs) are used in female athletes who have menstrual abnormalities, and are presumed to influence bone density. However, the correlation between OCP use and stress fracture risk reduction in this population is controversial [23,24,26,37]. Any individual who has a known bone disease or is at risk for low bone mass should undergo the appropriate evaluation (eg, laboratory, consider DEXA scan) to assist in prescribing an appropriate treatment and exercise program.

Individuals presenting with a stress fracture should undergo nutritional evaluation to identify deficits or abnormal eating behaviors. Intervention with a sports nutritionist is often helpful when dealing with athletes. Proper calorie consumption, both amount and quality, for activity level should be emphasized. Women of all ages should be counseled about consuming adequate calcium and vitamin D for healthy bone development and maintenance. One study showed that a group of athletes with stress fractures had lower calcium intake than a control group [38]. Although not fully elucidated, in the setting of menstrual abnormalities, calcium intake is recommended to be 1500 mg/d [26]. Calcium absorption is improved when taken with adequate vitamin D dosage of 800 IU/d [39].

Summary

Stress fractures are a common yet preventable sports injury. Women are at highest risk for developing stress fractures. A comprehensive assessment of the female athlete presenting with a stress fracture must include a detailed training review, nutritional and menstrual history, and biomechanical analysis. Stress fractures can be clinically diagnosed but occasionally require confirmatory diagnostic imaging. Conservative treatment based on activity modification is typically effective; however, high-risk stress fractures may require sports medicine consultation and possible surgical intervention. Rehabilitation includes minimizing symptoms and cardiovascular deconditioning while restoring range of motion, strength, and neuromuscular control. In addition, normalizing biomechanical deficits and optimizing energy balance is critical for achieving ultimate return to play. In summary, a comprehensive approach to the active patient includes education, identifying and modifying risk factors, and incorporating prevention strategies to reduce the incidence of stress fractures.

References

[1] McBryde AM. Stress fractures in athletes. J Sports Med 1975;3:212–7.
[2] Brunet ME, Cook SD, Brinker MR, et al. A survey of running injuries in 1505 competitive and recreational runners. J Sports Med Phys Fitness 1990;30(3):307–15.
[3] Markey KL. Stress fractures. Clin Sports Med 1987;6(2):405–25.
[4] O'Toole ML. Prevention and treatment of injuries to runners. Med Sci Sports Exerc 1992; 24(9 Suppl):S360–3.
[5] Jones BH, Bovee MW, Harris JM, et al. Intrinsic factors for exercise-related injuries among male and female army trainees. Am J Sports Med 1993;21(5):705–10.
[6] Pester S, Smith SC. Stress fractures in the lower extremity of soldiers in basic training. Orthop Rev 1992;21(3):297–303.
[7] Protzman RR, Griffis CG. Stress fractures in men and women undergoing military training. J Bone Joint Surg 1977;59(6):825.
[8] Callahan LR. Stress fractures in women. Clin Sports Med 2000;19(2):303–14.
[9] Bennell K, Matheson G, Meeuwisse W, et al. Risk factors for stress fractures. Sports Med 1999;28(2):91–122.

[10] Giladi M, Milgrom C, Simkin A, et al. Stress fractures. Identifiable risk factors. Am J Sports Med 1991;19(6):647–52.

[11] Windsor RE, Chambers K. Overuse injuries of the leg. In: Kibler WB, Herring SA, Press JM, editors. Functional rehabilitation of sports and musculoskeletal injuries. Gaithersburg (MD): Aspen Publications; 1998. p. 186–7.

[12] Rauh MJ, Macera CA, Trone DW, et al. Epidemiology of stress fracture and lower-extremity overuse injury in female recruits. Med Sci Sports Exerc 2006;38(9):1571–7.

[13] Zeni AI, Street CC, Dempsey RL, et al. Stress injury to the bone among women athletes. Phys Med Rehabil Clin N Am 2000;11(4):929–47.

[14] Daffner RH, Pavlov H. Stress fractures: current concepts. AJR Am J Roentgenol 1992; 159(2):245–52.

[15] Stanitski CL, McMaster JH, Scranton PE. On the nature of stress fractures. Am J Sports Med 1978;6(6):391–6.

[16] Matheson GO, Clement DB, McKenzie DC, et al. Stress fractures in athletes. A study of 320 cases. Am J Sports Med 1987;15(1):46–58.

[17] Bennell KL, Malcolm SA, Thomas PR, et al. Risk factors for stress fractures in track and field athletes: A twelve month prospective study. Am J Sports Med 1996;24(6):810–8.

[18] Garrett WE Jr, Safran MR, Seaber AV, et al. Biomechanical comparison of stimulated and nonstimulated skeletal muscle pulled to failure. Am J Sports Med 1987;15(5):448–54.

[19] Micheli LJ, Sohn RS, Soloman R. Stress fractures of the second metatarsal involving Lisfranc's joint in ballet dancer. A new overuse injury of the foot. J Bone Joint Surg 1985; 67(9):1372–5.

[20] Bennell KL, Brukner PD. Epidemiology and site specificity of stress fractures. Clin Sports Med 1997;16:179–96.

[21] Hulkko A, Orava S, Peltokallio P, et al. Stress fracture of the navicular bone. Nine cases in athletes. Acta Orthop Scand 1985;56(6):503–5.

[22] Drinkwater BL, Nilson K, Chesnut CH, et al. Bone mineral content of amenorrheic and eumenorrheic athletes. N Engl J Med 1984;311(5):277–81.

[23] Marcus R, Cann C, Madvig P, et al. Menstrual function and bone mass in elite women distance runners. Endocrine and metabolic factors. Ann Intern Med 1985;102(2):158–63.

[24] Barrow G, Saha S. Menstrual irregularity and stress fracture in collegiate female distance runners. Am J Sports Med 1998;16:209–16.

[25] Marx RG, Saint-Phard D, Callahan LR, et al. Stress fracture sites related to underlying bone health in athletic females. Clin J Sport Med 2001;11(2):73–6.

[26] Nattiv A, Armsey TD Jr. Stress injury to bone in the female athlete. Clin Sports Med 1997; 16(2):197–224.

[27] Frusztajer NT, Dhuper S, Warren MP, et al. Nutrition and the incidence of stress fractures in ballet dancers. Am J Clin Nutr 1990;51(5):779–83.

[28] Geslien GE, Thrall JH, Espinosa JL, et al. Early detection of stress fractures using 99mTc-polyphosphate. Radiology 1976;121(3 Pt.1):683–7.

[29] Arendt EA, Griffith HJ. The use of MR imaging in the assessment and clinical management of stress reactions of bone in high-performance athletes. Clin Sports Med 1997;16: 291–306.

[30] Fredericson M, Bergman AG, Hoffman KL, et al. Tibial stress reaction in runners. Correlation of clinical symptoms and scintigraphy with a new magnetic resonance imaging grading system. Am J Sports Med 1995;23(4):472–81.

[31] Whitelaw GP, Wetzler MJ, Levy AS, et al. A pneumatic leg brace for the treatment of tibial stress fractures. Clin Orthop Rel Res 1991;207:301–5.

[32] Rettig AC, Shelbourne KD, McCarroll JR, et al. The natural history and treatment of delayed union stress fractures of the anterior cortex of the tibia. Am J Sports Med 1988; 16(3):250–5.

[33] Boden BP, Osbahr DC. High risk stress fractures: evaluation and treatment. J Am Acad Orthop Surg 2000;8(6):344–53.

[34] Lee S, Anderson RV. Stress fractures of the tarsal navicular. Foot Ankle Clin 2004;9(1): 85–104.

[35] Finestone A, Giladi M, Elad H, et al. Prevention of stress fractures using custom biomechanical shoe orthoses. Clin Orthop Rel Res 1999;360:182–90.

[36] Cleek TM, Whalen RT. Effect of activity and age on long bones using a new densitometric technique. Med Sci Sports Exerc 2005;37(10):1806–13.

[37] Bennell K, White S, Crossley K. The oral contraceptive pill: a revolution for sportswomen? Br J Sports Med 1999;33(4):231–8.

[38] Myburgh KH, Bachrach LK, Lewis B, et al. Low bone mineral density at axial and appendicular sites in amenorrheic athletes. Med Sci Sports Exerc 1993;25(11):1197–202.

[39] NIH consensus conference. Optimal calcium intake. NIH Consensus Development Panel on Optimal Calcium Intake. JAMA 1994;272(24):1942–8.

ELSEVIER
SAUNDERS

Phys Med Rehabil Clin N Am
18 (2007) 417–438

PHYSICAL MEDICINE
AND REHABILITATION
CLINICS OF
NORTH AMERICA

ACL Tears in Female Athletes

Danica N. Giugliano, BA[a],
Jennifer L. Solomon, MD[a,b,*]

[a]Women's Sports Medicine Center, Hospital for Special Surgery, 535 East 70th Street,
New York, NY 10021, USA
[b]Weill Medical College of Cornell University, 1300 York Avenue, New York, NY 10021, USA

Epidemiology

Since the enactment of Title IX in 1972, the number of females involved in athletics has grown considerably. In the United States the percentage of girls participating in sports at the high school level increased almost tenfold from 1971 (3.7%) to 1998 (33%) [1]. By 1998, females represented 40% of all high school and college athletic participants [1].

With the growing number of athletes, the number of sport-related injuries has also increased greatly. Seventy percent of anterior cruciate ligament (ACL) injuries occur during athletic participation [2–4]. They are most common in sports that require rapid stopping, cutting, and changing direction, such as basketball, soccer, and team handball [5]. In the United States, the overall ACL injury rate for the general population is approximately 100,000 tears per year, corresponding to 1 in 3000 individuals [6,7]. Athletes who are injured may potentially miss an entire season or more of sports, lose scholarship funding, suffer psychologically and academically, or experience post-traumatic arthritis in the injured knee later in life [8].

The National Collegiate Athletic Association (NCAA) statistics have shown that, when compared with male athletes who participate in activities with similar rules and equipment, female athletes are two to eight times more likely to sustain an ACL injury [9]. Environmental, anatomic, hormonal, neuromuscular, and biomechanical risk factors of the female athlete have been studied to predict injury and determine ways to prevent tears. Experts believe that multiple factors are most likely involved in predisposing the female athlete to ACL injuries, but further research is necessary to

* Corresponding author. Women's Sports Medicine Center, Hospital for Special Surgery, 535 East 70th Street, New York, NY 10021.
  E-mail address: solomonj@hss.edu (J.L. Solomon).

determine methods of preventing injury. Reducing the ACL injury rate would improve the physical, psychological, and financial health of female athletes worldwide.

The role of the anterior cruciate ligament

The knee joint consists of the patellofemoral and tibiofemoral joints. The patellofemoral joint is the articulation between the patella and anterior femoral plateaus, and the tibiofemoral joint is the articulation between the proximal tibia and the distal femur. Within the tibiofemoral joint, on the distal end of the femur, are the large medial and lateral condyles, which make up the proximal articular surface. The intercondylar notch separates these plateaus and is where the ACL passes laterally to the posterior cruciate ligament (PCL) [10]. The articular surfaces of the proximal tibia that correspond to the femoral articular surfaces are two shallow concave medial and lateral plateaus [10]. The distal articular surface of the femur articulates with the patella anteriorly and with the tibia posteriorly and inferiorly. Shallow grooves of the lateral and medial condyle separate the anterior and inferior articulations.

The tibiofemoral joint is dynamically stabilized by the quadriceps, hamstrings, and triceps surae muscles and is passively stabilized by the joint capsule, lateral and medial menisci, and four ligaments (lateral collateral ligament, medial collateral ligament, ACL, and PCL). The hamstrings and ACL resist forward movement of the medial and lateral plateaus, preventing anterior dislocation of the tibia relative to the femur. During deeper flexion angles, the quadriceps, hamstrings, and ACL resist forward movement of the plateaus. Backward movement of the plateaus is resisted by the PCL and quadriceps, preventing posterior dislocation of the tibia relative to the femur. The PCL and ACL also help prevent hyperextension of the tibiofemoral joint, medial and lateral displacement of the tibia relative to the femur, and internal rotation of the tibia relative to the femur [10].

The ACL can also be described as consisting of two bundles: the anteromedial bundle and the posterolateral bundle, which are named for the orientation of their tibial insertions [11,12]. The anteromedial bundle is tight in flexion and resists anterior drawer (forward movement of the tibia) between 60° and 90° of flexion [12]. The posterolateral bundle is tight in extension and resists anterior subluxation near full extension [12]. A partial ACL tear can be caused by damage to either one of the two bundles [13,14]. Anterior force when the knee is close to full extension can damage the posterolateral bundle, whereas anterior force when the knee is in greater flexion can damage the anteromedial bundle [15].

Noncontact ACL injuries, which account for 70% of all ACL injuries in both male and female athletes [16], commonly occur during planting and cutting, and landing maneuvers [17]. Many different factors have been related to noncontact ACL injuries during these types of movements, including those that are more easily controlled (environmental factors) and those that are less easily controlled and innate to the female athlete (anatomic, hormonal, neuromuscular, and biomechanical factors).

Environmental factors

Shoe and surface type

With the proper ground–shoe surface interface during athletic events, female athletes may be able to reduce their risk for an ACL injury. Surfaces that increase friction between the player and the field of play can modify movement patterns in athletes, increasing their risk for ACL injuries. Drier playing surfaces, which increase the amount of friction between the surface and shoe, have been shown to have a greater ACL injury rate than wet surfaces [18]. ACL tears experienced by Australian football players were most frequent during high-evaporation and low-rainfall periods [19]. The effect of artificial playing surfaces on injury rate remains controversial. Synthetic turf has been shown to be a less-safe surface to play on than outdoor grass [20]. By contrast, ACL injury rate decreased by 50% for a group of Texas football teams who played on "FieldTurf," an artificial turf, rather than natural grass [21]. Artificial indoor floors have also been shown to be more dangerous than natural wood floors [22].

Torg and Quendenfeld [23] observed that the number and size of the cleats on a shoe correlated with the occurrence of knee and ankle injuries in American football players, with fewer injuries corresponding to smaller and fewer cleats. Lambson and colleagues [24] examined the effects of four different cleat designs on knee injury risk for 3119 high school football players. The shoes with cleats placed at the peripheral margin of the sole and smaller, pointed cleats positioned interiorly were associated with higher torsional resistance and a significantly higher ACL injury rate than the other three designs combined.

A complete understanding of the complex interaction at the shoe–surface interface remains elusive [23,24]. Livesay and colleagues [25] studied peak torque and rotational stiffness for different combinations of cleat types and surface types. They found that highest peak torques were developed by a grass shoe–FieldTurf combination and a turf shoe–Astroturf combination. The grass shoe consisted of fewer cleats than the turf shoe, but each cleat was higher and wider. For both types of shoes, a grass surface provided the least amount of torque compared with the synthetic surfaces (FieldTurf, Astroturf, and Astroplay). The rotational stiffness was also greatest for the turf shoe–Astroturf combination. The authors concluded that a grass shoe-grass surface may be closest to ideal in preventing ACL injuries, but deciding which shoe–surface combination also depends on other factors, such as the sport, age of the players, and level of play.

Knee bracing

Prophylactic, functional, and postoperative or rehabilitative knee braces have been used to prevent ACL injuries or reinjuries. However, their effects on the knee injury rate remain controversial. Prophylactic bracing has been shown to protect the ACL during a controlled, direct lateral blow [26] and does not add valgus pressure to the knee [27]. It has also been shown to provide 20% to 30% greater resistance to a lateral blow that is sufficiently large enough to cause a medial joint-line opening [27]. By contrast, a study of a college football team showed that the braced knees had a higher knee injury rate than nonbraced knees [28]. Other studies have shown that prophylactic bracing has no effect on injury rate [29,30].

Findings on the benefits of rehabilitative and functional knee braces remain mixed. Studies have shown that functional knee bracing on nonoperative patients may provide psychological [31] and subjective benefits, including a sense of stability [32]. It can also increase coordination [32], reduce anterior tibial translation under low loading conditions [33], and reduce anterior–posterior laxity [34]. A study using a functional knee brace that constrained knee extension showed an increase in knee flexion angle of athletes who performed stop-jump tasks [35]. Fleming and colleagues [36] showed that functional knee bracing protected the ACL during internal torques in the non–weight-bearing knee and during anterior–posterior shear loading in both the non–weight-bearing and weight-bearing knee.

Several studies have shown that the use of bracing for an extended period may have negative consequences, including reduced quadriceps strength. Houston and Goemans [37] found that bracing decreased quadriceps muscle strength by 12% to 30%. Risberg and colleagues [33] reported that postoperative patients who used bracing 1 to 2 years after the ACL tear had quadriceps strength values of less than 80% of the strength values of postoperative patients who only wore a brace for 3 months.

Several studies have shown that functional bracing does not protect the knee. Studies have shown that it does not decrease anterior tibial displacement relative to the femur [38–40] or influence ACL strain values for external torques and varus and valgus moments [36]. Studies have also shown no differences in strength, laxity, or function in the braced and nonbraced knee 2 years after surgery [41]. In addition, Risberg and colleagues [33] showed that bracing did not reduce the risk for further injuries to the meniscus or cartilage in the tibiofemoral joint.

The possible benefits of knee bracing remains controversial. Further studies that include a large sample size with a homogenous population are necessary to determine the effectiveness of knee bracing on ACL injury risk.

Anatomic factors

Bone lengths

The increase in torque on the knee joint that accompanies the growing tibia and femur in children can cause instability in the knee [42]. Men have been shown to compensate for this through increasing their power, strength, and coordination more than women, which may help to explain the increased risk for ACL tears in women [42,43].

Ireland reported that the hip width to femoral length ratio is a better predictor of ACL injury risk than the absolute lengths and widths of the lower extremities [5]. However, this ratio may not explain the difference in ACL injury rate between the genders, because the ratio has been shown to be roughly equal in men and women (0.73 and 0.77, respectively) [44].

Q angle and knee valgus

The quadriceps femoris angle, or Q angle, is the acute angle between the line that connects the anterior superior iliac spine to the midpoint of the patella and the line that connects the tibial tubercle to the same reference point on the patella [45]. Studies have shown that Q angles are larger in women than in men [5,44,46] and are larger in athletes who sustained a knee injury than in noninjured athletes [47]. A larger Q angle increases the lateral pull on the quadriceps muscle that is connected to the patella, adding medial stress to the knee and increasing the risk for an ACL tear [47]. A larger Q angle has been shown to predict 32.4% to 46% of variance in valgus–varus knee position [48], with valgus knee positioning predictive of future ACL injury risk [34]. Despite these findings, the effects of a large Q angle and knee valgus remain controversial, with other studies reporting that static Q angle measures are not predictive of knee valgus or ACL injury risk during dynamic movements [49,50].

Femoral notch width and shape

In men and women, as height increases, total condylar width also increases. Studies have shown that, as height increases, notch width increases in men but not in women [51]. Uhorchak and colleagues [52] reported that women who had a narrow intercondylar notch (<13 mm) had a 16.8 times grater risk ratio for an ACL injury than those who had a larger notch. Other studies have shown that a small notch width is associated with an increased risk for an ACL injury and can increase the severity of the tear [53,54]. Arendt [55] reported that notch width is smaller in women sustaining bilateral ACL tears than those who had a unilateral tear. In addition, those who sustained a unilateral tear had a smaller notch width than those who had no tears [55]. The effects of notch width size on ACL injury risk remains controversial, with Teitz and colleagues [56] reporting no difference in notch width size in injured and noninjured knees.

The *notch width index* (NWI), which is the width of the intercondylar notch divided by the width of the distal femur at the level of the popliteal groove, has also been studied to determine whether it can predict ACL injury risk. A study by Souryal and colleagues [57] reported no difference in NWI between noninjured subjects and those who experienced unilateral ACL injury. In addition, differences in NWI between the genders remain controversial. Griffin and colleagues [16] reported that NWI is greater in women than in men, but several studies have reported no statistically significant gender-related differences in notch width indices [54] and rate of ACL tears [56,58].

The shape of the femoral notch may also affect the ACL injury rate. Femoral notch shapes can be categorized as *reverse U-* or *side C-shaped*, *H-shaped*, or *A-shaped* [59]. A decreased notch width and an A-shaped notch might put a female athlete at a higher risk for a noncontact ACL injury [60]. However, evidence continues to conflict as to whether notch shape differs with gender [61] and whether shape affects ACL injury rate.

Anterior cruciate ligament size and mechanical properties

Female ACLs are smaller than male ACLs when normalized for body weight [61]. Several studies have shown a positive correlation between small ACLs and injury risk [51,52]. A smaller ACL encounters a greater amount of stress when force is applied to a knee joint. However, whether this stress is high enough to cause injury to the ACL is unclear [34]. In addition, women typically have a narrow notch width relative to the size of the ACL [51], which can cause impingement when the knee is in full extension, such as when landing from a jump or performing a cutting maneuver [59].

Mechanical property of the ACL may influence its ability to sustain increased loads. A cadaveric study by Chandrashekar and colleagues [62], which measured mechanical property by strain at failure, stress at failure, and modulus of elasticity, showed that female ACLs have a lower mechanical quality than male ACLs. Differences in material properties of female and male ACLs may prove important in determining why women have a higher risk for injury than men.

Laxity

Laxity, the combination of joint hypermobility and musculotendinous flexibility, is more prevalent in women than in men and may increase the risk for an ACL injury [63]. After puberty, flexibility has been shown to increase in girls and decrease in boys, leading to greater generalized laxity in adult women than in adult men [64]. Muscle stiffness is an important component in maintaining knee stability and injury prevention [59]. When force is applied to the knee, the muscles surrounding the knee contract and the knee stiffens, dissipating the force that the ACL carries [59]. Hamstring laxity can delay hamstring activation, decreasing the co-contraction between the quadriceps and hamstrings during foot strike and increasing the risk for an ACL injury [65]. Joint laxity in the knee can potentially strain the ACL by increasing sagittal knee motion (hyperextension), coronal knee motion (valgus), and anterior tibial translation [64]. Joint laxity in the foot is greater in women [64] and may affect the ACL by increasing ligamentous laxity and navicular drop [66,67]. Navicular drop has been shown to be a predictor of anterior tibial translation, which can strain the ACL [67].

Despite the greater laxity and flexibility in women [17,68,69], whether laxity predisposes a female athlete to an ACL injury remains controversial. Uhorchak and colleagues [52] reported that women who have greater anterior–posterior knee laxity had a 2.7 times greater risk for an ACL injury. Boden and colleagues [70] reported that the hamstring muscles were more lax in ACL-injured athletes when compared with noninjured athletes, whereas a study of individuals who had bilateral ACL ruptures reported that laxity was not a factor in ACL injury risk [71].

Body mass index

The effects of body mass index (BMI) on ACL injury rate remains controversial and inconsistent. Increased BMI can be associated with a decrease in relative strength. This can decrease the hip flexion angle and knee flexion velocity and increase the peak knee extension moment when landing from a jump, increasing the risk for an ACL injury [72]. In a study of cadets at the U.S. Military Academy, women who had a higher-than-normal BMI had a higher risk for a noncontact ACL injury than those who had a lower BMI [52]. However, in a study of men and women in basic combat training, Knapik and colleagues [73] showed that BMI is not associated with overall injury risk in either sex.

Hormonal factors

An increased level of estrogen in women relative to men is believed to be an underlying cause of female ACL injuries [49,74]. Estrogen receptors are present in human ACL fibroblasts [64], which produce the collagen that performs the major load-bearing function of the ACL [59]. When estrogen is present, the synthesis of collagen by the fibroblasts is reduced [64], which can reduce the strength of the ACL and increase the risk for an ACL injury [75]. Studies on nonhuman ACLs have shown that estradiol does not affect fibroblast proliferation and collagen synthesis [76]. However, in vitro studies on human ACLs have shown that an increase in sex hormone concentrations may influence ACL metabolism and collagen synthesis in an interactive, dose-dependent, and time-dependent manner [77,78].

High levels of estrogen have also been shown to decrease the neuromuscular control of the knee [64] and increase knee laxity [79–81]. Posthuma and colleagues [82] reported that motor skill ability decreases as estrogen levels increase during the premenstrual phases. Sarwar and colleagues [83] reported that during the ovulatory phase, when estrogen levels peak, quadriceps strength increases and muscle relaxation decreases. Several studies have shown greater laxity during the luteal phase of the cycle [79,80,84]. Other studies showed no difference in laxity during the different phases of the menstrual cycle [85,86] or when estradiol levels are high [87].

The effects of fluctuating estrogen levels on ACL injury rate during the different phases of the menstrual cycle also remains controversial. Wojtys and colleagues [88] reported the greatest incidence of ACL injury during the ovulatory phase, whereas several studies have shown a greater incidence of injury during the luteal phase [89,90] and follicular phase [91]. However, inconsistencies exist regarding menstrual phase definitions and sex steroid measurements, which likely impacts the variance in findings.

The effect of oral contraceptives on female ACL injury risk is unclear. Oral contraceptives lower the levels of estrogen in the female body [64]. Several studies reported lower traumatic injury rates for athletes who take oral contraceptives [9,89], but a study of college varsity athletes sustaining noncontact ACL injuries showed that the use of oral contraceptives did not influence risk for injury [92]. Until further research is conducted, no recommendations have been made to alter participation of female athletes using oral contraceptives [5].

Neuromuscular factors

Several studies have shown differences in neuromuscular development between men and women after the onset of puberty. Unlike girls, boys have neuromuscular spurts that match their growth spurts [42]. The rapid increase in size and weight, with the absence of increased neuromuscular power and control, in girls at or near puberty may contribute to the higher incidence rate of ACL injuries [42].

Female knees also have shorter activation duration in the gastrocnemius and gluteus muscles, which initiate and maintain knee and lower extremity stiffness [93]. In addition, females show leg dominance [34]. *Leg dominance* is the imbalance among muscle strength, flexibility, and coordination between the lower extremities and can predict future ACL injury risk [34]. Coactivation of the hamstrings and quadriceps muscles is important in protecting the knee against dynamic lower extremity valgus and excessive anterior drawer and abduction [64]. Women have been shown to have quadriceps-dominant contraction during landing and cutting [34], which can increase the anterior displacement of the tibia relative to the femur and increase the risk for an ACL tear [64]. Female athletes also have a low ratio of medial-to-lateral quadriceps recruitment and increased lateral hamstring firing [50]. These neuromuscular mechanisms compress the lateral joint, opens the medial joint, and increases the anterior shear force, which could increase the risk for an ACL injury [63,94].

When landing from a jump, women have increased rectus femoris firing and decreased gluteal muscle firing compared with men [95]. Using less hip musculature increases the force placed on the lower extremities, causing valgus collapse [64]. Decreased hip muscle activation also reduces maximal possible quadriceps and hamstring activation, altering optimal load-bearing capacity, and increasing the risk for an ACL injury [16]. Maneuvers performed with insufficient hip control in the transverse plane of motion have been shown to cause valgus collapse [64].

Mechanoreceptors in the ACL allow for a reflex response of hamstring activation when knee movements cause torque and elongation of the ACL, and can be indicators of anterior tibial translation on the femur [64]. Haycock and Gillette [96] found that uninjured women possessed lower single-leg sway measures than uninjured men, but after an ACL tear, women had increased single-leg sway. This finding may suggest trauma to the proprioceptive system in women who experience an ACL tear or that women who have decreased proprioception have a predisposition to ACL tears [96].

Fatigue can cause altered landing and cutting movements that can put the ACL at risk for a tear [97]. Wjotys and colleagues [98] reported that lower-extremity muscle fatigue increased anterior tibial translation by 32.5%. When performing stop-jump tasks while fatigued, a decrease in knee flexion angle, an increase in proximal tibial anterior shear force, and an increase in knee varus moment also occur [97]. Although fatigue may increase ACL injury risk, no research currently shows that women fatigue faster or are less conditioned than men.

Biomechanical factors

Noncontact female ACL injuries are most commonly caused during planting and cutting (29%), straight knee landing (28%), or one-step stop landing with knee hyperextended (26%) [17]. The posture and lower extremity alignment of women during these movements may predispose them to future ACL injuries. Women perform cutting maneuvers in a more erect position than men [99], which can cause decreased flexion in the knee and hip, increased valgus in the knee, and greater activation of the quadriceps muscles [100]. Performing actions in a more crouched position may reduce the risk for ACL injuries in female athletes [100].

Foot and ankle

Foot pronation, measured with navicular drop, can be caused by joint laxity of the foot and can affect tibial translation and lower extremity alignment [66,67]. Increased navicular drop moves the tibia forward [67] and increases internal tibial rotation [34]. Navicular drop has been shown to be greater in individuals who have sustained an ACL tear [101] and greater in women than in men [66,67]. However, further research is needed to determine whether navicular drop can predict ACL injury risk.

Variations in ankle joint angles have been shown to influence joint forces, moments, and muscular activation patterns in the knee [16,102]. Female athletes have a greater maximum ankle eversion than male athletes when performing cutting maneuvers [103], which may cause an ACL rupture by increasing valgus knee stress and tibial rotation.

Knee

Several studies have shown that specific knee biomechanics during landing and pivoting increase the risk for ACL injuries. When landing from a jump, female athletes are weaker in knee extension and muscle strength [69] and have greater adduction and abduction moments [104], which can alter the dynamic neuromuscular control of the lower extremity in the coronal plane [103]. Knee abduction moments (valgus torques) and angles have been shown to be significant predictors of ACL injuries (73% sensitivity and 78% specificity) [43].

McNair and colleagues [105] reported that ACL injury occurs between 20° of knee flexion and full extension, whereas Olsen and colleagues [106] and Boden and colleagues [70] reported injuries between 0° and 30° of flexion. At a knee flexion angle between 10° and 30°, the quadriceps muscles exert maximum anterior shear force, putting significant strain on the ACL [16]. No consensus has been reached as to whether female athletes land and cut with greater knee flexion than male athletes [64]. Yu and colleagues [107] found that, during ground contact, knee flexion angles decrease after the age of 12 years in girls but not boys. Other studies have also shown that women have less knee flexion than men [108]. However, Fagenbaum and Darling [109] reported that women land with greater knee flexion angles than men. Furthermore, many studies have reported that knee flexion angles are the same for both men and women [103,110].

Hip

Hip biomechanics during landing may also predispose a woman to ACL injury risk. Hewett and colleagues [43] reported that peak external hip flexion moments in the sagittal plane were greater in injured female athletes than in those who were uninjured. Lephart and colleagues [111] reported that, during landing, female athletes have greater hip internal rotation than male athletes. The gluteus maximus can control excessive hip rotation, but is activated less in women than in men [95]. In addition, women land with greater external hip adduction moments and smaller hip flexion angles on their dominant side [64]. Greater hip adduction can decrease hip control and imbalances in side-to-side neuromuscular strength, flexibility, and coordination of the hip can increase knee valgus, which can put strain on the ACL [64].

Core stability

The *core* is the strength and function of the abdominal, back extensor, and pelvic floor muscles that contribute to stability of the lumbopelvic–hip region complex. The core is where a person's center of gravity is located and where all movements begin [112]. A stable core can help stabilize the lower extremity, allowing it to function with optimal kinetic chain mechanics that reduce and stabilize forces [112]. Theoretically, if the core is weak, efficient movements cannot be produced, even if the lower extremities are strong. These inefficient movements can cause injury in the knee [112].

The effects of reduced core stability on ACL injury rates remain controversial. One study showed that men performed better than women on core strength tests and a positive correlation was seen between external rotation and abduction strength. However, a correlation did not exist between a weaker core and higher ACL injury rates in either men or women [5]. However, a different study showed that a weak core, demonstrated through hip abduction and external rotation weakness, increased the risk for lower extremity injury [5]. In addition, anecdotal observations show that athletes who sustained an ACL tear have weakness in the core [5]. More research using a large sample size and valid and reliable core stability measurements is necessary to elucidate the relationship between core stability and ACL injury risk.

Skill and level of exposure

The differences in skill level between the two genders have been studied to determine if women can decrease their risk for injury through training and experience. Skill level can be determined partially by an athlete's level of conditioning and amount of prior experience [113]. Harmon and Dick [114] studied injury rates among the different NCAA division levels and assumed that athletes who were more skilled played at higher levels. When comparing the same gender and sport, they reported that ACL injury rates were the same among the different levels. However, Bjordal and Arnoy [115] reported that the men in more skilled division levels of a soccer league had higher rates of ACL injuries.

Level of experience can reflect an athlete's mastery and competency in a given sport. Level of experience can be measured by the amount of previous participation in organized sports. Report have shown that the amount of prior experience among NCAA female basketball and soccer players has increased over the past decade, but the ACL injury rate among both male and female athletes has remained statistically stable [116,117]. Studies are limited, but a direct correlation between level of experience and ACL injury rate does not seem to exist among female athletes.

Athletes who are not well conditioned fatigue faster [118], resulting in decreased coordination, proprioception, and neuromuscular control [113], which can contribute to less joint stability and increased risk for an ACL injury [118]. Harmon and Ireland [113] reported no difference in the level of conditioning between noninjured male and female athletes or between male and female athletes who had ACL injuries. However, fatigue has been shown to affect proprioception, preactivation of muscle tension in anticipation of joint loading, and muscle-firing patterns in male and female athletes [118].

Preventative strategies

Research has shown that proper prevention programs may reduce the rate of injury in athletes [104,119]. Training strategies that address neuromuscular risk factors through increasing knee stiffness, improving balance, minimizing at-risk positions, and decreasing ACL strain can help prevent ACL tears [34]. One prospective study [104] showed that women who were not enrolled in an ACL tear prevention program had a 3.7 higher incidence rate of knee injury compared with female athletes who were enrolled. Untrained female athletes also had a 4.6 times higher rate of knee injury than untrained male athletes.

Markolf and colleagues [120] tested knee stiffness of men and women using a clinical testing apparatus designed to record anterior–posterior tibial force versus displacement and varus–valgus moment versus angulation during manual manipulation of the knee. They reported that athletes were capable of increasing knee stiffness by a factor of 10 through training that emphasized the hamstring and gastrocnemius muscle groups [120]. Griffis and colleagues [99] conducted a study of NCAA Division I female basketball players who were trained to perform cuts in a three-step movement pattern where the knee was kept flexed and the feet were kept under the hips. This training reduced ACL injuries by 89% over 2 years. Hewett and colleagues [121] studied a preseason training program teaching lower limb neuromuscular control during landing and strengthening the muscles surrounding the knee to increase joint stability. This program increased power in the hamstrings by 33% and the strength of the hamstrings by 20% in female athletes. It also decreased incidence of serious knee injury rates for women at high risk for these injuries.

Training programs that develop gender-specific modifications for female athletes may be able reduce the risk for female ACL tears. Most prevention programs should teach proper landing techniques that alter dynamic loading through neuromuscular control [34]. Plyometrics and agility-type exercises have been proven to improve muscle reaction time [122]. Increasing activation of the hamstrings [100] and using hip control [104] have also been shown to help prevent injuries.

Treatment options

Surgical and conservative treatment options are available for female athletes who experience an ACL tear. ACL injuries are often accompanied by other injuries, such as ligament sprains, meniscal tears, articular cartilage injuries, and bone bruises [123]. When determining which treatment is best for the injured athlete, these other injuries to the knee and the amount of rigorous activity that the athlete plans to participate in after treatment must be taken into account [123].

Surgical treatment is most often recommended when the athlete experiences an ACL tear in combination with other injuries, significant laxity is present in the knee, the ACL is vital for knee function, surgery would successfully restore the knee to normal function, or the athlete plans to participate in high-risk activities after treatment that cause repeated episodes of giving way (pivot–shift episodes). Nonsurgical treatment would be recommended for athletes whose ACL-deficient knee can function reasonably well under normal circumstances and who are not planning to participate in high-risk activities. Nonsurgical treatment may also be recommended for athletes who have advanced arthritis in the knee and who would develop osteoarthritis later in life despite reconstruction surgery. These guidelines may not be ideal for all female athletes and each athlete must be evaluated individually to determine the best treatment option [123].

Few studies have been designed to investigate the effect of age on operative versus nonoperative treatment. Barber and colleagues [124] found no difference in outcomes of ACL reconstruction in patients either younger or older than 40 years. From the current literature, age alone should not determine whether a person is a good candidate for ACL reconstruction [125].

Surgical reconstruction

Approximately 50,000 ACL reconstructions are preformed annually in the United States on men and women [7,126]. For athletes choosing surgical reconstruction, the timing of the surgery is not as important as the condition of the knee before surgery [123]. The knee should have full range of motion with minimal pain. In addition, the athlete must be mentally prepared for the reconstruction and postoperative rehabilitation required [123].

The most common technique for reconstructing the ACL is using an autograft arthroscopically. An autograft from the bone–patella–tendon bone (BPTB) or from the hamstring tendon is more common than one from the quadriceps tendon. Although the BPTB graft is known as the gold standard, more research is needed to determine if it produces better results than a hamstring graft in terms of knee laxity, knee pain, and return to play [127].

Using an allograft for ACL reconstruction is gaining popularity. The graft is most commonly used from the Achilles tendon, BPTB, and fascia lata. Allografts have been shown to have less donor-site morbidity, less surgical time, improved cosmetic results, and the possibility of an earlier and faster recovery. However, one main concern with using an allograft is disease transmission, because sterilization techniques are not used during surgery. Extensive donor screening and aseptic harvest techniques are the main mechanisms used to stop allograft disease transmission. Other concerns with using allografts are added costs to the surgical procedure, host immunogenic responses to the graft, delayed graft incorporation, and lack of long-term structural integrity. Sherman and Banffy [127] concluded that the benefits gained using the allograft do not outweigh the associated costs. However, an autograft may not be beneficial for everyone, and each athlete's individual needs must be considered when determining the type of graft used [127].

Few studies have compared outcomes of ACL reconstruction surgery based on gender. A study by Barber-Westin and colleagues [128] found no difference in complications or failure rate between men and women 26 months after autogenous ipsilateral central BPTB reconstructions. In addition, women averaged 6 more months of rehabilitation than men [128]. However, one study comparing men and women who had hamstring reconstruction surgery showed that women had more laxity and knee pain and did not return to the preinjury activity level [129]. Three other studies have shown similar results, but none of these studies on hamstring grafts have been prospective and controlled [130–132]. Other studies have also shown that BPTB autograft reconstruction is equally successful for men and women [128,133–135]. Harmon and Ireland [113] suggest that the desired activity level and potential for further injury should be the overriding concern over gender when deciding whether to undertake reconstruction surgery.

Conservative treatment

Nonsurgical treatment is possible for those patients who are less active, have minimal instability, or cannot follow the demanding postsurgical rehabilitation protocols [136]. Physical therapy includes strengthening of the quadriceps and hamstring muscles [137]. Patients may also use knee braces if they return to physical activity [137]. These braces may provide psychological benefits, but their effects on reinjury rate remains controversial [137].

Post-treatment

Rehabilitation is required postoperatively. No consensus has been reached regarding which variables should be used to characterize a rehabilitation program after reconstruction surgery. Rehabilitation programs can vary according to the use of cold therapy, immediate versus delayed motions, immediate versus delayed weight-bearing, closed versus open kinetic chain exercises, the use of bracing, home- versus clinic-based rehabilitation, neuromuscular electrical stimulation versus voluntary muscle contraction, specifics of exercise programs, and intensity and duration of rehabilitation [125].

Several studies have shown that most patients (65%–88%) can return to sport within 1 year after ACL reconstruction surgery [138–140]. A study by Fink and colleagues [141] of mixed-sport athletes 10 to 13 years after injury showed a 44% reduction in high-risk sports participation in those who were surgically treated and a 70% reduction in those who were nonsurgically treated. Some athletes are also able to return to high-level pivoting sports without surgery (19%–82%) [142,143]. These athletes most likely have functionally stable knees and a strong desire and motivation to return to a pivoting sport despite the ACL tear [144]. Myklebust and colleagues [142] also reported that, irrespective of treatment type, athletes who had sustained an ACL injury and returned to sport retired sooner than noninjured athletes. This finding may be because of significant knee problems sustained after the injury, such as instability, reduced range of motion, or pain [142].

The reinjury rate after reconstruction has been shown to range from 2.3% to 13%, depending on the intensity and level of risk of the postsurgical sport or activity [145–147]. Athletes who opt for nonoperative treatment and return to a pivoting sport may have a significantly higher risk for injury to the menisci and cartilage [148]. Myklebust and colleagues [142] reported that 22% of patients who were treated nonoperatively underwent surgery for an injured meniscus compared with 12% of patients who were treated operatively for their torn ACL.

Patients who have sustained an ACL injury also show a greater prevalence of osteoarthritis, irrespective of the type of treatment used [149]. ACL injury often causes acute bone bruises, meniscal injuries, and injuries to other ligaments and capsular tissue, which contribute to future osteoarthritis in the knee [150]. Furthermore, biomarkers often never return to normal function [151]. Myklebust and Bahr [148] reported that 10 years after injury, nearly half of patients display signs of osteoarthritis, and after 15 to 20 years, nearly all patients have osteoarthritis.

Summary

The rising number of women involved in athletics has brought a concomitant increase in sport-related injuries. Studies have shown that women are two to eight times more likely to experience an ACL tear than men. Environmental factors, such as knee bracing and ground–shoe surface interactions, can influence injury rates for women. In addition, anatomic, hormonal, neuromuscular, and biomechanical factors may predispose women to greater ACL injury risk. When considering the physical, psychological, and financial burden for the injured female athlete, determining those factors that increase women's risk for an ACL tear would be greatly beneficial. With much of the current studies showing conflicting and equivocal results, further research is necessary involving large sample sizes, reliable data, and the ability to explore the interrelationship between extrinsic and intrinsic risk factors in the female athlete.

References

[1] National Federation of State High School Associations and Department of Education Statistics. Women's Sports Foundation calculation; 1998.
[2] Feagin JA. Isolated anterior cruciate injury. In: Feagin JA, editor. The crucial ligaments. New York: Churchill Livingstone; 1988. p. 15–23.
[3] Johnson RJ. Prevention of anterior cruciate ligament injuries. In: Feagin JA, editor. The crucial ligaments. New York: Churchill Livingstone; 1988. p. 349–56.
[4] Smith BA, Livesay GA, Woo SLY. Biology and biomechanics of the anterior cruciate ligament. Clin J Sport Med 1988;12:637–46.
[5] Ireland ML. The female ACL: why is it more prone to injury? Orthop Clin North Am 2002; 33(4):637–51.
[6] Feagin JA, Lambert KL, Cunningham PR, et al. Consideration of anterior cruciate ligament injury in skiing. Clin Orthop Relat Res 1987;216:3–18.
[7] Miyasaka KC, Daniel DM, Stone ML, et al. The incidence of knee ligament injuries in the general population. Am J Knee Surg 1991;4:3–8.
[8] Freedman KB, Glasgow MT, Glasgow SG, et al. Anterior cruciate ligament injury and reconstruction among university students. Clin Orthop Relat Res 1998;356:208–12.
[9] Arendt E, Dick R. Knee injury patterns among men and women in collegiate basketball and soccer: NCAA data and review of literature. Am J Sports Med 1995;23:694–701.
[10] Hughes G, Watkins J. A risk-factor model for anterior cruciate ligament injury. Sports Med 2006;36(5):411–28.
[11] Zantop T, Petersen W, Fu F. Anatomy of the cruciate ligament. Operative Techniques in Orthopaedics 2005;15:20–8.
[12] Amis AA, Dawkins GP. Functional anatomy of the anterior cruciate ligament. Fiber bundle actions related to ligament replacements and injuries. J Bone Joint Surg Br 1991;73: 260–7.
[13] Eriksson E. Do we need to perform double-bundle anterior cruciate ligament reconstructions? Operative Techniques in Orthopaedics 2005;15:4.
[14] Furman W, Marshall JL, Girgis FG. The anterior cruciate ligament: a functional analysis based on postmortem studies. J Bone Joint Surg Am 1976;58:179–85.
[15] Petersen W, Zantop T. Partial rupture of the anterior cruciate ligament. Arthroscopy 2006; 22(11):1143–5.
[16] Griffin LY, Agel J, Albohm MJ, et al. Noncontact anterior cruciate ligament injuries: risk factors and prevention strategies. J Am Acad Orthop Surg 2000;8(3):141–50.
[17] Hutchinson MR, Ireland ML. Knee injuries in female athletes. Sports Med 1995;19: 288–302.
[18] Scranton PE Jr, Whitesel JP, Powell JW, et al. A review of selected noncontact anterior cruciate ligament injuries in the National Football League. Foot Ankle Int 1997;18:772–6.
[19] Orchard J, Seward H, McGivern J, et al. Rainfall, evaporation and the risk of non-contact anterior cruciate ligament injury in the Australian Football League. Med J Aust 1999;170: 304–6.
[20] Orchard JW, Powell JW. Risk of knee and ankle sprains under various weather conditions in American football. Med Sci Sports Exerc 2003;35:1118–23.
[21] Meyers MC, Barnhill BS. Incidence, causes, and severity of high school football injuries on FieldTurf versus natural grass: a 5-year prospective study. Am J Sports Med 2004;32: 1626–38.

[22] Olsen OE, Myklebust G, Engebretsen L, et al. Relationship between floor type and risk of ACL injury in team handball. Scand J Med Sci Sports 2003;13:299–304.

[23] Torg JS, Quendenfeld TC. Effect of shoe type and cleat length on incidence and severity of knee injuries among high school football players. Res Q 1971;42:203–11.

[24] Lambson RB, Barnhill BS, Higgins RW. Football cleat design and its effect on anterior cruciate ligament injuries: a three-year prospective study. Am J Sports Med 1996;24:155–9.

[25] Livesay GA, Reda DR, Nauman EA. Peak torque and rotational stiffness developed at the shoe-surface interface: the effect of shoe type and playing surface. Am J Sports Med 2006; 34(3):415–22.

[26] France EP, Paulos LE. In vitro assessment of prophylactic knee brace function. Clin Sports Med 1990;9(4):823–41.

[27] Albright JP, Saterbak A, Stokes J. Use of knee braces in sport: current recommendations. Sports Med 1995;20(5):281–301.

[28] Rovere GD, Haupt HA, Yates CS. Prophylactic knee bracing in college football. Am J Sports Med 1987;15(2):111–6.

[29] Martinek V, Friederich NF. [To brace or not to brace? How effective are knee braces in rehabilitation?]. Orthopade 1999;28(6):565–70 [in German].

[30] Millet CW, Drez DJ Jr. Principles of bracing for the anterior cruciate ligament-deficient knee. Clin Sports Med 1988;7(4):827–33.

[31] Rebel M, Paessler HH. The effect of knee brace on coordination and neuronal leg muscle control: an early postoperative functional study in anterior cruciate ligament reconstructed patients. Knee Surg Sports Traumatol Arthrosc 2001;9(5):272–81.

[32] Swirtun LR, Jansson A, Renstrom P. The effects of a functional knee brace during early treatment of patients with a nonoperated acute anterior cruciate ligament tear: a prospective randomized study. Clin J Sport Med 2005;15(5):299–304.

[33] Risberg MA, Holm I, Steen H, et al. The effect of knee bracing after anterior cruciate ligament reconstruction. A prospective, randomized study with two years' follow-up. Am J Sports Med 1999;27(1):76–83.

[34] Griffin LY, Albohm MJ, Arendt EA, et al. Understanding and preventing noncontact anterior cruciate ligament injuries: a review of the Hunt Valley II meeting, January 2005. Am J Sports Med 2006;34(9):1512–32.

[35] Yu B, Herman D, Preston J, et al. Immediate effects of a knee brace with a constraint to knee extension on knee kinematics and ground reaction forces in a stop-jump task. Am J Sports Med 2004;32:1136–43.

[36] Fleming BC, Renstrom PA, Beynnon BD, et al. The influence of functional knee bracing on the anterior cruciate ligament strain biomechanics in weightbearing and nonweightbearing knees. Am J Sports Med 2000;28(6):815–24.

[37] Houston ME, Goemans PH. Leg muscle performance of athletes with and without knee support braces. Arch Phys Med Rehabil 1982;63:431–2.

[38] Beynnon BD, Fleming BC, Churchill DL, et al. The effect of anterior cruciate ligament deficiency and functional bracing on translation of the tibia relative to the femur during nonweightbearing and weightbearing. Am J Sports Med 2003;31(1):99–105.

[39] Beynnon BD, Fleming BC, Labovitch R, et al. Chronic anterior cruciate ligament deficiency is associated with increased anterior translation of the tibia during the transition from non-weightbearing to weightbearing. J Orthop Res 2002;20(2):332–7.

[40] Ramsey DK, Lamontange M, Wrentenberg PF, et al. Assessment of functional knee bracing: an in vivo three-dimensional kinematic analysis of the anterior cruciate deficient knee. Clin Biomech (Bristol, Avon) 2001;16:61–70.

[41] Kartus J, Stener S, Kohler K, et al. Is bracing after anterior cruciate ligament reconstruction necessary? A 2-year follow-up of 78 consecutive patients rehabilitated with or without a brace. Knee Surg Sports Traumatol Arthrosc 1997;5(3):157–61.

[42] Hewett TE, Myer GD, Ford KR. Decrease in neuromuscular control about the knee with maturation in female athletes. J Bone Joint Surg Am 2004;86:1601–8.

[43] Hewett TE, Myer GD, Ford KR, et al. Biomedical measures of neuromuscular control and valgus loading of the knee predict anterior cruciate ligament injury risk in female athletes: a prospective study. Am J Sports Med 2005;33(4):492–501.

[44] Horton MG, Hall TL. Quadriceps femoris muscle angle: normal values and relationships with gender and selected skeletal measures. Phys Ther 1989;69(11):897–901.

[45] Hungerford DS, Barry M. Biomechanics of the patellofemoral joint. Clin Orthop Relat Res 1979;144:9–15.

[46] Hvid I, Anderson LB, Schmidt H. Chondromalacia patellae: the relation to abnormal patellofemoral joint mechanics. Acta Orthop Scand 1981;52:661–6.

[47] Shambaugh JP, Klein A, Herbert JH. Structural measures as predictors of injury in basketball players. Med Sci Sports Exerc 1991;23:522–7.

[48] Buchanan PA. Developmental perspectives on basketball players' strength, knee position in landing, and ACL injury gender differences [dissertation, research]. Bloomington (IN): Indiana University; 2003.

[49] Gray J, Taunton JE, McKenzie DC, et al. A survey of injuries to the anterior cruciate ligament of the knee in female basketball players. Int J Sports Med 1985;6:314–6.

[50] Myer GD, Ford KR, Hewett TE. The effects of gender on quadriceps muscle activation strategies during a maneuver that mimics a high ACL injury risk position. J Electromyogr Kinesiol 2005;15:181–9.

[51] Shelbourne KD, Davis TJ, Klootwyk TE. The relationship between intercondylar notch width of the femur and the incidence of anterior cruciate ligament tears. Am J Sports Med 1998;26(3):402–8.

[52] Uhorchak JM, Scoville CR, Williams GN, et al. Risk factors associated with noncontact injury of the anterior cruciate ligament: a prospective four-year evaluation of 859 West Point cadets. Am J Sports Med 2003;31:831–42.

[53] Souryal TO, Freeman TR. Intercondylar notch size and anterior cruciate ligament injuries in athletes: a prospective study. Am J Sports Med 1993;21:535–9.

[54] LaPrade RF, Burnett QM II. Femoral intercondylar notch stenosis and correlation to anterior cruciate ligament injuries: a prospective study. Am J Sports Med 1994;22:198–203.

[55] Arendt EA. Relationship between notch width index and risk of noncontact ACL injury. In: Griffin LY, editor. Prevention of noncontact ACL injuries. Rosemont (IL): American Academy of Orthopaedic Surgeons; 2001. p. 33–44.

[56] Teitz CC, Lind BK, Sacks BM. Symmetry of the femoral notch width index. Am J Sports Med 1997;25:687–90.

[57] Souryal TO, Moore HA, Evans P. Bilaterality in anterior cruciate ligament injuries: associated intercondylar notch stenosis. Am J Sports Med 1998;16:449–54.

[58] Schickendantz MS, Weiker GG. The predictive value of radiographs in the evaluation of unilateral and bilateral anterior cruciate ligament injuries. Am J Sports Med 1993;21: 110–3.

[59] Huston LJ, Greenfield ML, Wojtys EM. Anterior cruciate ligament injuries in the female athlete. Potential risk factors. Clin Orthop Relat Res 2000;372:50–63.

[60] Ireland ML. Special concerns of the female athlete. In: Fu FH, Stone DA, editors. Sports injuries: mechanisms, prevention, and treatment. 2nd edition. Baltimore (MD): Williams & Wilkins; 1994. p. 153–62.

[61] Anderson A, Dome DC, Gautam S, et al. Correlation of anthropometric measurements, strength, anterior cruciate ligament size, and intercondylar notch characteristics to sex differences in anterior cruciate ligament tear rates. Am J Sports Med 2001;29(1):58–66.

[62] Chandrashekar N, Mansouri H, Slauterbeck J, et al. Sex-based differences in tensile properties of the human anterior cruciate ligament. J Biomech 2006;39(16):2943–50.

[63] Rozzi SL, Lephart SM, Gear WS, et al. Knee joint laxity and neuromuscular characteristics of male and female soccer and basketball players. Am J Sports Med 1999;27:312–9.

[64] Hewett TE, Myer GD, Ford KR. Anterior cruciate ligament injuries in female athletes: Part 1, mechanisms and risk factors. Am J Sports Med 2006;34(2):299–311.

[65] Ford KR. A comparison of knee joint kinematics and related muscle onset patterns observed during a 180o cutting maneuver executed by male and female soccer players. In: Kinesiology and health promotion. Lexington (KY): University of Kentucky; 1997. p. 83.

[66] Loudon JK, Jenkins W, Loudon KL. The relationship between static posture and ACL injury in female athletes. J Orthop Sports Phys Ther 1996;24(2):91–7.

[67] Trimble MH, Bishop MD, Buckley BD, et al. The relationship between clinical measurements of lower extremity posture and tibial translation. Clin Biomech (Bristol, Avon) 2002;17:286–90.

[68] Grana WA, Moretz JA. Ligamentous laxity in secondary school athletes. JAMA 1978;240: 1975–6.

[69] Huston LJ, Wojtys EM. Neuromuscular performance characteristics in elite female athletes. Am J Sports Med 1996;19:288–302.

[70] Boden BP, Dean GS, Feagin JA, et al. Mechanisms of anterior cruciate ligament injury. Orthopedics 2000;23:573–8.

[71] Emerson RJ. Basketball knee injuries and the anterior cruciate ligament. Clin Sports Med 1993;12:317–28.

[72] Brown CN, Yu B, Kirkendall DT, et al. Effects of increased body mass index on lower extremity motion patterns in a stop-jump task: National Athletic Trainers Association annual meeting. Indianapolis, In, June 13–16, 2005. J Athl Train 2005;40(suppl 2):S32–3.

[73] Knapik JJ, Sharp MA, Canham-Chervak M, et al. Risk factors for training-related injuries among men and women in basic combat training. Med Sci Sports Exerc 2001;33:946–51.

[74] Zelisko JA, Noble HB, Porter M. A comparison of men's and women's professional basketball injuries. Am J Sports Med 1982;10:297–9.

[75] Slauterbeck JR, Narayan RS, Clevenger C, et al. Effects of estrogen level on the tensile properties of the rabbit anterior cruciate ligament. J Orthop Res 1999;17:405–8.

[76] Seneviratne A, Attia E, Williams RJ, et al. The effect of estrogen on ovine anterior cruciate ligament fibroblasts: cell proliferation and collagen synthesis. Am J Sports Med 2004;32: 1613–8.

[77] Yu WD, Liu S, Hatch JD, et al. Effect of estrogen on cellular metabolism of the human anterior cruciate ligament. Clin Orthop Relat Res 1999;366:229–38.

[78] Yu WD, Panossian V, Hatch JD, et al. Combined effects of estrogen and progesterone on the anterior cruciate ligament. Clin Orthop Relat Res 2001;383:268–81.

[79] Deie M, Sakamaki Y, Sumen Y, et al. Anterior knee laxity in young women varies with their menstrual cycle. Int Orthop 2002;26(3):154–6.

[80] Heitz NA. Hormonal changes throughout the menstrual cycle and increased anterior cruciate ligament laxity in females. J Athl Train 1999;343:144–9.

[81] Shultz SJ, Sander TC, Kirk SE, et al. Sex differences in knee joint laxity change across the female menstrual cycle. J Sports Med Phys Fitness 2005;45(4):594–603.

[82] Posthuma BW, Bass MJ, Bull SB, et al. Detecting changes in functional ability in women with premenstrual syndrome. Am J Obstet Gynecol 1987;156:275–8.

[83] Sarwar R, Beltran NB, Rutherford OM. Changes in muscle strength, relaxation rate and fatigability during the human menstrual cycle. J Physiol 1996;493:267–72.

[84] Shultz SJ, Kirk SE, Johnson ML, et al. Relationship between sex hormones and anterior knee laxity across the menstrual cycle. Med Sci Sports Exerc 2004;36(7):1165–74.

[85] Karageanes SJ, Blackburn K, Vangelos ZA. The association of the menstrual cycle with the laxity of the anterior cruciate ligament in adolescent female athletes. Clin J Sport Med 2000; 10(3):162–8.

[86] Belanger MJ, Moore DC, Crisco JJ 3rd, et al. Knee laxity does not vary with the menstrual cycle, before or after exercise. Am J Sports Med 2004;32(5):1150–7.

[87] Strickland SM, Belknap TW, Turner SA, et al. Lack of hormonal influences on mechanical properties of sheep knee ligaments. Am J Sports Med 2003;31(2):210–5.

[88] Wojtys EM, Huston LJ, Lindenfeld TN, et al. Association between the menstrual cycle and anterior cruciate ligament injuries in female athletes. Am J Sports Med 1998;26(5):614–9.

[89] Moller-Nielson J, Hammar M. Sports injuries and oral contraceptive use: is there a relationship? Sports Med 1991;12:152–60.

[90] Slauterbeck JR, Fuzie SF, Smith MP, et al. The menstrual cycle, sex hormones, and anterior cruciate ligament injury. J Athl Train 2002;37(3):275–8.

[91] Myklebust G, Engebretsen L, Braekken IH, et al. Prevention of anterior cruciate ligament injuries in female team handball players: a prospective intervention study over three seasons. Clin J Sports Med 2003;13:71–8.

[92] Arendt EA, Bershadsky B, Agel J. Periodicity of noncontact anterior cruciate ligament injuries during the menstrual cycle. J Gend Specif Med 2002;5:19–26.

[93] Kibler WB, Livingston B. Closed-chain rehabilitation for upper and lower extremities. J Am Acad Orthop Surg 2001;9(6):412–21.

[94] Sell T, Ferris CM, Abt JP, et al. Predictors of anterior tibia shear force during a vertical stop-jump: 2004 Combined Sections Meeting (CSM), In, Nashville, Tn, February 4–8, 2004. J Orthop Sports Phys Ther 2004;34(1):A56.

[95] Zazulak BT, Ponce PL, Straub SJ, et al. Gender comparison of hip muscle activity during single-leg landing. J Orthop Sports Phys Ther 2005;35:292–9.

[96] Haycock CE, Gillette JV. Susceptibility of women athletes to injury: myth vs. reality. JAMA 1976;236:163–5.

[97] Chappell JD, Herman DC, Knight BS, et al. Effect of fatigue on knee kinetics and kinematics in stop-jump tasks. Am J Sports Med 2005;33:1022–9.

[98] Wojtys EM, Wylie BB, Huston LJ. The effects of muscle fatigue on neuromuscular function and anterior tibial translation in healthy knees. Am J Sports Med 1996;24:615–21.

[99] Griffis ND, Vequist SW, Yearout KM, et al. Injury prevention of the anterior cruciate ligament. Presented at the American Orthopaedic Society for Sports Medicine. Traverse City (MI), June 1989.

[100] Kirkendall DT, Garrett WE. The anterior cruciate ligament enigma. Injury mechanisms and prevention. Clin Orthop Relat Res 2000;(372):64–8.

[101] Allen MK, Glasoe WM. Metrecom measurement of navicular drop in subjects with anterior cruciate ligament injury. J Athl Train 2000;35:403–6.

[102] Ford KR, Myer GD, Smith RL, et al. Use of an overhead goal alters vertical jump performance and biomechanics. J Strength Cond Res 2005;19:394–9.

[103] Ford KR, Myer GD, Toms HE, et al. Gender differences in the kinematics of unanticipated cutting in young athletes. Med Sci Sports Exerc 2005;37:124–9.

[104] Hewett TE, Lindenfeld TN, Riccobene JV, et al. The effect of neuromuscular training on the incidence of knee injury in female athletes: a prospective study. Am J Sports Med 1999; 27:699–706.

[105] McNair PJ, Marshall RN, Matheson JA. Important features associated with acute anterior cruciate ligament injury. N Z Med J 1990;103:537–9.

[106] Olsen OE, Myklebust G, Engebretsen L, et al. Injury mechanisms for anterior cruciate ligament injuries in team handball: a systematic video analysis. Am J Sports Med 2004;32: 1002–12.

[107] Yu B, McClure SB, Onate JA, et al. Age and gender effects on lower extremity kinematics of youth soccer players in a stop-jump task. Am J Sports Med 2005;33:1356–64.

[108] Malinzak RA, Colby SM, Kirkendall DT, et al. A comparison of knee joint motion patterns between men and women in selected athletic tasks. Clin Biomech (Briston, Avon) 2001;16: 438–45.

[109] Fagenbaum R, Darling WG. Jump landing strategies in male and female college athletes and the implications of such strategies for anterior cruciate ligament injury. Am J Sports Med 2003;31:233–40.

[110] McLean SG, Neal RJ, Myers PT, et al. Knee joint kinematics during the sidestep cutting maneuver: potential for injury in women. Med Sci Sports Exerc 1999;31:959–968.

[111] Lephart SM, Ferris CM, Riemann BL, et al. Gender differences in strength and lower extremity kinematics during landing. Clin Orthop Relat Res 2002;401:162–9.

[112] Biering-Sorensen F. Physical measurements as risk indicators for low-back trouble over a one-year period. Eur Spine J 1984;9:106–19.

[113] Harmon KG, Ireland ML. The athletic woman: gender differences in noncontact anterior cruciate ligament injuries. Clin Sports Med 2000;19(2):287–302.

[114] Harmon KG, Dick R. The relationship of skill level to anterior cruciate ligament injury. Clin J Sport Med 1998;8:260–5.

[115] Bjordal JM, Arnoy F. Epidemiology of anterior cruciate ligament injuries in soccer. Am J Sports Med 1997;25:341–5.

[116] Arendt EA, Agel J, Dick R. Anterior cruciate ligament injury patterns among collegiate men and women. J Athl Train 1999;34:86–92.

[117] NCAA Injury Surveillance System, 1989–1997. Overland Park, (KS), National Collegiate Athletic Association, 1997.

[118] Rozzi SL, Lephart SM, Fu FH. Effects of muscular fatigue on knee joint laxity and neuromuscular characteristics of male and female athletes. J Athl Train 1999;34(2): 106–14.

[119] Caraffa A, Cerulli G, Projetti M, et al. Prevention of anterior cruciate ligament injuries in soccer. A prospective controlled study of proprioceptive training. Knee Surg Sports Traumatol Arthrosc 1996;4:19–21.

[120] Markolf KL, Graff-Radford A, Amstutz HC. In vivo knee stability: a quantitative assessment using an instrumented clinical testing apparatus. J Bone Joint Surg Am 1978;60: 664–74.

[121] Hewett ET, Stroupe AL, Nance TA, et al. Plyometric training in female athletes. Am J Sports Med 1996;24:765–73.

[122] Wojtys EM, Huston LJ, Taylor PD, et al. Neuromuscular adaptations in isokinetic, isotonic, and agility training programs. Am J Sports Med 1996;24:187–92.

[123] Beynnon BD, Johnson RJ, Abate JA, et al. Treatment of anterior cruciate ligament injuries, part I. Am J Sports Med 2005;33(10):1579–602.

[124] Barber FA, Elrod BF, McGuire DA, et al. Is an anterior cruciate ligament reconstruction outcome age dependent? Arthroscopy 1996;12:720–5.

[125] Beynnon BD, Johnson RJ, Abate JA, et al. Treatment of anterior cruciate ligament injuries, part 2. Am J Sports Med 2005 Nov;33(11):1751–67.

[126] Frank CB, Jackson DW. The science of reconstruction of the anterior cruciate ligament. J Bone Joint Surg Am 1997;79(10):1556–76.

[127] Sherman OH, Banffy MB. Anterior cruciate ligament reconstruction: which graft is best? Arthroscopy 2004;20(9):974–80.

[128] Barber-Westin SD, Noyes FR, Andrews M. A rigorous comparison of results and complications between the sexes of results and complications after anterior cruciate ligament reconstruction. Am J Sports Med 1997;25:514–26.

[129] Barrett GR, Hartzog Jr CW, Ruff CG, et al. Clinical comparison of intra-articular anterior cruciate ligament reconstruction using autogenous semitendinosus tendon in males versus females [abstract]. Final Program Schedule and Book of Abstracts. In: ACL Study Group, Vail (CO), March 28-April 3, 1998.

[130] Corry IS, Webb JM, Clingeleffer AJ, et al. Arthroscopic reconstruction of the anterior cruciate ligament: a comparison of patellar tendon autograft and four-strand hamstring tendon autograft. Am J Sports Med 1999;27:444–54.

[131] Gobbi A, Domzalski M, Pascual J. Comparison of anterior cruciate ligament reconstruction in male and female athletes using the patellar tendon and hamstring autografts. Knee Surg Sports Traumatol Arthrosc 2004;12:534–9.

[132] Noojin FK, Barrett GR, Hartzog CW, et al. Clinical comparison of intraarticular anterior cruciate ligament reconstruction using autogenous semitendinosus and gracilis tendons in men versus women. Am J Sports Med 2000;28:783–9.

[133] Ferrari JD, Bach BR, Bush-Joseph CA, et al. Anterior cruciate ligament reconstruction in men and women: an outcome analysis comparing gender. Arthroscopy 2001;17:588–96.

[134] Ott SM, Ireland ML, Ballantyne BT, et al. Comparison of outcomes between males and females after anterior cruciate ligament reconstruction. Knee Surg Sports Traumatol Arthrosc 2003;11:75–80.

[135] Wiger P, Brandsson S, Kartus J, et al. A comparison of results after arthroscopic anterior cruciate ligament reconstruction in female and male competitive athletes: a two- to five-year follow-up of 429 patients. Scand J Med Sci Sports 1999;9:290–5.

[136] Dooley PJ, Chan DS, Dainty KN, et al. Patellar tendon versus hamstring autograft for anterior cruciate ligament rupture in adults. (Protocol) Cochrane Database of Syst Rev 2006; 210.1002/14651858:CD005960.

[137] Gerbino P, Nielson J. Knee injuries. In: Frontera WR, Herring SA, Micheli LJ, et al, editors. Clinical sports medicine: medical management and rehabilitation. 1st edition. Philadelphia: Elsevier Inc; 2007. p. 421–3.

[138] Siegel MG, Barber-Westin SD. Arthroscopic-assisted outpatient anterior cruciate ligament reconstruction using the semitendinosus and gracilis tendons. Arthroscopy 1998;14: 268–77.

[139] Gobbi A, Tuy B, Mahajan S, et al. Quadrupled bone-semitendinosus anterior cruciate ligament reconstruction: a clinical investigation in a group of athletes. Arthroscopy 2003;19: 691–9.

[140] Feller JA, Webster KE. A randomized comparison of patellar tendon and hamstring tendon anterior cruciate ligament reconstruction. Am J Sports Med 2003;31:564–73.

[141] Fink C, Hoser C, Hackl W, et al. Long-term outcome of operative or nonoperative treatment of anterior cruciate ligament rupture: is sports activity a determining variable? Int J Sports Med 2001;22:304–9.

[142] Myklebust G, Bahr R, Engebretsen L, et al. Clinical, functional and radiological outcome 6-11 years after ACL injuries in team handball players: a follow-up study. Am J Sports Med 2003;31:981–9.

[143] Roos H, Ornell M, Gardsell P, et al. Soccer after anterior cruciate ligament injury: an incompatible combination? A national survey of incidence and risk factors and a 7-year follow-up of 310 players. Acta Orthop Scand 1995;66:107–12.

[144] Eastlack ME, Axe MJ, Snyder-Mackler L. Laxity, instability, and functional outcomes after ACL injury: copers versus noncopers. Med Sci Sports Exerc 1999;31:210–5.

[145] Sandberg R, Balkfors B. Reconstruction of the anterior cruciate ligament. A 5-year follow-up of 89 patients. Acta Orthop Scand 1988;59:288–93.

[146] Otto D, Pinczewski LA, Clingeleffer A, et al. Five-year results of single-incision arthroscopic anterior cruciate ligament reconstruction with patellar tendon autograft. Am J Sports Med 1998;26:181–8.

[147] Bak K, Scavenius M, Hansen S, et al. Isolated partial rupture of the anterior cruciate ligament. Long-term follow-up of 56 cases. Knee Surg Sports Traumatol Arthrosc 1997;5: 66–71.

[148] Myklebust G, Bahr R. Return to play guidelines after anterior cruciate ligament surgery. Br J Sports Med 2005;39:127–31.

[149] Gillquist J, Messner K. Anterior cruciate ligament reconstruction and the long-term incidence of gonarthrosis. Sports Med 1999;27:143–56.

[150] Engebretsen L, Arendt E, Fritts HM. Osteochondral lesions and cruciate ligament injuries. MRI in 18 knees. Acta Orthop Scand 1993;64:434–6.

[151] Lohmander LS, Saxne T, Heinegard DK. Release of cartilage oligometric matrix protein (COMP) into joint fluid after knee injury and in osteoarthritis. Ann Rheum Dis 1994;53: 8–13.

ELSEVIER
SAUNDERS

Phys Med Rehabil Clin N Am
18 (2007) 439–458

PHYSICAL MEDICINE
AND REHABILITATION
CLINICS OF
NORTH AMERICA

Patellofemoral Pain

Jennifer E. Earl, PhD, ATC[a],
Carole S. Vetter, MD, ATC[b],*

[a]*Department of Human Movement Sciences, University of Wisconsin Milwaukee*
Athletic Training Education Program, Pavilion Room 350,
P.O. Box 413, Milwaukee, WI 53201, USA
[b]*Division Sports Medicine, Department of Orthopaedic Surgery,*
Medical College of Wisconsin, 9200 West Wisconsin Avenue,
Milwaukee, WI 53226, USA

Patellofemoral pain syndrome is defined as retropatellar or peripatellar pain. It is an extremely common diagnosis in the female athlete. However, obtaining an accurate diagnosis and outlining appropriate treatment are often challenging. Consensus is lacking in the literature regarding the cause and treatment of the syndrome [1]. The patellofemoral joint is complex and dependent on quadriceps function as well as on static and dynamic restraints. The etiology of patellofemoral pain is multifactorial with proposed causes including overuse, overload, biomechanical problems, and muscular dysfunction. Accurate diagnosis requires specific knowledge of the anatomy, biomechanics, and functional behavior of the patellofemoral joint [2]. Most patients are successfully treated by conservative means with the rare few requiring surgical intervention.

Epidemiology of patellofemoral pain

Patellofemoral pain syndrome is considered one of the most common disorders of the knee, accounting for 25% of all knee injuries treated in sports medicine clinics [1,3,4]. In clinics that manage patients who have musculoskeletal syndromes, patellofemoral pain syndrome accounts for almost 10% of all visits (76 of 814 visits) and for 20% to 40% of all knee problems (76 of 266 visits) [5]. DeHaven and Lintner [6] reported that among patients diagnosed with patellofemoral pain syndrome over a 7-year period, 18.1% were men and 33.2% were women. They also found an age predilection for the second and third decade of life. Fairbank and colleagues [7] reported

* Corresponding author.
E-mail address: cstreet@mcw.edu (C.S. Vetter).

on 446 randomly selected students age 13 to 19 years, finding 30% of them had experienced anterior knee pain in the last year and 18% of those in pain had stopped participating in sports because of the knee pain. Taunton and colleagues [8–11] retrospectively evaluated all patients presenting from 1998 to 2000 to a single health clinic for injuries related to running. Of the 2002 patients, the most common complaint was patellofemoral pain at 16.5%. Of those patients with patellofemoral pain related to running, 38% were men and 62% were women.

Biomechanical etiology of patellofemoral pain syndrome

In 1968, Hughston [12] wrote that the primary source of anterior knee pain was extensor mechanism malalignment. In 1979, James [13] coined the term "miserable malalignment syndrome" as the cause of anterior knee pain, describing a combination of factors, including femoral anteversion, squinting patella, patella alta, increased quadriceps angle (Q angle), and tibial external rotation (Fig. 1). These early observations form the foundation for research into the etiology of patellofemoral pain syndrome (PFPS). PFPS has a multifactorial etiology with factors ranging from

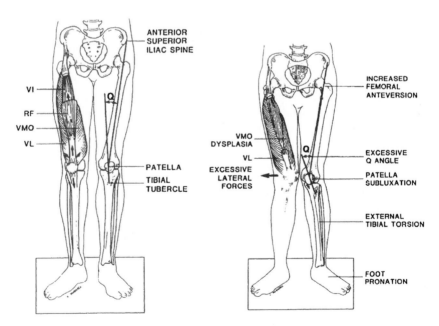

Fig. 1. The miserable malalignment syndrome. Increased femoral anterversion, increased genu valgum, external tibial torsion, and foot pronation. Q, quadriceps. RF, rectus femoris. VI, vastus intermedius VL, vastus lateralis. VMO, vastus medialis obliques. (*From* Fu FH, Stone DA, editors. Sports Injuries: Mechanism, prevention and treatment. 2nd edition. Baltimore: Williams & Wilkins, 1994:159; with permission.)

unsuitable playing surfaces and overtraining, to skeletal alignment abnormalities, to poor neuromuscular control of the lower extremity. The connection among these factors is that they are all assumed to alter the tracking of the patella within the trochlear groove. Proper tracking requires balanced forces acting on the patella (Fig. 2). If any force acting on the patella is too large or too small, then the movement of the patella may be altered, thereby placing additional stresses on the soft tissue of the joint. As the stress exceeds the tissues' mechanical strength, microdamage, inflammation, and pain result. After a comprehensive review of the literature, the authors have grouped the various etiological factors into three major groups: quadriceps dysfunction, static alignment, and dynamic alignment.

Quadriceps dysfunction

The patella is most directly stabilized by the distal quadriceps, especially the vastus medialis obliques and vastus lateralis. Lateral dynamic forces are produced by the vastus lateralis through the quadriceps tendon and by the biceps femoris, gluteal muscles, and tensor fascia latae through the iliotibial band and lateral retinaculum [14]. The vastus medialis obliques exclusively produce medial dynamic forces [15]. Weakness or delayed firing of the vastus medialis obliques is thought to cause the patella to track laterally,

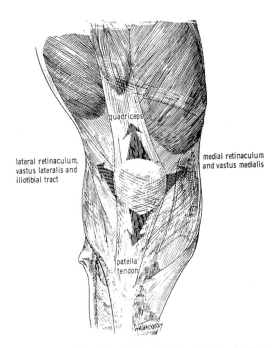

Fig. 2. Forces acting on the patella. (*From* Aglietti P, Buzzi R, Insall JN. Disorders of the patellofemoral joint. In: Insall JN, editor. Surgery of the Knee, 2nd edition. New York: Churchill Livingstone, 1993:243; with permission.)

irritating the soft tissues about the joint [16,17]. While some studies support a difference in vastus medialis oblique and/or vastus lateralis activity in PFPS patients [16,18–23], others have found no differences between those with PFPS and healthy controls [24–30]. Contradictory results may be explained by the variety of tasks analyzed and data collection methods used in these studies. Contradictory results may also mean that quadriceps dysfunction is not found in all patients with PFPS.

Static malalignment

The anatomical alignment of the pelvis and lower extremity may play a role in the development of PFPS in some individuals. This is referred to as "static alignment" because it is identifiable when the patient is not moving. These findings are also not easily modified with conservative rehabilitation.

A common clinical measurement of the alignment of the lower extremity is the Q angle. This is the angle formed by the intersection of two lines, one connecting the anterior superior iliac spine and the center of the patella and the other connecting the center of the patella to the tibial tuberosity. This angle is thought to represent the line of action of the quadriceps force. A larger Q angle indicates that a greater force is acting laterally on the patella, which may contribute to lateral patellar tracking [19]. Although many sources report that a Q angle greater than 15° to 20° is a risk factor for developing PFPS, the literature is inconsistent in supporting this finding [7,31]. A review of this literature by Livingston [32] describes how there is a consensus that the Q angle for a typical woman is 3° to 6° larger than the Q angle for a typical man, but there is limited evidence that a Q angle greater than 15° to 20° is related to extensor mechanism dysfunction. For example, only some PFPS patients have a Q angle greater than normal. The inconclusive findings may stem from inconsistent methods for measuring the Q angle. It is also possible that a larger than normal Q angle is just one of several contributing factors to PFPS.

Static malalignment, such as femoral neck anteversion, genu valgum, and external tibial torsion, are also theoretically related to PFPS because they would increase the Q angle. Anteversion, an increased angle between the frontal plane and the femoral neck, can lead to a lower extremity that rotates internally and a gait that toes in [33,34]. One cadaveric study of knees supports the theory that increased femoral internal rotation leads to increased contact pressure between the patella and the lateral trochlear groove, which would seemingly lead to symptoms of PFPS [35]. Although no difference in femoral anteversion between PFPS and control subjects has been found [7,34], it was reported that PFPS patients who failed conservative treatment had significantly more anteversion than those who were successfully treated conservatively [36]. Genu valgum also increases the Q angle and potentially increases the laterally directed forces on the patella [37]. However, when measured statically, there has been no difference in genu valgum between PFPS subjects and controls [7,38]. Genu valgum may play a more important role in the cause of PFPS during dynamic movement and is described in a later section. External tibial torsion can occur during development as a compensation for femoral anteversion [39]. This leads to the feet pointing outward when the knees are facing forward. The Q angle is larger in these individuals because of the lateral location of the tibial tuberosity. This static malalignment has been seen in some individuals with PFPS. Eckhoff and colleagues [40] reported that PFPS patients who had failed conservative treatment had approximately 6° more tibial external rotation than did those who had successful conservative treatment. Although the majority of PFPS patients have good outcomes with conservative rehabilitation, the studies by Eckhoff and colleagues illustrate that some patients have skeletal static malalignment that will not respond to conservative rehabilitation and may require surgical intervention [36,40].

It is often stated that hyperpronation of the foot is a causative factor for PFPS [41,42]. In theory, increased pronation causes the tibia to internally rotate during the weight acceptance phase of gait, thereby preventing the tibia from fully externally rotating during midstance. This prevents the knee from fully locking via the screw-home mechanism. To compensate, the femur internally rotates to allow the knee to fully lock. Femoral internal rotation during quadriceps contraction may cause a greater lateral force on the patella as it is compressed against the lateral trochlear groove [43]. While some studies have shown increased pronation in PFPS subjects [41,43], other studies show no such increase [31,44,45]. Despite the inconclusive findings of these studies, there is sufficient evidence that treating PFPS with foot orthotics improves patient outcomes [46–48]. The exact mechanism as to why foot orthotics are an effective treatment is still being investigated.

In conclusion, studies show that a small percentage of patients with PFPS have symptoms that are likely caused primarily by a static malalignment resulting in increased stress to the patellofemoral joint. For a large majority of PFPS patients, however, no static malalignment is present.

Dynamic malalignment

Examining for the static malalignment described above has a place in clinical and scientific evaluation. However, many of those malalignments change once movement is initiated. Furthermore, additional malalignment may exist during movement as a result of poor muscular control of the segments. For example, several investigators have shown that the static Q angle has no direct relationship to PFPS [7,31,49]. Rather, it is the "dynamic Q angle" that causes dysfunction, according to these investigators. The concept of poor dynamic alignment took form when clinicians observed a consistent pattern of excessive contralateral pelvic drop, hip adduction and internal rotation, knee abduction, and tibial external rotation and hyperpronation when patients performed a single-leg squat or step down

(Figs. 3 and 4). Several investigators have described this movement pattern and its link to PFPS [50–55]. It was previously thought that abnormal tracking of the patella was due to the abnormal movement of the patella within the trochlear groove. Recently, thinking has changed to the concept that abnormal patellar tracking may be due to abnormal movement of the femur beneath the patella. Dynamic MRI has shown that, during weight-bearing, PFPS subjects had greater femoral internal rotation than controls had [56]. This supports the idea that poor control of the femur may contribute to PFPS symptoms in some subjects.

The observed pattern of poor dynamic alignment has been quantified using kinematic analysis. The fact that a disproportionate number of females suffer noncontact anterior cruciate ligament (ACL) injuries has driven researchers to examine biomechanical differences between males and females during certain movements. Both noncontact ACL injury and PFPS are more prevalent in females and the underlying movement patterns that result in these injuries are similar. The difference is that noncontact ACL injuries occur when a load too large for the ligaments to handle is suddenly applied

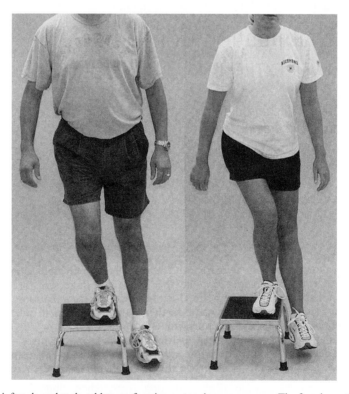

Fig. 3. A female and male athlete performing a step-down maneuver. The female on the right demonstrates hip adduction and internal rotation with tibial external rotation and foot pronation. (*From* Hutchinson MR, Ireland ML, Crook S. Rehabilitation concerns: lower extremity. In: Ireland ML, Nattiv A, editors. The female athlete. Philadelphia: WB Saunders; 2002.)

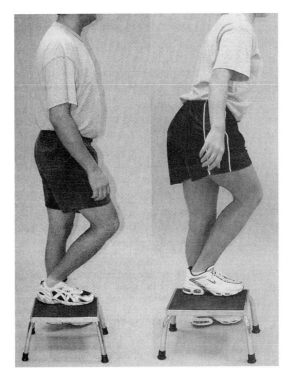

Fig. 4. A female and male athlete performing a step-down maneuver. The female on the right demonstrates anterior pelvic rotation. (*From* Hutchinson MR, Ireland ML, Crook S. Rehabilitation concerns: lower extremity. In: Ireland ML, Nattiv A, editors. The female athlete. Philadelphia: WB Saunders; 2002.)

to the lower extremity. In PFPS, the movement pattern causes increased loading of the tissues of the patellofemoral joint gradually, resulting in the overuse injury.

Three-dimensional video analysis shows that females compared to males have a greater peak knee abduction angle and less knee flexion during a side cutting maneuver [57–59], greater knee abduction during a bilateral drop-landing [60–62], and greater hip adduction [57,63] and hip internal rotation [57] during running and cutting. Zeller and colleagues [64] showed that females compared to males had greater foot dorsiflexion, foot pronation, hip adduction, hip flexion, and hip external rotation during a single-leg squat. Lephart and colleagues [65] had slightly different results when examining a single-leg landing. They found that females compared to males had greater hip internal rotation and less knee flexion and knee internal rotation.

Though slight differences in tasks and analysis prevent an absolute consensus on kinematic gender differences during functional tasks, the pattern of poor dynamic alignment in females is supported by objective data. The excessive frontal and transverse plane motion seen in females during functional tasks has been attributed to weakness in the hip abductors and external rotators [50–52,64,66]. During single-leg activities, the gluteus medius is essential in maintaining the position of the pelvis so that the lower extremity is properly aligned. It has been reported that 18.9% of the energy expended during running is used to control movement in the frontal plane [67]. Gluteus medius weakness allows the contralateral pelvis to drop, which puts the stance leg in an adducted position. This is accompanied by excessive internal rotation of the femur and tibia, as well as hyperpronation of the subtalar joint [49,54]. Weakness in contralateral hip, abdominal, and low back muscles has also been theorized as a factor in poor dynamic alignment [50,64,66,68,69].

Recent research has supported this theory that proximal muscle weakness is associated with lower-extremity injury [70–74]. Recreational runners with a variety of overuse injuries, including PFPS, were found to have significant hip abductor weakness on the injured side compared with the uninjured side and compared with uninjured controls [75]. Ireland and colleagues [50] showed that females with PFPS were significantly weaker in isometric hip abduction and external rotation than uninjured females. They suggested that this weakness may be a cause of the poor dynamic alignment pattern commonly seen in these patients. However, the investigators did not assess lower-extremity motion. In a separate study on hip strength and lower-extremity injury in collegiate athletes, Leetun and colleagues [66] reported that subjects who became injured during the season displayed weakness in hip abduction and external rotation during preparticipation examinations. They were also weaker in hip external rotation and abduction as well as in some of the core muscle endurance assessments. Both of the aforementioned studies hypothesize that the proximal weakness might explain why females display poor dynamic alignment and this may be a factor in both PFPS and noncontact ACL injury. Another study showed that healthy subjects with increased femoral anteversion had lower gluteus medius and vastus medialis oblique electromyographic activity during a clamshell exercise than those with normal hip rotation [76]. This may provide one explanation for how a static malalignment can influence muscle activity during a dynamic task. Although objective data on the prevalence of proximal muscle weakness in PFPS patients is not found in the literature, observations from clinical practice suggest that at least 50% of patients presenting with PFPS have observable weakness of the hip and/or core muscles. Additional research is needed to further understand the role of the hip and core musculature in the development of PFPS.

Conservative rehabilitation

In the vast majority of cases, PFPS is treated with conservative rehabilitation. However, studies show varying degrees of success. It has been reported that 70% of patients will be symptomatic again within 1 year following rehabilitation [4]. Many patients have successful short-term outcomes, but poor long-term outcomes. This may indicate that the cause of their symptoms was not adequately addressed. The multifactorial etiology of PFPS makes the task of isolating and treating the cause of the symptoms difficult. With a generalized rehabilitation program, the patients may experience short-term relief of symptoms, but it is common for symptoms to return when rehabilitation is terminated or when they return to their previous activity level [77,78].

Though a plethora of studies describe the effectiveness of particular rehabilitation techniques for PFPS, few meet the strict standards of evidence-based study or randomized controlled trial (RCT), making the development of clinical practice guidelines difficult. The RCT is the gold standard research design when attempting to compare the effectiveness of different treatment programs. Although there are many RCTs for a wide variety of treatment approaches to PFPS, no single intervention demonstrates a superior result to any other. In a systematic review of RCTs for PFPS rehabilitation, Bizzini and colleagues [79] found 20 studies between 1966 and 2000 met criteria for a RCT. They reported that most studies contained design flaws that drew into question the validity of the results or the ability to generalize to clinical practice. Many of the studies showed that patients in both treatment groups had good outcomes, but one treatment was not more effective than the other. Heintjes and colleagues [80] found 750 clinical trials focused on exercise therapy for PFPS. Of these, only 12 met their criteria for inclusion in the systematic review. They also concluded that more consideration must go into development of clinical trials for PFPS rehabilitation interventions.

Despite these limitations, moderately strong evidence indicates that some type of exercise intervention is effective in the treatment of PFPS [79–82]. It is less clear what specific type of intervention is best for each particular patient. Often the clinician uses a trial-and-error approach with multiple interventions until a positive outcome is achieved. Common interventional approaches include orthotic intervention, quadriceps-based strengthening, McConnell taping, bracing, and proximally focused exercise programs.

Orthotic intervention

Foot orthotics seem to be effective for treating patients with PFPS. Subjects who received orthotics in addition to an exercise program had better outcomes than did subjects on an exercise program without orthotics [46]. For PFPS subjects with excessive pronation, orthotics improved their symptoms and quality of life [47]. Sutlive and colleagues [82] determined that if a patient had greater than or equal to 2° of forefoot valgus, less than or equal to 78° of passive great-toe extension, and less than or equal to 3 mm of navicular drop, then the likelihood significantly increases that orthotics and restriction of activities will result in a successful outcome.

This is the first study in the literature giving specific measurable criteria to determine which patients are most likely to benefit from orthotic intervention.

Quadriceps-based exercise programs

The majority of PFPS exercise programs focus on strengthening the quadriceps muscle and many focus selectively on strengthening the vastus medialis obliques. There is some evidence that an exercise program for PFPS is more effective than no exercise program in reducing pain [80]. Closed-kinetic-chain–based exercise is preferred in many studies because, compared to open kinetic chain exercise, closed kinetic chain exercise produces less patellofemoral joint stress and is considered more functional [83]. Several RCTs conclude that there is no difference in patient outcome when comparing closed kinetic chain to open kinetic chain exercise programs [48,83–86]. A critical review of these studies concludes that an exercise program can reduce symptoms and improve function for PFPS patients, but there is not enough evidence to determine what specific exercise intervention is better than others [79,80].

McConnell taping

McConnell taping is commonly used in PFPS rehabilitation in an attempt to improve tracking by repositioning the patella. This treatment technique incorporates tape to realign the patella and closed kinetic chain exercises to strengthen the quadriceps [87]. It is difficult to evaluate the effects of taping alone in treating PFPS because many of the studies include taping with exercise intervention. Some studies have shown that there is no difference in outcomes between a taping-plus-exercise intervention and exercise intervention alone [88,89]. However, one study shows a benefit of taping in addition to exercise [90].

Bracing

Two types of braces are used in the treatment of PFPS. The first is a sleeve-type brace with a lateral buttress to prevent the patella from tracking laterally. Two studies using this type of brace were included in Bizzini and colleagues' systematic review [79,91–93]. Neither study found the use of the patellar brace improved outcomes more than not using the brace. There is conflicting evidence regarding the second type of brace for the treatment of PFPS. This brace is a progressive resistance brace called Protonics [92,94]. It is a long-leg brace with a hinged knee joint that can be set to provide varying resistance to knee flexion. The theory is that by providing resistance to the hamstring muscles, the pelvis will tilt posteriorly, thereby reducing symptoms of PFPS [94]. Overall, there is limited evidence of sufficient quality to determine if bracing is an effective treatment for PFPS.

Proximal-focused strengthening programs

It has been hypothesized that improving the function of the gluteus medius and other hip muscles may dynamically improve the alignment of the lower extremity, resulting in decreased soft tissue stresses and patellar pain [49,50,54,64,66,69]. Sahrmann [54] reported that exercise programs focusing on correcting dysfunctional movement patterns were effective in treating overuse injuries. However, no quantifiable measurements were taken. Mascal and colleagues [95] described a rehabilitation program that focused on proximal and core strengthening and that was effective for two patients with PFPS and notable proximal weakness. The 14-week program focused on recruitment and endurance training of the hip and trunk musculature. The patients had reduced symptoms and increased function. One patient evaluated kinematically showed improvement in dynamic alignment. A recent study by Tyler and colleagues [96] demonstrated that a 6-week treatment intervention focusing on closed kinetic chain hip strengthening and flexibility resulted in significant improvement of pain in men and women with PFPS. However, the study did not conduct any biomechanical analysis of movement.

Limitations of PFPS outcomes research

Although there are many published studies on various aspects of PFPS rehabilitation, few are of high enough quality to provide strong evidence that the interventions are effective. One reason studies often fail to show a specific intervention to be effective is because there are subgroups of PFPS etiologies, which means that some subjects in the study do not have the dysfunction that the intervention is attempting to correct. Other investigators have discussed this notion of subgroups based on etiologic factors [52,79,80,82]. As outlined previously, PFPS symptoms do not all stem from the same cause. For an RCT to be most successful, it is critical that the PFPS symptoms for all subjects in the study sample be related to the same cause. For example, a patient with PFPS may meet all inclusion criteria for a study on the effectiveness of foot orthotics. However, if the dysfunction causing that patient's knee pain is actually due to a weak quadriceps, that patient will probably not have a positive outcome from orthotic intervention, which will confound the results of the study. To avoid the trial-and-error approach, additional clinical decision rules need to be developed to guide clinicians more directly toward the intervention most appropriate for the patient.

A prospective cohort study design is often used in the development of clinical decision rules. Diagnostic tests are evaluated and compared with a reference standard and, in most cases, with the outcome of the intervention. In this design, history questions and assessment procedures are considered diagnostic tests. The clinician gathers data from these diagnostic tests, makes a clinical judgment, and then specifies a course of treatment. In reha-bilitation, an ideal diagnostic test is one that can effectively predict whether a patient will benefit from a particular treatment intervention [97]. This re-search design has recently been used to develop clinical decision rules for the use of orthotics in PFPS [82], and for the use of patellar taping in PFPS [98]. More studies of this design are needed to determine which subgroup of PFPS patients are most likely to benefit from a specific intervention. This will greatly strengthen the body of literature on the conservative rehabilita-tion of PFPS.

Surgical treatment of patellofemoral pain

Surgery for patellofemoral pain syndrome is indicated in those few pa-tients who have persistent symptoms in spite of appropriate rehabilitation and who have a problem that is genuinely correctable with surgery. Patient selection and postoperative rehabilitation are critical for improving chances of a favorable outcome. Patients whose conservative therapy has failed be-cause of noncompliance with rehabilitation are often not good surgical candidates. The decision to perform surgery for patellofemoral pain is based on the specific diagnosis of the pain. There must be a clear understanding of the contributing factors: malalignment, maltracking, cartilage degeneration, a combination of the three, or none of the three. Surgery for patellofemoral pain syndrome is considered a last resort and encompasses various specific procedures, each with specific indications, techniques, and results.

Lateral retinacular release

Lateral retinacular release is most often performed arthroscopically and is indicated for patellofemoral pain associated with isolated negative patellar tilt (tight lateral retinaculum) and minimal patellofemoral cartilage damage [99]. Patients should have lateral patellofemoral tenderness, lateral tracking without subluxation, and a normal Q angle. The procedure involves arthro-scopic evaluation of the patellofemoral compartment and cutting of the entire lateral retinaculum from the level of the vastus lateralis to the retro-patellar fat pad. During the procedure, if any articular cartilage issues are identified, they can be addressed at the same time. The most common artic-ular cartilage changes noted are fraying and fissuring of the cartilage. These areas are treated by smoothing the cartilage and removing loose fragments. This surgical technique is called a chondroplasty. Studies reveal the results of lateral release surgery can be variable and it is therefore not indicated for all anterior knee pain. When used for the strict indications outlined above, the results are good. Oglivie-Harris and Jackson [100] reported 85% good results in patients with minimal cartilage disease. Shea and Fulkerson reported [101] 92% good to excellent results in patients with isolated negative patellar tilt and minimal cartilage damage and 22% good results in those patients with more severe articular cartilage disease.

Proximal realignment procedures

Although most commonly indicated for the patient who has had a traumatic dislocation of the patella or recurrent subluxations, proximal imbrica-
tion of the medial retinaculum and vastus medialis obliques can be necessary
to balance the soft tissue restraints around the patella [101]. Indications for
this surgery are painful lateral patellar subluxation due to deficient medial
structures in patients with a normal Q angle. The procedure is most commonly paired with a lateral release and involves imbricating the proximal
medial patellar retinaculum and patellofemoral ligament and advancing the
vastus medialis obliques more distally on the patella. The later part of the
procedure effectively decreases the "functional" quadriceps angle, giving
the vastus medialis obliques a better mechanical advantage [102]. Early studies have shown 81% good results [103,104]. However, more recent literature
raises concerns about overpressure on the medial patella causing increased
articular load and pain to the medial patellofemoral compartment [105].

Distal realignment

There are several surgical techniques involving realignment of the tibial
tubercle. A straight medial tibial tubercle transfer (also known as a Roux-
Elmslie-Trillat procedure) is used to correct an abnormal Q angle (Fig. 5).

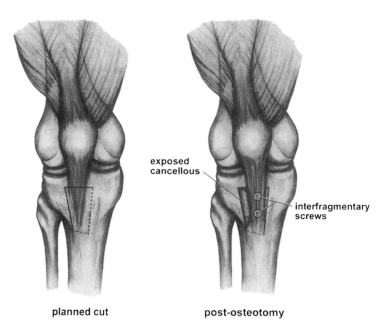

Fig. 5. Distal realignment procedure with straight medial transfer of the tibial tubercle. (*From*
Farr, J. Distal realignment for recurrent patellar instability. Operative Techniques in Sports
Medicine: Patellar Instability 2001;9(3):180; with permission.)

It is indicated for patients with malalignment and abnormal tracking due to a larger than normal Q angle [106,107]. Often the patients have a history of patella subluxation, dislocation, or both. A straight medial tibial tubercle transfer is often combined with a lateral release and, in some instances of instability, proximal realignment. For patients with patellofemoral pain syndrome, a straight medialization of the tubercle will unload overpressure and chondrosis of the lateral facet of the patella [108,109]. Cox [110] reports 77% good to excellent results with a 7% recurrence of instability.

An anterior and medial transfer of the tibial tubercle (also known as a Fulkerson osteotomy) is used to correct malalignment and abnormal tracking, as well as to decrease patellofemoral contact pressures [111]. Biomechanical studies have shown that elevation of the tibial tubercle by 1.2 cm can decrease the patellofemoral compression force by 57% [112]. The Fulkerson osteotomy is an oblique osteotomy of the tibial tubercle that allows anterior and medial transfer of the tubercle (Fig. 6). Similar to most distal realignment procedures, the Fulkerson osteotomy is often combined with a lateral release. It is indicated in patients with documented lateral and distal patellar chondral wear and lateral patellar tracking or subluxation. Lewallen and colleagues [113] found that with this osteotomy, the patellar contact area shifts proximally and medially, thereby unloading the lateral and

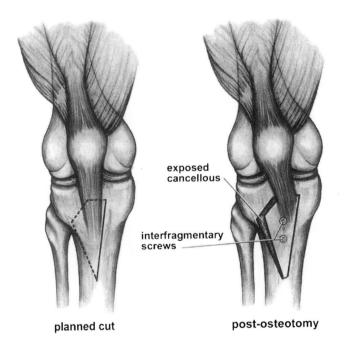

Fig. 6. Distal realignment procedure with anterior and medial transfer of the tibial tubercle. (*From* Farr, J. Distal realignment for recurrent patellar instability. Operative Techniques in Sports Medicine: Patellar Instability 2001;9(3):181; with permission.)

distal patella. They also found that total contact stress still decreases despite a decrease in total joint contact area. It is also theorized that anteromedialization of the tibial tubercle increases the quadriceps efficiency by increasing its lever arm [114]. Results of the Fulkerson osteotomy as reported by Fulkerson [115] are very good with 93% subjective excellent or good results and 89% objective excellent or good results with no deterioration of results noted at 5 years out.

A straight anteriorization of the tibial tubercle (also known as a Maquet procedure) is used to decrease patellar contact pressure when there is no malalignment or abnormal Q angle. It is best suited for middle and distal arthritic lesions of the patella. It is considered a salvage procedure for patellar arthrosis and has less satisfactory clinical results [116,117]. The procedure requires substantial elevation of the tubercle with bone grafting to hold the native tubercle elevated. Subsequently there is a resultant cosmetic and functional dissatisfaction due to the prominent tubercle.

Summary

Patellofemoral pain is an extremely common disorder with no true consensus as to the cause and appropriate treatment. However, the current standard of care is conservative treatment including physical therapy to address any and all biomechanical issues with quadriceps-based strengthening, iliotibial band stretching, hamstring stretching, and proximally focused exercise programs, as well as orthotic intervention, McConnell taping, and bracing. Surgery for patellofemoral pain syndrome is indicated in those few patients who have persistent symptoms in spite of appropriate rehabilitation and who have a problem that can genuinely be corrected by surgery.

References

[1] Cutbill JW, Ladly KO, Bray RC, et al. Anterior knee pain: a review. Clin J Sport Med 1997; 7:40–5.

[2] Fulkerson JP, Hungerford DS. Disorders of the patellofemoral joint. 2nd edition. Baltimore (MD): Williams & Wilkins; 1990.

[3] Baquie P, Brukner P. Injuries presenting to the Australian sports medicine centre: a 12-month study. Clin J Sport Med 1997;7:28–31.

[4] Devereaux MD, Lachmann SM. Patello-femoral arthralgia in athletes attending a sports injury clinic. Br J Sports Med 1984;18:18–21.

[5] Kannus P, Aho H, Jarvinen M, et al. Computerized recording of visits to an outpatient sports clinic. Am J Sports Med 1987;15:79–85.

[6] DeHaven KE, Lintner DM. Athletic injuries: comparison by age, sport, and gender. Am J Sports Med 1986;14:218–24.

[7] Fairbank JC, Pynsent PB, van Poortvliet JA, et al. Mechanical factors in the incidence of knee pain in adolescents and young adults. J Bone Joint Surg Br 1984;66(5):685–93.

[8] Taunton J, Ryan M, Clement D, et al. A retrospective case-control analysis of 2002 running injuries. Br J Sports Med 2002;36:95–101.

[9] Thomee R, Augustsson J, Karlsson J. Patellofemoral pain syndrome: a review of current issues. Sports Med 1999;28(4):245–62.

[10] Baker MM, Juhn MS. Patellofemoral pain syndrome in the female athlete. Clin Sports Med 2000;19(2):315–29.

[11] Fulkerson JP. Diagnosis and treatment of patients with patellofemoral pain. Am J Sports Med 2002;30(3):447–56.

[12] Hughston JC. Subluxation of the patella. J Bone Joint Surg Am 1968;50:1003–26.

[13] James S. Chrondromalacia of the patella in the adolsecent. In: Kennedy J, editor. The injured adolescent knee. Baltimore (MD): Williams & Wilkins; 1979. p. 205–51.

[14] Dye S, Vaupel G. Functional anatomy of the knee: bony geometric, static, and dynamic restraints, sensory and motor innervation. In: Lephart S, Fu F, ed. Proprioception and neuromuscular control in joint stability. Champaign (IL): Human Kinetics;2000:59–77.

[15] Moss R, DeVita P, Dawson M. A biomechanical analysis of the patellofemoral joint. J Athl Train 1992;27:64–9.

[16] Cowan SM, Bennell KL, Hodges PW, et al. Delayed onset of electromyographic activity of vastus medialis obliquus relative to vastus lateralis in subjects with patellofemoral pain syndrome. Arch Phys Med Rehabil 2001;82:183–9.

[17] Grabiner M, Koh T, Draganich L. Neuromechanics of the patellofemoral joint. Med Sci Sports Exerc 1994;26:10–21.

[18] Cowan SM, Hodges PW, Bennell KL, et al. Altered vastii recruitment when people with patellofemoral pain syndrome complete a postural task. Arch Phys Med Rehabil 2002; 83:989–95.

[19] Hungerford D, Barry M. Biomechanics of the patellofemoral joint. Clin Orthop Relat Res 1979;144:9–15.

[20] Murray M, Mollinger L, Gardner G, et al. Kinematic and EMG patterns during slow, free, and fast walking. J Orthop Res 1984;2:272–80.

[21] Owings TM, Grabiner MD. Motor control of the vastus medialis oblique and vastus lateralis muscles is disrupted during eccentric contractions in subjects with patellofemoral pain. Am J Sports Med 2002;30:483–7.

[22] Voight M, Wieder D. Comparative reflex response times of vastus medialis obliquus and vastus lateralis in normal subjects and subjects with extensor mechanism dysfunction; an electromyographical study. Am J Sports Med 1991;19:131–7.

[23] Witvrouw E, Sneyers C, Lysens R, et al. Reflex response times of vastus medialis oblique and vastus lateralis in normal subjects and subjects with patellofemoral pain syndrome. J Orthop Sports Phys Ther 1996;24:160–5.

[24] Gilleard W, McConnell J, Parsons D. The effect of patellar taping on the onset of vastus medialis obliquus and vastus lateralis muscle activity in persons with patellofemoral pain. Phys Ther 1998;78:25–32.

[25] Grabiner M, Koh T, Andrish J. Decreased excitation of vastus medialis oblique and vastus lateralis in patellofemoral pain syndrome. European Journal of Experimental Musculoskeletal Research 1992;1:33–9.

[26] Karst G, Willett G. Onset timing of electromyographic activity in the vastus medialis oblique and vastus lateralis muscles in subjects with and without patellofemoral pain syndrome. Phys Ther 1995;75:813–23.

[27] Mohr KJ, Kvitne RS, Pink MM, et al. Electromyography of the quadriceps in patellofemoral pain with patellar subluxation. Clin Orthop Relat Res 2003;415:261–71.

[28] Powers C, Landel R, Perry J. Timing and intensity of vastus muscle activity during functional activities in subjects with and without patellofemoral pain syndrome. Phys Ther 1996;76:946–55.

[29] Sheehy P, Burdett R, Irrgang J, et al. An electromyographic study of vastus medialis obliquus and vastus lateralis activity while ascending and descending steps. J Orthop Sports Phys Ther 1998;27:423–9.

[30] Worrell T, Crisp E, LaRosa C. Electromyographic reliability and analysis of selected lower extremity muscles during lateral step-up conditions. J Athl Train 1998;33: 156–62.

[31] Thomee R, Renstrom P, Karlsson J, et al. Patellofemoral pain syndrome in young women: a clinical analysis of alignment, pain parameters, common symptoms and functional activity level. Scand J Med Sci Sports 1995;5:237–44.

[32] Livingston L. The quadriceps angle: a review of the literature. J Orthop Sports Phys Ther 1998;28:105–9.

[33] Fabry G, Mac Ewen D, Shands A. Torsion of the femur. J Bone Joint Surg Am 1973;55: 1726–38.

[34] Reikeras O. Patellofemoral characteristics in patients with increased femoral anteversion. Skeletal Radiol 1992;21:311–3.

[35] Lee T, Anzel S, Bennett K, et al. The influence of fixed rotational deformities of the femur on the patellofemoral contact pressures in human cadaver knees. Clin Orthop Relat Res 1994;302:69–74.

[36] Eckhoff D, Montgomery W, Kilcoyne R, et al. Femoral morphometry and anterior knee pain. Clin Orthop Relat Res 1994;302:64–8.

[37] Dillon P, Updyke W, Allen W. Gait analysis with reference to chondromalacia patella. J Orthop Sports Phys Ther 1983;5:127–31.

[38] Kujala U, Friberg O, Aalot T, et al. Lower limb asymmetry and patellofemoral joint incongruence in the etiology of knee exertion injuries in athletes. Int J Sports Med 1987;8:214–20.

[39] Cooke T, Chir B, Price N, et al. The inwardly pointing knee: and unrecognized problem of external rotational malalignment. Clin Orthop Relat Res 1990;260:56–60.

[40] Eckhoff D, Brown A, Kilcoyne R, et al. Knee version associated with anterior knee pain. Clin Orthop Relat Res 1997;339:152–5.

[41] Powers C, Maffucci R, Hampton S. Rearfoot posture in subjects with patellofemoral pain. J Orthop Sports Phys Ther 1995;22:155–60.

[42] Woodall W, Welsh J. A biomechanical basis for rehabilitation programs involving the patellofemoral joint. J Orthop Sports Phys Ther 1990;11:535–42.

[43] Tiberio D. The effect of excessive subtalar joint pronation on patellofemoral mechanics: a theoretical model. J Orthop Sports Phys Ther 1987;9:160–5.

[44] Messier S, Davis S, Curl W, et al. Etiologic factors associated with patellofemoral pain in runners. Med Sci Sports Exerc 1991;23:1008–15.

[45] Powers C, Chen P, Reischl S, et al. Comparison of foot pronation and lower extremity rotation in persons with and without patellofemoral pain. Foot Ankle Int 2002;23:634–40.

[46] Eng J, Pierrynowski M. The effect of soft foot orthotics in the treatment of patellofemoral pain syndome. Phys Ther 1993;73:62–70.

[47] Johnston L, Gross M. Effects of foot orthoses on quality of life for individuals with patellofemoral pain syndrome. J Orthop Sports Phys Ther 2004;34:440–8.

[48] Stiene H, Brosky T, Reinking M, et al. A comparison of closed kinetic chain and isokinetic joint isolation exercise in patients with patellofemoral dysfunction. J Orthop Sports Phys Ther 1996;24:136–41.

[49] Host J, Craig R, Lehman R. Patellofemoral dysfunction in tennis players: a dynamic problem. Clin Sports Med 1995;14:177–203.

[50] Ireland M, Willson J, Ballantyne B, et al. Hip strength in females with and without patellofemoral pain. J Orthop Sports Phys Ther 2003;33:671–6.

[51] Perry J. Gait analysis: normal and pathological function. Thorofare (NJ): Slack; 1992.

[52] Powers C. The influence of altered lower-extremity kinematics on patellofemoral joint dysfunction: a theoretical perspective. J Orthop Sports Phys Ther 2003;33:639–46.

[53] Riegger-Krugh C, Keysor J. Skeletal malalignments of the lower quarter: correlated and compensatory motions and postures. J Orthop Sports Phys Ther 1996;2:164–70.

[54] Sahrmann S. Muscle imbalances in the female athlete. In: Pearl A, editor. The athletic female. Champaign (IL): Human Kinetics; 1993. p. 209–19.

[55] Wilk K, Davies G, Mangine R, et al. Patellofemoral disorders: a classification system and clinical guidelines for nonoperative rehabilitation. J Orthop Sports Phys Ther 1998;28: 307–22.

[56] Powers C, Ward S, Frederiscon M, et al. Patellofemoral kinematics during weight-bearing and non-weight bearing knee extension in persons with lateral subluxation of the patella: a preliminary study. J Orthop Sports Phys Ther 2003;33(11):677–85.

[57] Ferber R, Davis I, Williams D. Gender differences in lower extremity mechanics during running. Clin Biomech (Bristol, Avon) 2003;18:350–7.

[58] Malinzak R, Colby S, Kirkendall D, et al. A comparison of knee joint motion patterns between men and women in selected athletic tasks. Clin Biomech (Bristol, Avon) 2001; 16:438–45.

[59] McLean S, Myers P, Neal R, et al. A quantitative analysis of knee joint kinematics during the sidestep cutting maneuver. Bull Hosp Jt Dis 1998;57:30–8.

[60] Ford K, Myer G, Hewett T. Valgus knee motion during landing in high school female and male basketball players. Med Sci Sports Exerc 2003;35:1745–50.

[61] Hewett T, Myer G, Ford K. Decrease in neuromuscular control about the knee with maturation in female athletes. J Bone Joint Surg Am 2004;86:1601–8.

[62] Kernozek T, Torry M, Van Hoof H, et al. Gender differences in frontal and sagittal plane biomechanics during drop landings. Med Sci Sports Exerc 2005;37:1003–12.

[63] Pollard C, McClay Davis I, Hamill J. Influence of gender on hip and knee mechanics during a randomly cued cutting maneuver. Clin Biomech (Bristol, Avon) 2004;19: 1022–31.

[64] Zeller B, McCrory J, Kibler B, et al. Differences in kinematics and electromyographic activity between men and women during the single-legged squat. Am J Sports Med 2003; 31:449–56.

[65] Lephart S, Ferris C, Riemann B, et al. Gender differences in strength and lower extremity kinematics during landing. Clin Orthop Relat Res 2002;401:162–9.

[66] Leetun D, Ireland M, Willson J, et al. Core stability measures as risk factors for lower extremity in athletes. Med Sci Sports Exerc 2004;36:926–34.

[67] McClay I, Manal K. Three-dinemsional kinetic analysis of running: significance of secondary planes of motion. Med Sci Sports Exerc 1999;31:1629–37.

[68] Nadler S, Malanga G, DePrince M, et al. The relationship between lower extremity injury, low back pain, and hip strength in male and female collegiate athletes. Clin J Sport Med 2000;10:89–97.

[69] Powers C, Heino J, Rao S, et al. The influence on patellofemoral pain on lower limb loading during gait. Clin Biomech (Bristol, Avon) 1999;14:722–8.

[70] Beckman S, Buchanan T. Ankle inversion injury and hypermobility: effect on hip and ankle muscle electromyogaphy onset latency. Arch Phys Med Rehabil 1995;76:1138–43.

[71] Buchanan T, Kim A, Lloyd D. Selective muscle activation following rapid varus/valgus perterbations at the knee. Med Sci Sports Exerc 1996;28:870–6.

[72] Frederiscon M, Cookingham C, Chaudhari A, et al. Hip abductor weakness in distance runners with iliotibial band syndrome. Clin J Sport Med 2000;10:169–75.

[73] Friel K, McLean N, Myers C, et al. Ipsilateral hip abductor weakness after inversion ankle sprain. J Athl Train 2006;41:74–8.

[74] Jaramillo J, Worrell T, Ingersoll C. Hip isometric strength following knee surgery. J Orthop Sports Phys Ther 1994;20:160–5.

[75] Niemuth P, Johnson R, Myers M, et al. Hip muscle weakness and overuse injuries in recreational runners. Clin J Sport Med 2005;15:14–21.

[76] Nyland J, Kuzemchek S, Parks M, et al. Femoral anteversion influences vastus medialis and gluteus medius EMG amplitude: composite hip abductor EMG amplitude ratios during isometric combined hip abduction-external rotation. J Electromyogr Kinesiol 2004;14: 255–61.

[77] Blond L, Hansen L. Patellofemoral pain syndrome in athletes: a 5.7 year retrospective follow-up study of 250 athletes. Acta Orthop Belg 1998;64:393–400.

[78] Hoch A, Pepper M, Akuthota V. Stress fractures and knee injuries in runners. Phys Med Rehabil Clin N Am 2005;16:749–77.

[79] Bizzini M, Childs J, Piva S, et al. Systematic review of the quality of randomized controlled trials for patellofemoral pain syndrome. J Orthop Sports Phys Ther 2003;33:4–20.

[80] Heintjes E, Berger M, Bierma-Zeinstra S, et al. Exercise therapy for patellofemoral pain syndrome [review]. Cochrane Database Syst Rev 2003;4:1–34:CD003472.

[81] Crossley K, Bennell K, Green S, et al. A systematic review of physical interventions for patellofemoral pain syndrome. Clin J Sport Med 2001;11:103–10.

[82] Sutlive T, Mitchell S, Maxfield S, et al. Identification of individuals with patellofemoral pain whose symptoms improved after a combined program of foot orthosis use and modified activity: a preliminary investigation. Phys Ther 2004;84:49–61.

[83] Witvrouw E, Lysens R, Bellemans J, et al. Open versus closed kinetic chain exercises for patellofemoral pain: a prospective, randomized study. Am J Sports Med 2000;28:687–94.

[84] Gaffney K, Fricker P, Dwyer T, et al. Patellofemoral joint pain: a comparison of two treatment programmes. Excel 1992;8:179–89.

[85] Wijnen L, Lenssen A, Kuys-Wouters Y, et al. McConnell therapy versus Coumans bandage for patellofemoral pain—a randomised pilot study. Nederlands Tijdschrift voor fysiotherapie [in Dutch] 1996;12–7.

[86] Witvrouw E, Danneels L, Van Tiggelen D, et al. Open versus closed kinetic chain exercises in patellofemoral pain: a 5 year prospective randomized study. Am J Sports Med 2004;32: 1122–30.

[87] McConnell J. The management of chondromalacie patellae: a long term solution. Aust J Physiother 1986;32:215–33.

[88] Clark D, Downing N, Mitchell J, et al. Physiotherapy for anterior knee pain: a randomised controlled trial. Ann Rheum Dis 2000;59:700–4.

[89] Kowall M, Kolk G, Nuber G, et al. Patellar taping in the treatment of patellofemoral pain. a prospective randomized study. Am J Sports Med 1996;24:61–6.

[90] Whittingham M, Palmer S, Macmillan F. Effects of taping on pain and function in patellofemoral pain syndroms: a randomized controlled trial. J Orthop Sports Phys Ther 2004;34: 504–10.

[91] Finestone A, Radin E, Lev B, et al. Treatment of overuse patellofemoral pain. Prospective randomized controlled clinical trial in a military setting. Clin Orthop Relat Res 1993;293: 208–10.

[92] Miller M, Hinkin D, Wisnowski J. The efficacy of orthotics for anterior knee pain in military trainees. A preliminary report. Am J Knee Surg 1997;10:10–3.

[93] Denton J, Willson JD, Ballantyne BT, et al. The addition of the Protonics brace system to a rehabilitation protocol to address patellofemoral joint syndrome. J Orthop Sports Phys Ther 2005;35:210–9.

[94] Timm K. Randomized controlled trial of Protonics on patellar pain, position, and function. Med Sci Sports Exerc 1998;23:665–70.

[95] Mascal C, Landel R, Powers C. Management of patellofemoral pain targeting hip, pelvis, and trunk muscle function: 2 case reports. J Orthop Sports Phys Ther 2003;33:642–60.

[96] Tyler T, Nicholas S, Mullaney M, et al. The role of hip muscle function in the treatment of patellofemoral pain syndrome. Am J Sports Med 2006;34:630–6.

[97] Fritz J, Wainner R. Examining diagnostic tests: an evidence based practice perspective. Phys Ther 2001;81:1546–64.

[98] Lesher J, Sutlive T, Miller G, et al. Development of a clinical prediction rule for classifying patients with patellofemoral pain syndrome who respond to patellar taping. J Orthop Sports Phys Ther 2006;36:854–66.

[99] Fulkerson JP. Patellofemoral pain disorders: evaluation and management. J Am Acad Orthop Surg 1994;2:124–32.

[100] Oglivie-Harris DJ, Jackson RW. The arthroscopic treatment of chondromalacia patellae. J Bone Joint Surg Br 1984;66:660–5.

[101] Shea KP, Fulkerson JP. Preoperative computerized tomography scanning and arthroscopy in predicting outcome after lateral retinacular release. Arthroscopy 1992;8:327–34.

[102] Insall J, Bullough PG, Burstein AH. Proximal "tube" realignment of the patella for chondromalacia patellae. Clin Orthop Relat Res 1979;144:63–9.

[103] Insall J, Falvo KA, Wise DW. Chondromalacia patellae: a prospective study. J Bone Joint Surg Am 1976;58:1–8.

[104] Scuderi G, Cuomo F, Scott WN. Lateral release and proximal realignment for patellar subluxation and dislocation: a long-term follow-up. J Bone Joint Surg Am 1988;70(6): 856–61.

[105] Sallay PI, Poggi J, Speer KP, et al. Acute dislocation of the patella: a correlative pathoanatomic study. Am J Sports Med 1996;24:52–60.

[106] Muneta T, Yamamoto H, Ishibashi T, et al. Computerized tomographic analysis of tibial tubercle position in the painful female patellofemoral joint. Am J Sports Med 1994;22: 67–71.

[107] Shelbourne KD, Porter DA, Rozzi W. Use of a modified Elmslie-Trillat procedure to improve abnormal patellar congruence angle. Am J Sports Med 1994;22:318–23.

[108] Post WR, Fulkerson JP. Distal realignment of the patellofemoral joint: indications, effects, results, and recommendations. Orthop Clin North Am 1992;23:631–43.

[109] Myers P, Williams A, Dodds R, et al. The three-in-one proximal and distal soft tissue patellar realignment procedure: results and its place in the management of patellofemoral instability. Am J Sports Med 1999;27:575–9.

[110] Cox JS. Evaluation of the Roux-Elmslie-Trillat procedure for knee extensor realignment. Am J Sports Med 1982;10:303–10.

[111] Fulkerson JP, Becker GJ, Meaney JA, et al. Anteromedial tibial tubercle transfer without bone graft. Am J Sports Med 1990;18:490–7.

[112] Ferguson AB Jr, Brown TD, Fu FH, et al. Relief of patellofemoral contact stress by anterior displacement of the tibial tubercle. J Bone Joint Surg Am 1979;61(2):159–66.

[113] Lewallen DG, Riegger CL, Myers ER, et al. Effects of retinacular release and tibial tubercle elevation in patellofemoral degenerative joint disease. J Orthop Res 1990;8(6):856–62.

[114] Maquet P. Advancement of the tibial tuberosity. Clin Orthop Relat Res 1979;144:16–26.

[115] Fulkerson JP. Anteromedialization of the tibial tuberosity for patello-femoral malalignment. Clin Orthop Relat Res 1983;177:176–81.

[116] Radin EL, Pan HQ. Long term follow-up study on the Maquet procedure with special reference to the causes of failure. Clin Orthop Relat Res 1993;290:253–8.

[117] Schepsis AA, DeSimone AA, Leach RE. Anterior tibial tubercle transposition for patellofemoral arthrosis: a long-term study. Am J Knee Surg 1994;7:13–20.

ELSEVIER
SAUNDERS

Phys Med Rehabil Clin N Am
18 (2007) 459–476

PHYSICAL MEDICINE
AND REHABILITATION
CLINICS OF
NORTH AMERICA

Musculoskeletal Disorders of Pregnancy, Delivery and Postpartum

Joanne Borg-Stein, MD[a,b,c],*, Sheila A. Dugan, MD[d,e]

[a]*Physical Medicine and Rehabilitation, Harvard Medical School,
25 Shattuck Street, Boston, MA 02115, USA*
[b]*Spaulding-Wellesley Rehabilitation Center, 65 Walnut Street, Wellesley, MA 02481, USA*
[c]*Newton Wellesley Hospital Spine Center, 2014 Washington Street, Newton, MA 02462, USA*
[d]*Department of Physical Medicine and Rehabilitation, Rush University Medical Center,
1725 W. Harrison Street, Suite 970, Chicago, IL 60612, USA*
[e]*Chicago Institute of Neurosurgery and Neuroresearch, Elmhurst Memorial
Center for Health, Elmhurst, IL 60126, USA*

A 32-year-old woman, who has given birth after her first pregnancy, presents with a 2-month history of postpartum anterior pelvic/groin pain. She relates a prolonged second stage of labor resulting in normal vaginal delivery. No significant lacerations were noted. Postpartum evaluations by her obstetrician and a consulting urologist reveal no pathology that would explain her pain. She had functional limitations secondary to pain, which included difficulty with stair climbing and lifting her baby. Pertinent physical examination findings at the time of presentation included normal lower-extremity neurologic examination including all branches of the lumbosacral plexus. Pelvic rock test, pelvic compression, and palpation over the pubic symphysis, adductor tubercles, and adductor muscles all reproduced her pain.

Introduction

Gender-specific care of musculoskeletal impairments is an increasingly important topic in women's health. It is estimated that virtually all women experience some degree of musculoskeletal discomfort during pregnancy, and 25% have at least temporarily disabling symptoms. Lower back pain is the most common impairment, affecting 50% of pregnant women. Other common disorders include pelvic pain, upper- and lower-extremity pain, and peripheral neuropathy. This article provides a guide for appropriate

---

* Corresponding author. Spaulding-Wellesley Rehabilitation Center, 65 Walnut Street, Wellesley, MA 02481.

E-mail address: jborgstein@partners.org (J. Borg-Stein).

1047-9651/07/$ - see front matter © 2007 Elsevier Inc. All rights reserved.
doi:10.1016/j.pmr.2007.05.005

differential diagnosis, evaluation, and management of these regional musculoskeletal and peripheral neurologic disorders that affect women during pregnancy and the postpartum period. The article describes the relevant regional musculoskeletal anatomy, the hormonal and biochemical changes of pregnancy, specific conditions, and their management, as well as recommendations for exercise and physical therapeutics. The article reviews the current knowledge and evidence-based medical research available on the topic of musculoskeletal diagnoses in pregnancy. Much of the available literature is based on case series and on expert opinion from clinical practice experience. Given the high prevalence of these diagnoses, it is imperative for physicians treating musculoskeletal disorders to be familiar with appropriate management.

Physiologic changes of pregnancy

Soft-tissue edema during pregnancy is reported by approximately 80% of women, with findings most notable during the last 8 weeks of pregnancy [1]. Increased fluid retention can predispose to tenosynovial or nerve entrapment. Ligamentous laxity is another physiologic change of pregnancy. It is related to the production of the hormones relaxin and estrogen. In animal studies, relaxin is associated with remodeling from large-diameter to small-diameter collagen fibers [2]. Relaxin is known to remodel pelvic connective tissue and activate the collagenolytic system [3]. There may be a correlation between mean serum relaxin levels during pregnancy and low back pain or symphyseal pain. There is an initial increase of relaxin levels until a peak value at the 12th week followed by a decline until the 17th week. Thereafter, stable serum levels around 50% of the peak value are recorded [4].

Symphysis pubis widening begins during the 10th to 12th week of pregnancy under the influence of relaxin. This can be associated with tenderness and pain and is usually exacerbated by exercise. Normal antepartum widening does not exceed 10 mm [5].

Weight gain during pregnancy is normal. In combination with ligamentous laxity, there may be increased joint discomfort. A 20% weight gain during pregnancy may increase the force on a joint by as much as 100%. Hyperlordosis of pregnancy may be seen as the result of forces induced by a gravid uterus and may be seen as an accentuation of an anterior pelvic tilt. The sacroiliac joints resist this forward rotation. As the pregnancy progresses, both forward rotation and hyperlordosis increase as the sacroiliac ligaments become lax. These factors contribute to increasing mechanical strain on the low back, sacroiliac, and pelvis [1].

Pelvic pain of pregnancy

There is a spectrum of disorders affecting the pubic symphyseal region during pregnancy and parturition. Pubic symphysis regional pain occurs as a result of increased motion related to the ligamentous laxity as mentioned above. In an older European study, it was estimated that the prevalence of this condition is 1 in 36 women [6]. More recent studies found higher rates. A study from Denmark found an incidence rate of 20.1% [7]. A study from Iran found an incidence rate of 28% [8]. Risk factors for developing pregnancy-related pelvic girdle pain include history of previous low back pain, trauma of the back or pelvis, multiparae, high weight, high levels of stress, and low job satisfaction [9]. Mild cases of symphysis inflammation generally respond to rest and ice.

Osteitis pubis

Osteitis pubis is characterized by bony resorption about the symphysis followed by spontaneous resossification (Fig. 1) [1]. The pregnant or postpartum woman has a gradual onset of pubic symphysis pain, followed by rapid progression over the course of a few days, leading to excruciating pain radiating down the inside of both thighs, exacerbated by any movement of the limbs. The prognosis for recovery is generally good, with a self-limited course that lasts from several days to weeks before gradually subsiding [10,11].

Occasionally, the course of groin/pubic pain may be quite prolonged and should be treated with initial bed rest followed by ambulation with a walker as tolerated. Anti-inflammatory agents can be given to affected women after parturition. Intrasymphyseal injection of lidocaine and steroid may shorten the duration of symptoms [12]. Ultrasound imaging may identify the pubic symphysis and accurately guide injection [13].

Acupuncture stimulation may be a valuable treatment to ameliorate pain in the condition of pelvic pain in late pregnancy and postpartum [14]. The

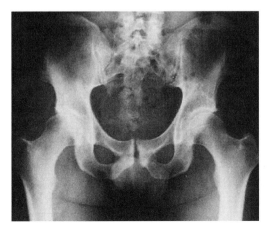

Fig. 1. Osteitis pubis. Plain radiograph of the pelvis revealing a slight widening and small amount of adjacent sclerosis of the symphysis pubis. (*From* Scott K, Carek P. Osteitis pubis: a diagnosis for the family physician. J Am Board Fam Pract 1998;11(4):291–5, with permission from the American Board of Family Medicine.)

application of a pelvic belt may reduce pubic symphyseal pain or sacroiliac pain [15].

Specific stabilizing exercises for pelvic pain of pregnancy have demonstrated benefit and should be incorporated as well [16].

Rupture of the symphysis pubis

Rupture of the symphysis pubis, a true rupture of the ligaments supporting the symphysis pubis, is only rarely reported. This is believed to occur as a result of the wedge effect of the forceful descent of the fetal head against the pelvic ring, usually during delivery, creating a separation of approximately 1 cm [17]. Another case series suggested that symphyseal rupture can occur as a result of forceful and excessive abduction of the thighs during labor [18]. Characteristically, there is a sudden pain in the region of the symphysis pubis, sometimes an audible crack, followed by radiation of pain to the back or thighs. A gap may be palpable with associated soft-tissue swelling. Treatment is generally conservative. Initial bed rest in a lateral decubitus position with a pelvic binder is indicated. Progression to weight bearing as tolerated with a walker is appropriate when symptoms permit [19].

Complications are rare, and subsequent vaginal delivery is possible [20]. In extremely rare circumstances, persistence of symptoms may warrant surgical stabilization with open reduction and internal fixation [21].

Pelvic dislocation of pregnancy

Severe pelvic dislocation of pregnancy is extremely rare. Cases reported are associated with difficult parturition. Patients sustain simultaneous rupture of the symphysis pubis and sacroiliac joints, with resultant pelvic dislocation. All patients in a series from Boston developed persistent sacroiliac pain after being managed with closed reduction. Based on the evidence, an operative approach should be considered for patients with symphyseal diastasis of 4.0 cm or more [22].

Low back pain of pregnancy

Epidemiology

The epidemiology of low back pain in pregnancy demonstrates incidence rates of approximately 50% among retrospective reviews [6,23]. Low back pain rates have been found to increase with advancing maternal age, with a history of back pain during a previous pregnancy, with successive births, with a higher body mass index, and with a history of hypermobility [6,24]. A recent study by Wang and colleagues [25] demonstrated increased low back pain in younger women. No consistent relationship has been found between rate of back pain with the height of the mother, with the mother's weight gain, or with the weight of the baby [17]. It is reported that only 32% of women with low back pain during pregnancy report this to their prenatal providers, and only 25% of prenatal care providers recommend a specific treatment for their patients. Nearly 30% of women are forced to stop performing at least one daily activity because of low back pain over the course of their pregnancy [25].

Low back pain is also reported in 30% to 45% of women in the postpartum period [26]. The main factors associated with development of postpartum back pain are previous episodes of back pain. Risk factors associated with persistent back pain after 24 months seem to be the onset of severe pain early during gestation, the inability to reduce weight to prepregnancy levels, high body mass index, and history of hypermobility [26,27].

Previous physical activity decreases the risk of low back pain and pelvic pain during pregnancy [28]. Exercise during the second half of pregnancy significantly reduces the intensity of low back pain [29].

Etiology

Low back pain during pregnancy has multiple causes, and the relative frequency of these causes has not been fully established. These causes include mechanical strain, pelvic ligamentous laxity, sacroiliac pain, vascular compression, spondylolisthesis, discogenic pain, and hip pathology (discussed later in this article). One popular theory for the cause of nonspecific low back pain of pregnancy posits that the enlarging gravid uterus and accompanying compensatory lumbar lordosis contribute to substantial mechanical strain on the lower back. In addition, the tendency for pelvic rotation is increased as the lumbar lordosis increases. These altered biomechanics, in combination with relaxation of the pelvic and sacroiliac joints under the influence of relaxin, may further increase strain on the pelvis and low back [1,17,23].

Lumbar disk herniations of pregnancy, although relatively uncommon, are estimated to occur in approximately 1 in 10,000 cases of lumbosacral pain of pregnancy [30]. During pregnancy, noncontrast MRI can be performed to identify the pathology. To date, no recognized adverse biological effects of MRI on the developing fetus have been identified, although the long-term effects of MRI on the developing fetus have not been fully evaluated [31].

Another hypothesis suggests that the vascular system may play an important role in the pathogenesis of back pain during pregnancy. In a 1992 study, Fast and Hertz [32] hypothesize that prolonged time in the supine position leads to obstruction of the vena cava. They further suggest that increased pressure and venous stasis in combination with a decrease in basal oxygen saturation may lead to hypoxemia and compromise the metabolic supply of the neural structures, resulting in pain.

In susceptible women, pregnancy may be a factor for the development of degenerative spondylolisthesis [33]. In women with previously diagnosed spondylolisthesis, no increase in low back pain or increase in slippage during pregnancy was found [34]. As in other individuals with spondylolisthesis, low back pain may be unrelated to the presence of this anatomic finding and may be caused by disk, facet joint, or muscle abnormalities.

History and physical exam

The pregnant woman with low back pain generally reports lumbar, pelvic, or sacroiliac pain aggravated by weight bearing and activity. Sitting, resting, recumbency, and use of a supportive pillow often ameliorate the symptoms. Occasionally, there is a vague accompanying posterior thigh or inguinal radiation of pain into the leg. True nerve root pain is uncommon. The physical examination of the pregnant woman with back pain should begin with a standard neuromuscular exam that includes observation, palpation, range-of-motion tests, tests for muscle imbalances, and a thorough neurological examination. In addition, the examiner should assess posture and degree of lordosis. Occasionally, a "step-off" sign will be appreciated in the lumbar spine and may suggest spondylolisthesis. Tenderness is often present over the sacroiliac joints and lumbar paraspinal muscles. Sacroiliac compression tests, bimanual compression over the iliac crests, and Patrick's test all may elicit sacroiliac pain. A careful examination of the hip should be performed as well.

Treatment

Most patients with low back pain respond to activity and postural modifications. Scheduled rest with elevation of the feet to flex the hips and decrease the lumbar lordosis helps relieve muscle spasm and acute pain [17]. A regular exercise program before pregnancy reduces the risk for back pain during pregnancy [35]. During pregnancy, exercise may be initiated once the acute pain is controlled. Sitting pelvic-tilt exercises and aquatic exercise have been shown to decrease pain intensity [36,37]. Exercise to increase strength of the abdominal and back muscles is also recommended [38].

Lumbar support binders may also provide pain relief (Fig. 2). A recent study looked at women with lower back pain who were at least 20 weeks gestation and who wore a maternity support binder during waking hours for 2 straight weeks. They had significant reduction in mean pain scores and effect of pain on daily activities, including those related to family, house and yard, recreation, exercise, and sleep. The maternity binders were well accepted by the women [39]. Furthermore, the lumbar and abdominal support has not been shown to adversely affect the hemodynamics of the fetus or mother [40].

A recent retrospective, observational study of 167 patients with low back and pelvic pain of pregnancy demonstrated improvement in 72% of patients treated with acupuncture administered during the second and third trimesters. No significant adverse effects were noted [41]. In addition, a study by Guthrie and Martin [42] looked at a group of 500 pregnant women with lower back pain and demonstrated that osteopathic manipulative treatment (specific techniques included muscle energy, myofascial release, ligamentous articular strain, high-velocity–low-amplitude thrust) to the lumbar area

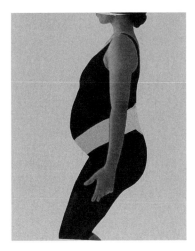

Fig. 2. Back-A-Line maternity support binder. (*Courtesy of* Back-A-Line, Inc., San Francisco, CA; with permission.)

during the third trimester significantly reduced back pain experienced during labor and delivery, as measured by amount of analgesic medication requested.

A recent survey study from Wang and colleagues [43] found that both providers of prenatal health care and pregnant women in New Haven County are likely to use complementary and alternative treatments for pregnancy-related low back pain. Massage (61.4%), acupuncture (44.6%), relaxation (42.6%), yoga (40.6%), and chiropractic (36.6%) were the most common complementary and alternative medical therapies recommended for low back pain in pregnancy by the providers of prenatal health in that sample.

The medication of choice for pain relief is acetaminophen because antiprostaglandins (aspirin and nonsteroidal anti-inflammatory drugs) are relatively contraindicated in pregnancy because they can cause premature closure of the ductus arteriosis in the fetus if given at or near term. Other medications that the US Food and Drug Administration rates class B (no evidence of risk in humans during pregnancy) may be considered for pain control during pregnancy. These include cyclobenzaprine, oxycodone (if used for short periods not near term), and prednisone.

There is no literature examining the safety or efficacy of epidural steroid injections during pregnancy. In the authors' clinical experience, interlaminar epidural steroid injections, performed without any fluoroscopic guidance, can be administered safely by an interventional pain specialist with extensive experience in epidural injections in pregnancy. Surgery for lumbar disk herniation during pregnancy with cauda equina syndrome or progressive neurologic deficit can be safely undertaken if clinical circumstances dictate. Brown and Levi [44] report a case series of three pregnant women who were successfully treated this way. Care should be carefully coordinated with the obstetrician.

Acquired compressive nerve and root disorders of pregnancy and puerperium

Introduction

Peripheral nerves are susceptible to injury in the pregnant, laboring, and postpartum woman by several mechanisms: compression, traction, ischemia, and, less commonly, laceration. As would be expected biomechanically, labor and delivery are more likely to compromise the lumbosacral plexus and lower-limb peripheral nerves, whereas activities of daily living and child care, especially those requiring repetitive or prolonged positioning of the upper limb, are associated with upper-limb peripheral nerve injury. Upper-limb neuropathies (eg, median neuropathy at the wrist) can also occur during pregnancy because of peripheral edema.

Mechanisms of peripheral nerve injury

Compression and traction are the most common mechanisms of peripheral nerve entrapment in pregnancy and the puerperium. Compression neuropathies are most common in anatomic locations where excessive pressure can occur (median nerve in the carpal tunnel) or in superficial nerves (common peroneal nerve at the fibular head). The endoneurium, a connective tissue matrix of collagen and fatty tissue, surrounds individual nerve fascicles, absorbing shock and dissipating pressure. Nerves with tightly packed fasciculi and thin endoneurium are more susceptible to compression. Pregnancy-related swelling and prolonged positioning increase compressive forces, resulting in increased prevalence of compression neuropathies in pregnancy and postpartum child-care activities. Labor and delivery are also associated with compressive mononeuropathies and lumbosacral plexopathies [45–47]. Traction neuropathies result when the stretch applied to the nerve exceeds the elastic capacity of the neural and connective tissue. Intrinsic nerve characteristics, such as the amount of perineurium, the lamellated sheaths of perineural cells, and collagen fibrils, have been implicated in differential risk of traction injury [48]. A combination of compression and stretch may result in decreased perineural blood flow and ischemic injury. Less severe injuries that cause focal demyelination and conduction block are the most common type in pregnancy and the puerperium. These neuropathies are generally short-lived and have a good recovery [49].

Carpal tunnel syndrome (median neuropathy at the wrist)

Hand pain is the second most frequent musculoskeletal symptom of pregnancy, with carpal tunnel syndrome (CTS) frequently the cause [17]. The median nerve can be entrapped at the wrist in the enclosed space formed by the carpal bones and the overlying transverse carpal ligament. CTS typically presents with pain and paresthesias in the first three digits of the hand, often bilaterally, and is most frequently diagnosed during the third trimester

[50]. The rate of CTS varies from 2% to 25% in pregnant women [51,52]. The pain can worsen at night or during the day with repetitive wrist flexion or extension.

Peripheral edema has been implicated in pregnancy-related CTS and is most common in older, primiparous women [51,53]. Prolactin and fluid retention coupled with prolonged, awkward positioning of the wrist and hand may cause CTS related to nursing. The symptoms of CTS frequently resolve within days to weeks after labor and delivery. Forty-three percent to 95% of women have resolution of symptoms within 2 weeks postpartum [17,54]. In one study, women with onset of CTS symptoms early during pregnancy had prolonged recovery time after delivery [55]. Nonsurgical management of CTS is appropriate in pregnant women because most patients obtain relief after delivery. In pregnant women symptomatic enough to require treatment, splinting of the wrist in a neutral position is recommended. More than 80% of women had good relief of symptoms using thermoplastic night splints for 2 weeks [51]. Serial electrophysiologic studies done before and after splinting in one case study demonstrated rapid improvement in physiologic measures, mirroring clinical improvement [56]. Education on correct positioning of the hand and wrist for occupational and child-care activities should be provided to women with CTS during and after pregnancy. Steroid injections are useful in patients with recalcitrant symptoms [50,57]. Infrequently, surgery is indicated during pregnancy or the postpartum period for patients with ongoing severe symptomatology and positive electrodiagnostic studies [57,58].

Meralgia paresthetica (lateral femoral cutaneous neuropathy)

The lateral femoral cutaneous nerve is a pure sensory nerve supplying sensation to the anterolateral thigh. It passes slightly medial and inferior to the anterior superior iliac spine after exiting the pelvis by traveling under the inguinal ligament. Injury to the nerve causes burning, pain, or numbness in the region of innervation, referred to as meralgia paresthetica syndrome. Pregnancy, along with obesity, diabetes mellitus, trauma, belt pressure, and anatomic variation, is a risk factor for meralgia paresthetica [59]. One recent study found that pregnant women had 12 times the likelihood of meralgia paresthetica compared with nonpregnant patients in a primary-care setting [60]. Lateral femoral cutaneous neuropathy was the most common finding in a prospective study of postpartum lumbosacral spine and lower-limb nerve injuries resulting from labor and delivery [26]. Cesarean delivery may infrequently lead to meralgia paresthetica from a wide incision, stretching, or retractor placement, although the prevalence does not vary substantially with method of delivery [26,61]. As with CTS, pregnancy-related meralgia paresthetica syndrome typically resolves after delivery. The diagnosis is typically clinical; the nerve conduction study of the lateral femoral cutaneous nerve can be difficult to obtain, even in healthy, asymptomatic individuals.

Pregnant patients are advised not wear clothes that fit tightly along the hips and to avoid as much as possible carrying older children on the ipsilateral hip. Several investigators postulate that intrapartum nerve injury can be reduced by attention to laboring practices [26,62]. Consideration of frequent position changes for laboring, with avoidance of prolonged hip flexion, may reduce compression on the lateral femoral nerve. In addition, shortening pushing time by allowing the fetus to descend into the perineum without active maternal pushing may reduce nerve compression or traction.

Femoral neuropathy and other intrapartum maternal nerve injuries

The incidence of lumbosacral spine and lower-limb nerve injuries related to labor and delivery varies in studies, depending on sample size and study methodology. A retrospective study using codes for nerve injury from the International Classification of Diseases, Ninth Edition, examined charts over 16 years for 140,000 women and found 0.08% incidence of nerve injury [63]. The investigators concluded that improvements in modern obstetric practice might be responsible for a reduction in nerve injury rates of almost 5% since the turn of the century [64]. A more recent prospective study of 6000 women who delivered in a 1-year period found an almost 1% (0.92%) rate of injury [26]. Injury rate was not associated with obstetric anesthesia but rather nulliparity and prolonged pushing. Many studies are limited by lack of electromyographic documentation because the injuries are frequently of limited duration and new mothers may not follow up for an electrodiagnostic study before symptom resolution. Most nerve injuries resolve over weeks to months.

Femoral neuropathy has been documented as a consequence of labor and delivery. During a prolonged second stage of labor, compression of the femoral nerve under the inguinal ligament may occur. Stretch or ischemia of the intrapelvic, poorly vascularized portion of the femoral nerve may be another mechanism of injury, as the femoral nerve does not descend through the true pelvis [45]. However, in cases in which the iliopsoas muscle, along with the quadriceps, is found to be weak, the lesion may be proximal to the inguinal ligament, where branches to the iliopsoas arise [65]. Femoral neuropathy can result in significant functional impairment, particularly in ascending and descending stairs, walking, and transferring from sitting to standing. Physical therapy evaluation and assistive-device training is mandatory before hospital discharge. Treatment is supportive, and prognosis is good. Demyelinating lesions typically recover in 6 months or less [54].

Lumbosacral plexopathies

Lumbosacral plexopathies resulting in proximal or distal lower-limb weakness can occur. Plexus-associated foot drop can result from compression of the peroneal division of the sciatic nerve in the pelvis or compression of the common peroneal nerve at the head of the fibula [66]. Common peroneal nerve compression at the fibular head was documented in laboring women both from hand placement and squatting [67–70]. Obturator nerve palsies have been described as related to labor and delivery. The nerve crosses the pelvic brim and may be compressed by the descending fetal head or instrumentation used for fetal evacuation [64,66].

Upper-limb pain of pregnancy and postpartum

DeQuervain's tenosynovitis

DeQuervain's tenosynovitis is an inflammatory condition of the abductor pollicis longus and extensor pollicis brevis tendons of the first dorsal compartment of the wrist. It can develop in pregnancy or during the postpartum period, with localized pain along the radial aspect of the wrist. Fluid retention related to hormonal status is suspected in the pathophysiology in pregnant and lactating women. Overuse during childcare activities is also implicated [71,72]. Symptoms may persist until nursing is discontinued [73]. The clinical diagnosis is based on history, symptom location, and local tenderness over the first dorsal compartment. Provocative maneuvers include Finkelstein's test, in which the pain is provoked with ulnar deviation of the wrist with the thumb flexed inside a closed fist. Symptoms are usually self-limited and respond to conservative management, including thumb spica splints, icing, and activity modification. Oral anti-inflammatory medications can be used in the postpartum patient, and corticosteroid injections to the tendon sheath are used in pregnancy and postpartum. Local corticosteroid injections were shown to be more efficacious than splinting in a study of 18 patients [74]. Occasionally, operative treatment is necessary in the postpartum period [75].

Lower-extremity pain of pregnancy and postpartum

Hip pain of pregnancy

Hip pain in the pregnant woman can present with progressive symptoms and can lead to significant disability. Several rare but worrisome entities must be considered when a pregnant woman presents with complaints of hip pain. As noted earlier, conditions of the low back and pelvic girdle can present with associated hip pain and should be included in the differential diagnosis. Likewise, intraarticular hip pathology can refer pain to the pelvis and back and can be misdiagnosed as pelvic instability. It is important to test hip range of motion with the pelvis and lower spine maintained in a stable position so as to differentiate intraarticular hip pathology from referred pain [17]. In any pregnant woman presenting with antalgic gait, transient osteoporosis of the hip or osteonecrosis of the femoral head must be considered.

Transient osteoporosis of the hip is a rare condition that presents with weight-bearing hip pain, usually in the third trimester of pregnancy. Plain anteroposterior radiography of the pelvis with properly positioned lead shielding may reveal osteoporosis of the femoral head and neck with preserved joint space [76,77]. MRI reveals high-intensity signal in the bone marrow on T2-weighted images [78,79]. Early recognition and treatment with protective weight bearing will allow the condition to be self-limited and without long-term sequelae [1]. Antiresorptive bone agents, including calcitonin and bisphosphonates, shortened the duration of the symptoms both in pregnant and postpartum patients [80,81]. However, the use of bisphosphonates during pregnancy is controversial. Several groups have found that gestational exposure to bisphosphonates was associated with decreased fetal bone growth. Bisphosphonates may have an effect on fetal serum calcium levels. If clinicians choose to start treatment before delivery, serum calcium levels should be monitored closely. To reports of congenital abnormalities associated with use of bisphosphonates have appeared in animal teratology studies [82]. The prognosis for natural recovery is good if the osteoporosis is associated with pregnancy and not related to preexisting osteoporosis predating the pregnancy [83]. Failure to diagnose this condition can result in fracture, which may precipitate the need for surgical intervention [84].

Avascular necrosis of the femoral head has been reported in pregnant women with no additional risk factors for avascular necrosis (Fig. 3) [85]. Several theories regarding the pathogeneses have been proposed, including higher adrenocortical activity combined with weight gain and higher levels of female sex hormones in conjunction with increased intraosseous pressures [86,87]. The symptoms typically occur in the third trimester, with weight-bearing pain in the hip, pelvis, or groin. At times, the pain radiates to the knee [17]. MRI can delineate the pathology, with partial femoral head involvement in most cases. Restricted weight bearing is initiated to prevent progression of femoral head necrosis, with definitive treatment after delivery as appropriate. Postpartum treatment may include medications, such as bisphosphonates, or surgical management, depending on the severity and stage of osteonecrosis.

Other causes of lower-extremity pain during pregnancy

In a case-controlled study, about 100 postpartum and matched nulliparous controls were surveyed regarding lower-extremity pain complaints [88]. The postpartum subjects were twice as likely as the nulliparous controls to have symptoms of leg and foot pain. Most postpartum women noted the onset of lower-limb pain during the second or third trimester of pregnancy. History of regular exercise was not protective or causative of pain related to pregnancy. Ligamentous laxity may be associated with lower-limb injury. A case study documented transient laxity of the anterior cruciate ligament in a pregnant woman during her third trimester and postpartum period.

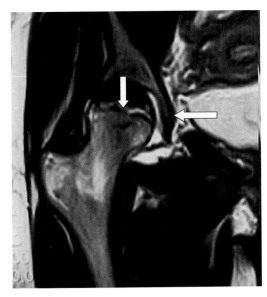

Fig. 3. Avascular necrosis. MRI of the right hip shows an osteonecrotic lesion in the anterosuperior portion of the femoral head that is well demarcated but is inhomogeneous. Arrows point to the "double line sign," which is a classic radiologic sign of avascular necrosis and is made up of two concentric low and high signal bands. (*From* Wheeless textbook of orthopaedics. Data Trace Internet Publishing, LLC 2006. Available at http://www.wheelessonline.com/image7/avnn4.jpg. Accessed January 10, 2007; with permission.)

This patient's anterior cruciate ligament reconstruction was performed 2 months before conception [2]. Relaxin-related dissociation of large collagen fibrils was thought to be causative. The mechanism of ligamentous pain production may be secondary to strain. Ligaments, especially at the site of bony insertion, lie on a bed of well-vascularized and highly innervated insertional angle fat. Numerous nerve endings are at the attachment sites [89].

The differential diagnosis in pregnant and postpartum women with musculoskeletal pain should include other bone, joint, and soft-tissue structures, in addition to ligaments. For instance, the labrum of the hip or meniscus of the knee may be at greater risk of injury during pregnancy. Two cases of pregnant women presenting with acute locking of the knee were reported. One of these required urgent arthroscopic repair of a torn meniscus [90]. History of previous injury in the area, current injury in adjacent areas, or systemic metabolic conditions, such as pregnancy-related osteoporosis, could be associated with an acute musculoskeletal injury in pregnant women. Sacral and tibial stress fractures, rib fractures, and vertebral fractures related to osteoporosis are documented in pregnant women [91–94]. In a case study of a pregnant woman with normal lumbar and femoral bone density, bilateral sacral stress fractures were related to unaccustomed loading in the last trimester [95]. Recurrent ankle sprains or patellofemoral symptoms are theoretical risks during pregnancy that women should consider in their exercise planning.

Local treatment of acute lower-limb musculoskeletal injury includes rest, ice, compression, and elevation. Protected mobility with orthoses or protected weight bearing with assistive devices should be employed in relation to injury with clinical reasoning similar to that for the nonpregnant population. Careful observation of women who become pregnant within a few months after anterior cruciate ligament reconstruction is recommended [2]. As with other medical conditions, surgery is done during pregnancy only in the setting of acute, debilitating musculoskeletal conditions. If surgery is deemed necessary, local and regional anesthetics are used due to their better safety profile. First-trimester general anesthesia is associated with a slightly increased risk of spontaneous abortion [90].

Case presentation: management

In the case described at the beginning of this article, the initial diagnostic impression was of osteitis pubis. MRI was obtained and confirmed the diagnosis of osteitis pubis. There was no evidence of pelvis stress fracture, pubic symphysis rupture, or avascular necrosis of the hips.

Management consisted of local injection of Depo-Medrol with lidocaine to the pubic symphyseal region to reduce local pain. Acupuncture was added for adjunctive pain management. The patient chose not to use any medications because she was still nursing. A pelvic binder was provided for short-term use for support and to reduce pain from ambulating, climbing stairs, and lifting the baby. A physical therapist clinically experienced in this area provided gentle manual therapy, and progressive pelvic, hip girdle, and abdominal stabilization exercises. Conditioning, endurance, and strength training progressed as per patient tolerance. The patient improved over the course of 3 to 4 months.

Summary

Virtually all women experience some degree of musculoskeletal discomfort during pregnancy with approximately 25% having disabling symptoms. Additionally, many women develop musculoskeletal disorders postpartum due to the continued hormonal influences of lactation on the musculoskeletal system and the biomechanical and ergonomic stresses of child-care–related activities.

Accurate and prompt diagnosis and comprehensive management are important for a good outcome and prevention of chronic pain and disability. Prognosis is often good as many of the conditions are self-limited. Treatment often includes a combination of local injection, bracing, therapeutic exercise, manual therapy, and functional rehabilitation. Reassurance and patient education are critical.

References

[1] Ritchie JR. Orthopedic considerations during pregnancy. Clin Obstet Gynecol 2003;46: 456–66.

[2] Blecher AM, Richmond JC. Transient laxity of an anterior cruciate ligament-reconstructed knee related to pregnancy. Arthroscopy 1998;14:77–9.

[3] Weiss M, Nagelschmidt M, Struck H. Relaxin and collagen metabolism. Horm Metab Res 1979;11:408–10.

[4] Kristiansson P, Svardsudd K, von Schoultz B. Serum relaxin, symphyseal pain, and back pain during pregnancy. Am J Obstet Gynecol 1996;175:1342–7.

[5] Young J. Relaxation of the pelvic joints in pregnancy: pelvic arthropathy of pregnancy J Obstet Gynaecol Br Emp 1940;47:493.

[6] Mantle MJ, Greenwood RM, Currey HL. Backache in pregnancy. Rheumatol Rehabil 1977; 16:95–101.

[7] Albert HB, Godskesen M, Westergaard JG. Incidence of four syndromes of pregnancy-related pelvic joint pain. Spine 2002;27:2831–4.

[8] Mousavi SJ, Parnianpour M, Vleeming A. Pregnancy related pelvic girdle pain and low back pain in an Iranian population. Spine 2007;32:E100–4.

[9] Albert HB, Godskesen M, Korsholm L, et al. Risk factors in developing pregnancy-related pelvic girdle pain. Acta Obstet Gynecol Scand 2006;85:539–44.

[10] Gonik B, Stringer CA. Postpartum osteitis pubis. South Med J 1985;78:213–4.

[11] Kubitz RL, Goodlin RC. Symptomatic separation of the pubic symphysis. South Med J 1986;79:578–80.

[12] Schwartz Z, Katz Z, Lancet M. Management of puerperal separation of the symphysis pubis. Int J Gynaecol Obstet 1985;23:125–8.

[13] Adler RS, Sofka CM. Percutaneous ultrasound-guided injections in the musculoskeletal system. Ultrasound Q 2003;19:3–12.

[14] Lund I, Lundelberg T, Lonnberg L, et al. Decrease of pregnant women's pelvic pain after acupuncture: a randomized controlled single-blind study. Acta Obstet Gynecol Scand 2006;85:12–9.

[15] Mens JM, Damen L, Snijders CJ, et al. The mechanical effect of a pelvic belt in patients with pregnancy-related pelvic pain. Clin Biomech (Bristol, Avon) 2006;21:122–7.

[16] Stuge B, Laerum E, Kirkesola G, et al. The efficacy of a treatment program focusing on specific stabilizing exercises for pelvic girdle pain after pregnancy: a randomized controlled trial. Spine 2004;29:351–9.

[17] Heckman JD, Sassard R. Current concepts review: musculoskeletal considerations in pregnancy. J Bone Joint Surg Am 1994;76:1720–30.

[18] Cappiello GA, Oliver BC. Rupture of symphysis pubis caused by forceful and excessive abduction of the thighs with labor epidural anesthesia. J Fla Med Assoc 1995; 82:261–3.

[19] Jain N, Sternberg LB. Symphyseal separation. Obstet Gynecol 2005;105:1229–32.

[20] Culligan P, Hill S, Heit M. Rupture of the symphysis pubis during vaginal delivery followed by two subsequent uneventful pregnancies. Obstet Gynecol 2002;100:1114–7.

[21] Rommens PM. Internal fixation in postpartum symphysis pubis rupture: report of three cases. J Orthop Trauma 1997;11:273–6.

[22] Kharrazi FD, Rodgers WB, Kennedy JG, et al. Parturition-induced pelvic dislocation: a report of four cases. J Orthop Trauma 1997;11:277–81.

[23] Carlson HL, Carlson NL, Pasternak BA, et al. Understanding and managing the back pain of pregnancy. Curr Womens Health Rep 2003;3:65–71.

[24] Mogren IM, Pohjanen AI. Low back pain and pelvic pain during pregnancy: prevalence and risk factors. Spine 2005;30:983–91.

[25] Wang SM, Dezinno P, Maranets I, et al. Low back pain during pregnancy: prevalence, risk factors, and outcomes. Obstet Gynecol 2004;104:65–70.

[26] To WW, Wong MW. Factors associated with back pain symptoms in pregnancy and the persistence of pain 2 years after pregnancy. Acta Obstet Gynecol Scand 2003;82:1086–91.

[27] Mogren IM. BMI, pain and hypermobility are determinants of long-term outcome for women with low back pain and pelvic pain during pregnancy. Eur Spine J 2006;15:1093–102.

[28] Mogren IM. Previous physical activity decreases the risk of low back pain and pelvic pain during pregnancy. Scand J Public Health 2005;33:300–6.

[29] Garshasbi A, Faghih Zadeh S. The effect of exercise on the intensity of low back pain in pregnant women. Int J Gynaecol Obstet 2005;88:271–5.

[30] LaBan MM, Viola S, Williams DA, et al. Magnetic resonance imaging of the lumbar herniated disc in pregnancy. Am J Phys Med Rehabil 1995;74:59–61.

[31] LaBan MM, Rapp NS, von Oeyen P, et al. The lumbar herniated disk of pregnancy: a report of six cases identified by magnetic resonance imaging. Arch Phys Med Rehabil 1995;76:476–9.

[32] Fast A, Hertz G. Nocturnal low back pain in pregnancy: polysomnographic correlates. Am J Reprod Immunol 1992;28:251–3.

[33] Sanderson PL, Fraser RD. The influence of pregnancy on the development of degenerative spondylolisthesis. J Bone Joint Surg Br 1996;78:951–4.

[34] Saraste H. Spondylolysis and pregnancy: a risk analysis. Acta Obstet Gynecol Scand 1986; 65:727–9.

[35] Ostgaard HC, Zetherstrom G, Roos-Hansson E, et al. Reduction of back and posterior pelvic pain in pregnancy. Spine 1994;19:894–900.

[36] Kihlstrand M, Stenman B, Nilsson S, et al. Water-gymnastics reduced the intensity of back pain in pregnant women. Acta Obstet Gynecol Scand 1999;78:180–5.

[37] Suputtitada A, Wacharapreechanont T, Chaisayan P. Effect of the "sitting pelvic tilt exercise" during the third trimester in primigravidas on back pain. J Med Assoc Thai 2002; 85(Suppl 1):170–9.

[38] Spankus JD. The cause and treatment of low back pain during pregnancy. Wis Med J 1965; 64:303–4.

[39] Carr CA. Use of a maternity binder for the relief of pregnancy-related back pain. J Obstet Gynecol Neonatal Nurs 2003;32:459–502.

[40] Dolan L, Ashe RG, Walsh D, et al. Does urinary incontinence in a primigravida affect quality of life? Proceeding of the 32nd Annual Meeting of the International Continence Society. Heidelburg (Germany) 28-30 August 2002. Neurourol Urodyn 2002;21:316–7.

[41] Ternov NK, Grennert L, Albert A, et al. Acupuncture for lower back pain and pelvic pain in late pregnancy: a retrospective report on 167 consecutive cases. Pain Med 2001; 2:204–7.

[42] Guthrie RA, Martin RH. Effect of pressure applied to the upper thoracic (placebo) versus lumbar areas (osteopathic manipulative treatment) for inhibition of lumbar myalgia during labor. J Am Osteopath Assoc 1982;82:247–51.

[43] Wang SM, DeZinno P, Fermo L, et al. Complementary and alternative medicine for low back pain in pregnancy: a cross-sectional survey. J Altern Complement Med 2005;11:459–64.

[44] Brown MD, Levi AD. Surgery for lumbar disc herniation during pregnancy. Spine 2001;26: 440–3.

[45] Al Hakim M, Katirji MB. Femoral neuropathy induced by lithotomy position: a report of 5 cases with a review of the literature. Muscle Nerve 1993;16:891–5.

[46] Holdcroft A, Gibberd FB, Hargrove RL, et al. Neurological complications associated with pregnancy. Br J Anaesth 1995;75:522–6.

[47] Wong CA, Scavone BM, Dugan S, et al. Incidence of postpartum lumbosacral spine and lower extremity nerve injuries. Obstet Gynecol 2003;101:279–88.

[48] Bonney G. Iatrogenic injuries of nerves. J Bone Joint Surg Br 1986;68:9–13.

[49] Wilbourne AJ. Iatrogenic nerve injuries. Neurol Clin 1998;16:55–82.

[50] Stolp-Smith KA, Pascoe MK, Ogburn PL. Carpal tunnel syndrome in pregnancy: frequency, severity and prognosis. Arch Phys Med Rehabil 1998;79:1285–7.

[51] Ekman-Ordeberg G, Salgeback S, Ordeberg G. Carpal tunnel syndrome in pregnancy: a prospective study. Acta Obstet Gynecol Scand 1987;66:233–5.

[52] Voitk AJ, Mueller JC, Farlinger DE, et al. Carpal tunnel syndrome in pregnancy. Can Med Assoc J 1983;128:277–81.

[53] Wand JS. Carpal tunnel syndrome in pregnancy and lactation. J Hand Surg [Br] 1990;15:93–5.

[54] Sax TW, Rosenbaum RB. Neuromuscular disorders in pregnancy. Muscle Nerve 2006;34: 559–71.

[55] Padua L, Aprile I, Caliandro P, et al. Carpal tunnel syndrome in pregnancy: multiperspective follow-up of untreated cases. Neurology 2002;59:1643–6.

[56] Weimer LH, Yin J, Lovelace RE, et al. Serial studies of carpal tunnel syndrome during and after pregnancy. Muscle Nerve 2002;25:914–7.

[57] Wand JS. The natural history of carpal tunnel syndrome in lactation. J R Soc Med 1989;82: 349–50.

[58] Assmus H, Hashemi B. Surgical treatment of carpal tunnel syndrome in pregnancy: results from 314 cases. Nervenarzt 2000;71:470–3.

[59] Haerer AF. DeJong's the neurologic examination. Philadelphia: JB Lippincott; 1992.

[60] van Slobbe AM, Bohnen AM, Bernsen RM, et al. Incidence rates and determinants in meralgia paresthetica in general practice. J Neurol 2004;251:294–7.

[61] Redick LF. Maternal perinatal nerve palsies. Postgraduate Obstetrics & Gynecology 1992; 12:1–5.

[62] Hansen SL, Clark SL, Foster JC. Active pushing versus passive fetal descent in the second stage of labor: a randomized controlled trial. Obstet Gynecol 2002;99:29–34.

[63] Vargo MM, Robinson LR, Nicholas JJ, et al. Postpartum femoral neuropathy: relic of an earlier era? Arch Phys Med Rehabil 1990;71:591–6.

[64] Donaldson JO. Neurology of pregnancy. Philadelphia: Saunders; 1989.

[65] Biemond A. Femoral neuropathy. In: Vinken PJ, Bruyn GW, editors. Handbook of clinical neurology. New York: John Wiley and Sons; 1977. p. 303–10.

[66] Aminoff MJ. Neurological disorders and pregnancy. Obstet Gynecol 1978;132:325–35.

[67] Colachis SC III, Pease WS, Johnson EW. A preventable cause of foot drop during childbirth. Am J Obstet Gynecol 1994;171:270–2.

[68] Adornato BT, Carlini WG. "Pushing palsy": a case of self-induced bilateral peroneal palsy during natural childbirth. Neurology 1992;42:936–7.

[69] Reif ME. Bilateral common peroneal palsy secondary to prolonged squatting in natural childbirth. Birth 1988;15:100–2.

[70] Babayev M, Bodack MP, Creature C. Common peroneal neuropathy secondary to squatting during childbirth. Obstet Gynecol 1998;91:830–2.

[71] Schned ES. DeQuervain's tenosynovitis in pregnant and postpartum women. Obstet Gynecol 1986;68:411–4.

[72] Shumacher HR Jr, Dorwart BB, Korzeniowski OM. Occurrence of DeQuervain's tendonitis during pregnancy. Arch Intern Med 1985;145:2083–4.

[73] Johnson CA. Occurrence of DeQuervain's disease in postpartum women. J Fam Pract 1991; 32:325–7.

[74] Avci S, Yilmaz C, Sayli U. Comparison of nonsurgical treatment measure for DeQuervain's disease of pregnancy and lactation. J Hand Surg [Am] 2002;27:322–4.

[75] Skoff HD. "Postpartum/newborn" DeQuervain's tenosynovitis of the wrist. Am J Orthop 2001;30:428–30.

[76] Bramlett KW, Killian JT, Nasca RJ, et al. Transient osteoporosis. Clin Orthop 1987;222: 197–202.

[77] Beaulieu JG, Razzano CD, Levine RB. Transient osteoporosis of the hip in pregnancy: review of the literature and a case report. Clin Orthop 1976;115:165–8.

[78] Bloem JL. Transient osteoporosis of the hip: MR imaging. Radiology 1988;167:753–5.

[79] Takatori Y, Kokubo T, Ninomiya S, et al. Transient osteoporosis of the hip: magnetic resonance imaging. Clin Orthop 1991;271:190–4.

[80] Arayssi TK, Tawbi HA, Usta IM, et al. Calcitonin in the treatment of transient osteoporosis of the hip. Semin Arthritis Rheum 2003;32:388–97.

[81] La Montagna G, Malesci D, Tirri R, et al. Successful neridronate therapy in transient osteoporosis of the hip. Clin Rheumatol 2005;24:67–9.

[82] French AE, Kaplan N, Lishner M, et al. Taking bisphosphonates during pregnancy. Can Fam Physician 2003;49:1281–2.

[83] Phillips AJ, Ostlere SJ, Smith R. Pregnancy-associated osteoporosis: does the skeleton recover? Osteoporos Int 2000;11:449–54.

[84] Wood ML, Larson CM, Dahners LE. Late presentation of a displaced subcapital fracture of the hip in transient osteoporosis of pregnancy. J Orthop Trauma 2003;17:582–4.

[85] Pellicci PM, Zolla-Pazner S, Rabhan WM, et al. Osteonecrosis of the femoral head associated with pregnancy: report of three cases. Clin Orthop 1984;185:59–63.

[86] Cheng N, Burssens A, Mulier JC. Pregnancy and post-pregnancy avascular necrosis of the femoral head. Arch Orthop Trauma Surg 1982;100:199–210.

[87] Lausten GS. Osteonecrosis of the femoral head during pregnancy. Arch Orthop Trauma Surg 1991;110:214–5.

[88] Vullo VJ, Richardson JK, Hurvitz EA. Hip, knee and foot pain during pregnancy and the postpartum period. J Fam Pract 1996;43:63–8.

[89] Benjamin M, Redman S, Milz S, et al. Adipose tissue at entheses: the rheumatologic implications of insertional distribution. A potential site of pain and stress dissipation? Ann Rheum Dis 2004;63:1549–55.

[90] Flik K, Anderson K, Urmey W, et al. Locked knee during pregnancy. Arthroscopy 2004;20:191–5.

[91] Thienpont E, Simon JP, Fabry G. Sacral stress fracture during pregnancy: a case report. Acta Orthop Scand 1999;70:525–6.

[92] Clemetson IA, Popp A, Lippuner K, et al. Postpartum osteoporosis associated with proximal tibial stress fracture. Skeletal Radiol 2004;33:96–8.

[93] Amagada JO, Joels L, Catling S. Stress fracture of rib in pregnancy: what analgesic? J Obstet Gynaecol 2002;22:559.

[94] Sarikaya S, Ozdolap S, Acikgoz G, et al. Pregnancy-associated osteoporosis with vertebral fractures and scoliosis. Joint Bone Spine 2004;71:84–5.

[95] Schmid L, Pfirrmann C, Hess T, et al. Bilateral fracture of the sacrum associated with pregnancy: a case report. Osteoporos Int 1999;10:91–3.

PHYSICAL MEDICINE
AND REHABILITATION
CLINICS OF
NORTH AMERICA

ELSEVIER
SAUNDERS

Phys Med Rehabil Clin N Am
18 (2007) 477–496

Recognizing and Treating Pelvic Pain and Pelvic Floor Dysfunction

Heidi Prather, DO[a,*],
Theresa Monaco Spitznagle, PT, DPT, MHS[b],
Sheila A. Dugan, MD[c]

[a]Section, Physical Medicine and Rehabilitation, Washington University Orthopedics,
One Barnes Jewish Hospital Plaza, Suite 11300, Saint Louis, MO 63110, USA
[b]Program In Physical Therapy Washington University School of Medicine,
4444 Forest Park Blvd, Suite 1101, St. Louis, MO 63108, USA
[c]Department of Physical Medicine and Rehabilitation, 1725 W. Harrison St.,
Ste 970, Chicago, IL 60612, USA

Reported prevalence rates of pain within the pelvis range from 3.8% to 24% in women aged 15 to 73 years [1–3]. Despite the significant number of women affected, pelvic floor pain and dysfunction are commonly overlooked in women seeking medical care. This oversight may be attributed to changes in medical practice that restrict time spent with patients, the often embarrassing and personal nature of the subject, the social stigmas for some cultures, or the perceived notion that no effective treatment exists. Overlap exists among medical specialists who treat patients who have pelvic pain, including gynecologists, urologists, gastroenterologists, and colorectal surgeons. Physiatrists are uniquely qualified to manage patients who have pelvic pain because of their knowledge of the musculoskeletal and nervous systems and their awareness of the relationships among pain, physiology, and function. Their approach is also nonsurgical. As with many other conditions, a procedure does not always exist that fits the disorder, and the physiatrist can offer that missing link for some patients.

Early recognition or prevention of pelvic floor dysfunction may literally change the trajectory of individual's life, especially late in life. The top three reasons for nursing home admission (reduced mobility, urinary incontinence, and fecal incontinence) have pelvic floor dysfunction as a common theme [4]. This article introduces pelvic floor anatomy, neurophysiology,

* Corresponding author.
E-mail address: pratherh@wudosis.wustl.edu (H. Prather).

and function and provides an overview of pelvic floor dysfunctions and their recognition and treatment.

Anatomy of the pelvic floor

The pelvic floor is a dome-shaped striated muscular sheet or sling that, together with the endopelvic fascia, supports the bladder, uterus, and rectum (Fig. 1). Specialized smooth muscular urinary and anal sphincters allow for storage and evacuation of urine and stool. Pelvic floor muscles attach to

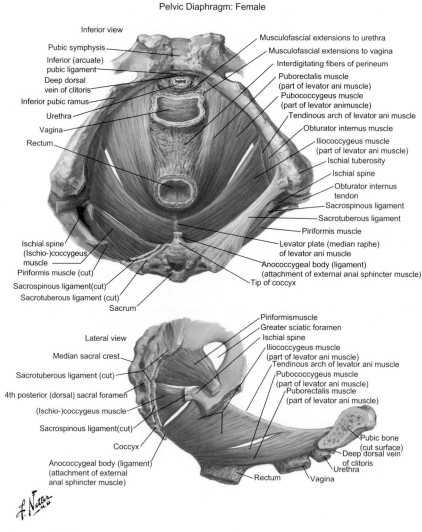

Fig. 1. Pelvic floor musculature from below. (*Reprinted from* Netter Anatomy Illustration Collection, © Elsevier Inc. All rights reserved.)

local pelvic bony structures along the inner surface of the lesser pelvis. However, global muscles from the lumbar spine and lower extremities and their fascia play a large supportive role in lumbopelvic stability and mobility. The pelvic floor muscles include the levator ani (iliococcygeus, pubococcygeus, and puborectalis) muscles and the coccygeus. The paired levator ani and coccygeus muscles, together with the fascia above and below, are sometimes referred to collectively as the diaphragm of pelvis [5,6]. The levator ani arises from the posterior surface of the superior ramus of the pubis, lateral to the symphysis, and attaches to the inner surface of the spine of the ischium along with the obturator fascia and tendinous arch of the pelvic fascia. The fibers of the levator ani pass downward and backward toward the middle of the pelvis with attachments to the coccyx and anococcygeal raphe. The latter extends between the coccyx and anus. Midline fibers insert into the rectum and blend with fibers of the sphincter muscles, whereas anterior fibers can invest in the sides of the prostate in men and the vagina in women. At the central tendinous portion of the perineum, the levator ani joins the fibers of the more superficial pelvic floor muscles, the transversus perinea (transversus perinea superficialis and profundus).

Structure of the pelvic walls

The pelvic walls are formed by bones and ligaments partly lined with muscles and covered with fascia. The anterior pelvic wall is a shallow wall formed by the posterior surfaces of the pubic bones and symphysis pubis. This landmark is easily identified with palpation on most patients. The posterior pelvic wall is a more extensive wall, consisting of the sacrum, coccyx, and piriformis muscle.

The lateral pelvic wall is a component of the pelvis formed by part of the innominate bone, the obturator foramen, the sacrotuberous and sacrospinous ligaments, and the obturator internus muscle and fascia. The inferior pelvic wall or pelvic floor consists of the levator ani muscles, coccygeus, and pelvic fascia and is accessible to palpation only through internal pelvic or rectal examination.

Joints of the pelvis

The pelvis is a ring and the base of support for the upper and lower torso and extremities. Forces are ultimately distributed through the pelvis directly and indirectly. Located in the posterior pelvic ring are the sacroiliac joints. These are synovial joints inferiorly, have anterior and posterior capsules, and are surrounded by ligaments. The anterior sacroiliac ligament acts as a sling. The dorsal longitudinal sacroiliac joint (SIJ) ligament crosses the joint and attaches to the dorsal surface of the sacrum and ilium in three layers lying in oblique planes to one another. In isolation, this ligament is believed to contribute to posterior pelvic pain because it contains both pain receptors and proprioceptors and absorbs forces directly from the SIJ and indirectly from the hip [7] The interosseous sacroiliac ligaments are short ligaments within the SIJ and connect the sacrum to the ilium. They are believed to be among the strongest ligaments in the body. Ligaments extrinsic to the SIJ but that contribute to posterior pelvic pain include the iliolumbar and sacrotuberous ligaments. The iliolumbar ligament absorbs and distributes forces from the lumbar spine and ilium. The sacrotuberous ligament absorbs and distributes forces from the lower extremity through direct and fascial attachments to the hamstrings and thoracodorsal fascia [8,9]. All of these ligaments are important for joint stability [10,11].

The symphysis pubis is a cartilaginous joint between the two pubic bones. It is surrounded by ligaments that allow subtle motion in frontal (inferior and superior sheer motion) and rotational planes. This joint is subjected to substantial mechanical stresses during pregnancy.

The sacrococcygeal joint is a cartilaginous joint that is joined by ligaments. Much movement is possible at this joint, although this varies among individuals. Women who have a previous history of direct trauma to the coccyx region may have healed in an asymmetric alignment or may continue to have increased mobility of the segment that may be symptomatic with routines activities of daily living, direct pressure at the site, gluteal contraction, defecation, or intercourse. These should all be investigated in women whose presentation of pelvic pain includes coccyx pain.

Nerves of the pelvis and perineum

The lumbosacral trunk passes into the pelvis and joins the sacral nerves as they emerge from the anterior sacral foramina. From a clinical perspective, the important nerve branches associated with clinical syndromes at or near the pelvic floor include sciatic, obturator, femoral, lateral femoral cutaneous, and pudendal. The clinical anatomy of the pudendal nerve and its branches make it prone to damage during complicated vaginal childbirth and surgical interventions. The pudendal nerve arises from the sacral plexus from the ventral branches S2, S3, and S4. It passes between the piriformis and coccyges muscles as it travels from the pelvis through the greater sciatic foramen and then passes over the spine of the ischium to reenter the pelvis through the lesser sciatic foramen. This nerve supplies sensation to the external genitalia and motor function to the urinary and external anal sphincters and muscles responsible for ejaculation in men and orgasm in both genders (Fig. 2).

Because of its complex and comprehensive function, the pudendal nerve is implicated in pelvic floor dysfunction related to pain, incontinence, and sexual dysfunction. In one study [12], a pudendal nerve block decreased vaginal pressures, increased the length of the urogenital hiatus, and decreased electromyography activity of the puborectalis muscle, suggesting that the pudendal nerve innervates the levator ani muscle [12]. Other studies [13,14] show that the motor branch to the levator ani, the levator ani nerve, approaches the

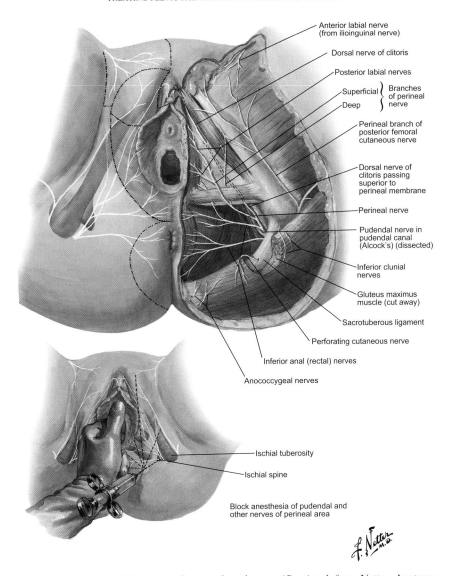

Fig. 2. Innervation of the pelvic floor and perineum. (*Reprinted from* Netter Anatomy Illustration Collection, © Elsevier Inc. All rights reserved.)

pelvic floor muscles on their visceral side. Near the ischial spine, the levator ani nerve and the pudendal nerve lie above and below the levator ani muscle, respectively. The median distance between the levator ani nerve and the point of entry for a pudendal block into the levator ani muscle is 5 mm. Therefore, a transvaginal pudendal nerve blockade will probably block both nerves simultaneously [13,14]. Other authors [15] disagree that the pudendal nerve sends a branch to the levator ani. Gross dissections of cadavers suggest that innervation of the female levator ani muscle ias not provided by the pudendal nerve but rather originates directly from the sacral nerve roots (S3–S5) that travel on the superior surface of the pelvic floor. Because definitive studies involving nerve transection and neural tracer studies cannot be performed in living humans, further investigations using appropriate animal models may delineate the neuroanatomy [15].

Hip and pelvis injuries

Pelvic and hip injuries can be divided into bony and soft tissue causes. Bony causes include but are not limited to osteoarthritis, stress fractures, avulsion injuries, acetabular labral tears, femoral acetabular impingement, osteitis pubis, and avascular necrosis of the head of the femur. Soft tissue conditions include muscle strains, tendonitis, bursitis, and nerve entrapment. As in other areas of the body, local splinting of the pelvic floor diaphragm may result from painful hip and pelvis injuries. Conversely, prolonged maladaptive hypertonic or hypotonic pelvic floor dysfunction may change joint loading, leading to musculoskeletal sequela such as degenerative joint disease of the hip. This article briefly mentions these disorders, because each may refer pain to the pelvic floor. Pelvic floor pain may develop secondary to spine or pelvic trauma and should be incorporated into the treatment plan.

Urinary continence

Urinary continence depends on central and local neurologic and musculo-skeletal control along with an adequate level of cognition and physical functioning. A full review of continence is beyond the scope of this article, although continence issues related to the pelvic floor are briefly discussed [16]. Increases in abdominal pressure during activities of daily living challenge continence. Supportive and sphincteric structures must be functional to prevent incontinence and prolapse of genital organs [17]. Urethral closure pressure is maintained higher than bladder pressure through the combined action of the urethral sphincter and a supportive hammock under the urethral and vesical neck. This supporting layer consists of (1) the anterior vaginal wall and the connective tissue that attaches it to the pelvic bones, (2) the pubovaginal portion of the levator ani muscle, and (3) the uterosacral and cardinal ligaments constituting the tendinous arch of the pelvic fascia. The number of striated muscle fibers of the sphincter decreases with age and parity. Computer models indicate that vaginal birth places the levator ani under tissue stretch ratios of up to 3.3 and the pudendal nerve under strains of up to 33%.

Anorectal continence

The internal and external anal sphincters are primarily responsible for maintaining fecal continence [18]. Defecation is a somatovisceral reflex regulated by dual nerve supply, including somatic and autonomic to the anorectum. The net effects of sympathetic and cholinergic stimulation are to increase and reduce anal resting pressure, respectively, and to allow for storage or voiding as appropriate. Fecal incontinence and functional defecatory disorders may result from structural changes or functional disturbances in the mechanisms of fecal continence and defecation.

Viscerosomatic reflex

Viscerosomatic reflexes result from afferent stimuli from viscera affecting somatic tissues. Visceral receptors send afferent impulses through the dorsal horn of the spinal cord to synapse on interconnecting neurons. These neurons convey impulses to the sympathetic and peripheral motor efferents, resulting in sensory and motor changes in muscle, skin, and fascia of the trunk, including the pelvic floor. Persistent muscle contraction of the pelvic floor related to noxious visceral stimulation, such as that associated with endometriosis or irritable bowel syndrome, can cause splinting and pain with reduction of normal pelvic floor muscle function. The body adapts by recruiting nearby muscles, such as the psoas and iliacus, which can cause related symptoms such as posterior pelvic and lower back pain. Manual treatment may be advocated to address the restrictions in the somatic structures that may be secondary to a primary visceral disorder. Treatment of local muscle and joint dysfunction will also treat the viscerosomatic reflexes that may cause the symptoms [19], resulting in reduced pain, increased mobility and muscle excursion, and enhanced lymphatic and venous drainage. The ultimate goal is to restore normal pelvic floor neuromuscular control to allow for normal voiding.

Pelvic floor dysfunction overview

Pelvic floor dysfunction describes pain or abnormal function of the muscular sling within the bony pelvis. Box 1 provides examples of additional dysfunctions associated with pelvic pain. The pelvic floor supports viscera, sphincter function, hip and trunk movement, and sexual function. Dysfunctions are commonly divided into hypertonic and hypotonic. *Hypertonic*, or high-tone, dysfunctions include pain and excessive muscle tension and can present with associated constipation and dyspareunia (pain with intercourse). *Hypotonic*, or low-tone, dysfunctions can present with incontinence and may be related to collagen changes, previous childbirth or gynecological surgery, or peripheral nerve injury. Women who exercise may describe their pelvic floor pain as acute or insidious at onset. These women often seek medical advice when their athletic performance declines or they are no longer able to exercise. In these circumstances, health care providers must acknowledge the woman's desire to return to or continue with sports or exercise and should

---

Box 1. Examples of dysfunctions associated with pelvic pain

Dyspareunia

Dysmenorrhea

Vulvodynia
- Hyperpathia
- Burning
- Itching

Involuntary spasms of muscles
- Vaginismus
- Pelvic floor tension myalgia
- Levator ani syndrome

Defecation dysfunction
- Constipation
- Diarrhea
- Fecal incontinence
- Rectal itching and burning

Voiding dysfunction
- Urinary urgency
- Urinary frequency
- Painful urination

Sexual dysfunction
- Anorgasmia

Coccygodynia

Lower back pain and upper leg pain

Mood disturbances
- Anxiety
- Depression

Fatigue (mental and physical)

---

offer an alternative form or intensity of exercise during evaluation and treatment of the pelvic floor dysfunction.

As in other regions of the body, gender differences exist in the anatomy of the hips and pelvis, such as those listed in Box 2. Women have broader pelvises than men, and those who have even broader and shallower pelvises may have greater hip range of motion. Women are more likely to have mild to severe developmental dysplasia of the hip, which may also contribute to greater degrees of hip motion and thereby increased need for balanced muscle strength and length to provide joint stability [20,21]. The

---

Box 2. Gender differences of the pelvis

Female pelvis is broader
Female pelvic inlet is oval compared with the heart shape
  in the male
Female pelvic cavity is roomier
Female pelvic outlet is larger, with everted ischial tuberosities
Female sacrum is shorter, wider, and flatter
Female pubic arch is more rounded and wider

---

combination of greater femoral neck anteversion and shorter limb length leads to a lower center of gravity for women compared with men [22]. Neuromuscular differences in firing patterns of motor units may arise from these anatomic differences, but have not been proven to increase injury risk [23]. The ligaments, fascia, and muscles of the pelvic girdle support the force closure (muscles and ligaments that surround the joint to provide stability) of the SIJ working in concert with form closure (bony congruency of joint surfaces) [10]. Alterations in force closure occur during pregnancy because of increasing abdominal girth, changes in load transfer, and deconditioning, in addition to ligamentous laxity caused by the shift in levels of hormones, including relaxin and estrogen. Inadequate closure may cause increased SIJ pain in pregnant women [24].

Although no specific studies have been performed in female athletes, imbalances in muscle flexibility and strength may predispose female athletes to pelvic girdle and hip pain. Form closure is less congruent in women because of the shape of the pelvis and less-extensive joint surfaces, which may make women more reliant on muscles and ligaments for stability. The muscular system may be unable to withstand the added forces, especially during extensive periods of training or with repetitive unidirectional loading, which can lead to injury or incontinence, depending on the individual.

The myriad tissues that refer pain to the pelvic floor must be considered in the differential diagnosis of patients presenting with pelvic pain. This list includes but is not limited to the genitourinary or colorectal systems, intra-articular hip pathology (such as acetabular labral tears), lumbosacral radiculopathy, plexopathy, or peripheral neuropathy, including the pudendal nerve and its division, or muscles of the abdominal wall or lumbar spine.

Physical examination of the pelvic floor

Examiners should first discuss the purpose of the external and internal physical examination with their patients. Patients must be informed that the palpatory examination is not a substitute for a general pelvic examination. The latter should be performed before referral to a physiatrist to assure that all other causes, including mass and infection, have been excluded. A room with expected privacy is essential. A male physician should consider having a female health care provider present for the internal examination.

The examiner first evaluates the external genitalia for changes in color, obvious discharge, scars, and asymmetries in the labial folds (Fig. 3). Light palpation of the gluteals, peroneal body, and labia helps determine the presence of allodynia. A sensory examination using a cotton swab to assess light

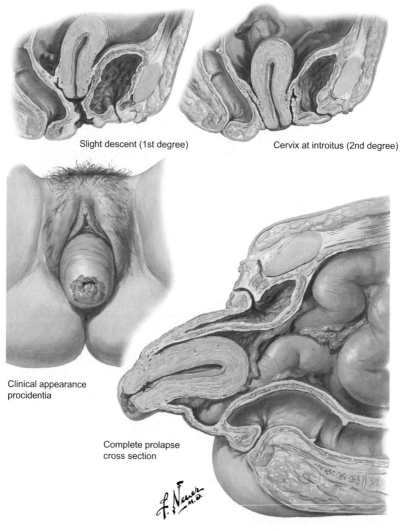

Slight descent (1st degree)

Cervix at introitus (2nd degree)

Clinical appearance procidentia

Complete prolapse cross section

Fig. 3. Uterine prolapse. (*Reprinted from* Netter Anatomy Illustration Collection, © Elsevier Inc. All rights reserved.)

touch and pinprick sensation is often then performed. A positive swab test shows allodynia when light stroking with the cotton end causes pain. Parting the labial folds, the examiner can then visualize pelvic floor elevation by asking the patient to contract. A lift should be noted. Gross observation of a cystocele, or uterine prolapse (Fig. 4), may be visualized at this time.

Gentle palpation of the perineal body and superficial pelvic floor should then be completed to assess for pain and tone. The next step is to advance palpation to the deep pelvic floor musculature (PFM). Patients can be queried for local and referred pain patterns. Assessment for pain and function will then help determine a treatment plan.

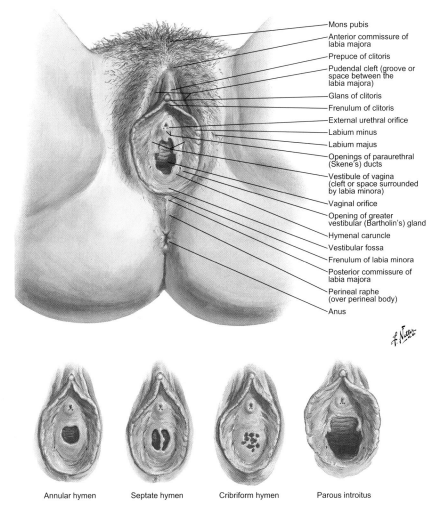

Fig. 4. External genitalia and vulva. (*Reprinted from* Netter Anatomy Illustration Collection, © Elsevier Inc. All rights reserved.)

Pelvic floor muscle performance assessment

To fully determine the function of the PFM, several properties of muscle performance should be considered. The first property of muscle to consider is the ability to generate a force. Clinically, PFM strength testing is performed through subjectively assessing the force of contraction felt on the palpating digit, the presence of a perceivable lift of the palpating digit, the number of contractions performed, and the duration of the contractions [25]. The contribution of the contractile properties of the muscle fibers should also be considered. Two basic types of skeletal muscle fibers exist: type 1 (slow twitch) and type 2 (fast twitch). Type 1 skeletal muscle fibers are fatigue-resistive, whereas type 2 skeletal muscle fibers are easily fatigued [26]. The skeletal muscle fiber type of the PFM is 30% type 2 and 70% type 1 [27]. The type 1 fibers are needed for tonic support, whereas the type 2 fibers are necessary for dynamic closure of the outlet of the pelvis in response to rapid changes in intra-abdominal pressure. Fiber type has been found to be varied in individuals who have supportive pelvic floor muscle dysfunction [28]. Thus, support-related and non–support-related muscular impairments should be differentiated when prescribing pelvic floor exercise. For individuals who have decreased motor recruitment of the PFM, fast contractions with short duration to address the fast twitch fibers and slow longer-duration contractions to address slow twitch fibers are needed.

Muscle stiffness, defined as the change in tension per unit change in length [29], is tested by passive range of motion of a specific joint. Resistance to passive movement, or *stiffness*, is a property of the elastic and nonelastic connective tissue components constituting a joint [30]. Clinically, pelvic muscle stiffness is assessed during the palpation component of the PFM examination. *Baseline muscle stiffness*, defined as the tissue resistance felt during manual stretch of the musculature, should not be confused with muscular tone palpated during rest. When muscle hypertrophy occurs, an increase occurs in the number of sarcomeres in parallel [26]. Clinically, increased muscle stiffness caused by hypertrophy, a relative increase in thickness of the muscle, should not be confused with increased tone caused by a neural impairment.

Muscle length has a direct impact on the force that can be generated in a muscle. Based on the length–tension curve, a muscle that is either too short or too long will test weak [26]. Thus, considering the relative length of a muscle at contraction is critical to understanding its force-generating properties. Clinically, PFM length is determined through the resting position of the musculature. Assessment is based on the depth of the palpating digit. If the most superficial edge of the levator ani is palpated by the examiner at the depth of their distal interphalangeal joint, the muscle length is considered shortened. In contrast, if the examiner must insert the digit beyond the proximal interphalangeal joint, the muscle is considered lengthened. Childbirth and habitual Valsalva during functional activities [31,32] can help increase PFM length. In contrast, PFM hypertonus dysfunction, an impairment in which the musculature is habitually contracted, causes a decrease in PFM length, with subsequent weakness caused by the habitual shortened position of the muscle.

Myofascial pain syndromes may develop primary or secondary to trauma of muscle imbalance. Travell and Simons [33] have outlined specific pelvic floor muscles that can be involved. Trigger points within these muscle groups have the potential to refer pain (Table 1). Muscles with attachments to the pelvis that are susceptible to trigger point formation and subsequent pelvic pain floor pain include the adductor magnus, coccygeus, levator ani, oblique abdominals, obturator internus, and piriformis. Muscles that are susceptible to trigger point formation with referral to the lower abdominal, inguinal, or posterior pelvis include the coccygeus, levator ani, gluteus maximus, gluteus medius, multifidi, quadratus lumborum, rectus abdominus, and soleus.

Further investigation into the social history regarding life stressors is important. A history of sexual abuse, emotional abuse, anxiety, depression, and general lifestyle stress can cause or contribute to muscle tension [34]. Women must be informed that treating the concomitant psychosocial problems will facilitate their progress regarding pain control. When increased muscle tone is determined to be a contributing cause of pelvic pain, a pelvic floor, musculoskeletal, neurologic, and posture evaluation involving the spine, hip, and pelvis will help determine a comprehensive approach to treatment. The external and internal pelvic examinations identify specific muscles with increased tone and pain and areas of allodynia. The musculoskeletal and neurologic examinations of the spine, pelvis, and hips help determine primary or secondary causes of pain. Biofeedback using electromyelography can help determine baseline muscle activity with the woman at rest. This tool is also useful in identifying muscle tone changes that occur with position changes, exercise, or functional activities of daily living.

Another cause of pain related to muscles of the pelvic floor is muscle dyssynergia. If the muscles are unable to coordinate contraction and relaxation at the appropriate times during micturition, defecation, and intercourse, dysfunctions can occur, referred to as *pelvic floor dyssynergia*. This symptom complex has several causes. Pudendal nerve injury can result in sensory and motor deficits and inhibit appropriate muscle contraction and relaxation. If improper technique during exercise causes a bearing down on the pelvic floor rather than lifting, dyssynergia may occur. Other neurologic disorders

Table 1
Trigger point referral patterns

Trigger point locations	Neural innervation	Referred pain sites
Levator ani muscles	S1, S2, S3, S4	Pelvic floor, vagina, rectum, buttocks
Piriformis muscle	L5–S3	Low back, buttocks, pelvic floor
Obturator internus and externus	L3–S2	Pelvic floor, buttocks, anterior thigh

that cause an inability to isolate pelvic floor muscle contractions can also facilitate dyssynergia [34].

After specific muscle pain and tone, muscle strength should be examined. Both tone and strength on each side of the pelvis must be compared. Several grading systems are used to describe muscle strength, ranging from absent to strong. Laycock [27] developed a grading system describing muscle strength in values from 0 to 5 (0 = none, 1 = flicker, 2 = weak, 3 = moderate, 4 = good, and 5 = strong). The examiner measures the contraction up to 10 seconds, counts the number of repetitions up to 10, and records the number of fast 1-second contractions.

Chiarelli [34] developed another pelvic floor muscle strength grading system, also with a numbering system from 0 to 5 (0 = no contraction; 1 = flicker, only with the muscle stretched; 2 = a weak squeeze, 2-second hold; 3 = a fair squeeze, definite lift; 4 = good squeeze, good squeeze with lift repeatable; 5 = a strong squeeze, good lift, repeatable). Using this system to measure strength, the examiner observes the patient's ability to contract the pelvic floor muscles without using accessory muscles and without bearing down. Both methods can be used to help determine if strengthening exercises should be part of the therapeutic program. Patients who have increased tone and normal strength will not benefit from strengthening exercises but rather from relaxation techniques and activity modification [35].

Vulvodynia

Vulvodynia is a clinical condition defined by the International Society for the Study of Vulvovaginal Diseases (ISSVD) in 1984 as "chronic vulvar discomfort that is characterized by the complaint of burning, stinging, irritation, or rawness in the absence of skin disease or infection" [36]. It can begin acutely and frequently becomes chronic. Although described in the late 1880s [37] as "excessive sensitivity" of the vulva, many health care providers are not familiar with the condition. The ISSVD recently revised the definition to include two subgroups: localized and generalized vulvar dysesthesia. Each subgroup is further categorized as provoked, spontaneous, or mixed [38]. The ISSVD also suggested a change in terminology regarding *vestibulitis*, which is inflammation of the vestibule, or the area that surrounds the entrance to the vagina containing vestibular and bartholin's glands that provide lubrication (Fig. 5) [39]. Vulvodynia does not always include an inflammatory component, but is frequently accompanied by physical disabilities, limitation of daily activities, sexual dysfunction, and psychological distress [40]. Diagnosing vulvodynia requires a comprehensive assessment that rules out local neurologic and musculoskeletal dysfunction. However, when recognized, desensitization techniques used by a physical therapist and integrated early into the patient's home program can deter this condition from becoming chronic. Medications that affect neuropathic pain through the central nervous system usually facilitate recovery.

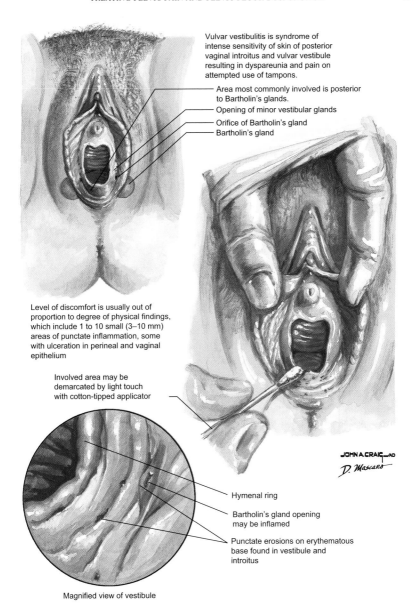

Vulvar vestibulitis is syndrome of intense sensitivity of skin of posterior vaginal introitus and vulvar vestibule resulting in dyspareunia and pain on attempted use of tampons.

Area most commonly involved is posterior to Bartholin's glands.

Opening of minor vestibular glands

Orifice of Bartholin's gland

Bartholin's gland

Level of discomfort is usually out of proportion to degree of physical findings, which include 1 to 10 small (3–10 mm) areas of punctate inflammation, some with ulceration in perineal and vaginal epithelium

Involved area may be demarcated by light touch with cotton-tipped applicator

Hymenal ring

Bartholin's gland opening may be inflamed

Punctate erosions on erythematous base found in vestibule and introitus

JOHN A. CRAIG—AD
D. Mascaro

Magnified view of vestibule

Fig. 5. Vulvar vestibulitis. (*Reprinted from* Netter Anatomy Illustration Collection, © Elsevier Inc. All rights reserved.)

Treatment of pelvic pain

A multidisciplinary approach to treatment is advantageous for women who have pelvic floor pain. This patient population lends itself well to collaborative medicine across multiple disciplines, including physicians who have surgical and other specialties that provide medical management. Again, physiatrists are well suited to help direct patient care, such as medical management of pain related to endometriosis once medication regimes and surgical needs have been met, and pelvic pain in females who have moderate to severe hip osteoarthritis. Physiatrists can help patients identify functional goals and ways to reduce pain. Determining what lifestyle modifications may be necessary to achieve these functional goals should be investigated and implemented during treatment.

After infection and serious medical causes for pain have been excluded, pelvic floor pain should be managed through addressing psychological, neurochemical, and mechanical factors that are determined to contribute to the disorder. Working with a physical therapist; prescribing medications to modify pain, anxiety, and facilitate restorative sleep patterns; aerobic conditioning; and lifestyle modifications are all part of a comprehensive treatment program. When appropriate, further referral for psychological counseling and intervention should be considered.

Medications

Medications can be very helpful in modifying pain, but must be specific for the problem. For example, patients who have recent onset or exacerbation of pain related to muscle, joints, or nerves will likely respond well to consistent anti-inflammatory medication use for a set period. Conversely, patients who have experienced insidious onset of pelvic pain for several months may not respond to the same medication, and therefore medications should be tailored to the presumed type of pain. Myofascial pain often responds well to tricyclic antidepressants (TCAs) or similar agents, such as trazodone and cyclobenzaprine. Anti-inflammatories may be helpful and should be tried but should also be discontinued if no added benefit is achieved. Pain that seems to have a neurogenic component can be treated with anti-inflammatories in the acute and subacute phase of treatment. TCAs are specific for neurogenic pain, and similar agents, including trazodone and cyclobenzaprine, can also be effective. Antiepileptic medications can also be helpful, but these agents have various side effects, such as dizziness and sedation, that can impair function.

Some medications also require monitoring. The authors use gabapentin and pregabalin for patients who have pelvic floor pain with a neurogenic component. The complexity of risk–benefit issues must be considered when prescribing the agent. A recent retrospective review of gabapentin use for vulvodynia showed that two thirds of patients experienced response to treatment [41], whereas one quarter of patients experienced side effects, with fatigue the most common, causing 11% of patients to discontinue the medication.

Narcotics and related medications such as tramadol can help reduce moderate to severe pain, but again, only for a set period. The physician should remember that pain that does not respond well to a narcotic may not need more narcotic but another agent to address the type of pain. Neurogenic pain often does not entirely respond to narcotic medication, and therefore an agent that addresses neurogenic pain may provide more satisfactory pain reduction when used with the narcotic. Muscles relaxants may help reduce overall muscle tone but are not selective for the pelvic floor. Patients often find that these medications are sedative and inhibit function, and therefore nightly use may be the best option for patients who find the effects beneficial.

Topical agents, including estrogen creams, may be helpful in patients who have vaginal atrophy related to menopause. A topical anesthetic used for dental procedures may also help desensitize the vulvar area.

Sleep regulation is important for any patient who has pain, especially chronic pain. Medications that help patients fall asleep and maintain it through all stages are important for patients to feel rested the following day and to reduce myofascial pain. TCAs and TCA-like medications may provide this benefit.

Physical therapy

An individualized therapeutic exercise directed by a physical therapist who has training and expertise in pelvic floor pain is vital to treatment programs. As with many musculoskeletal dysfunctions, the first step in determining treatment strategies is to identify the type of tissue alterations that have occurred with repeated movements and sustained postures [30]. Tissues potentially involved with pelvic pain include nerves, muscles, ligaments, and cartilaginous structures within the spine, pelvis, and hips [42]. Several trunk and hip muscles are synergists of the PFM [43,44]. Commonly, treatment of the pelvic musculature impairments and the corresponding synergist improves symptomatology that is mediated by the neural and mechanical tissues in the region.

When treating pain syndromes in the pelvis, attention should be given to the extrinsic tissues of the hip, spine, and SIJ [45]. In addition, intrinsic muscle and neural impairments must be treated. Specific soft tissue mobilization has been suggested to address adhesions, diminish trigger points, and desensitize tissues [46–48]. Because of the multiple pain-sensitive structures within the pelvis, treatment should focus on the cause of the dysfunction rather than simply the source. Thus, pain with palpation of the PFM should not be the sole finding determining the course of care. With a soft tissue dysfunction such as tension myalgia of the pelvic floor muscles, treatment without regard to the specific physiologic properties of muscle and other pelvic structures greatly impairs treatment outcomes. Trigger points that respond only transiently to soft tissue techniques may be treated with injections of short-acting anesthetics agents, such as 2% lidocaine, in conjunction with manual treatment. Botulinum toxin type A injections have been used clinically, with increasing literature reporting their effectiveness in reducing pain, constipation, and dyspareunia [49–51].

The goal of therapy is to address muscle imbalances through muscle stretching and strengthening exercises as necessary. Various techniques, including scar release, myofascial release, acupressure, muscle energy, strain–counterstrain, joint mobilization, posture, and gait education, can also help reduce pain. Biofeedback can also be incorporated to help reduce muscle tone and improve muscle firing patterns, and is especially helpful for patients who have pain related to dyssynergia. Educating patients is made easier with biofeedback because they are able to receive objective information on muscle firing patterns at rest and with activities of daily living. Instruction in proper breathing techniques while performing exercises and activities is essential in assuring that the muscle tone level in the pelvic floor is not inadvertently raised. An important goal is controlling pelvic floor contraction during exhalation to allow the pelvic and respiratory diaphragms to act in synergy. Hypotonic pelvic floor muscles can be treated with electrical stimulation using surface electrode or vaginal or rectal probes as appropriate. A physical therapist can facilitate training the pelvic floor to contract before lifting, laughing, and coughing. Modalities including heat and cold may facilitate pain management and muscle relaxation [35].

Summary

Pelvic floor dysfunction can have debilitating effects on women. Greater recognition of the disorder by the health care community is the first step in reducing impairments and disability that many women experience. Understanding the role of muscle and nerve dysfunction locally and the likelihood of associated mood disorders and functional decline will facilitate collaborative care by experts across the operative, nonoperative, psychological, and rehabilitation spectrum. Short- and long-term goals include improving treatments based on evidence-based medicine and research in this area. Physiatrists are uniquely qualified to manage patients who have pelvic pain and to develop and implement innovative research because of their knowledge of the musculoskeletal system, the nervous system, and awareness of the relationships among pain, physiology, and function. This much-needed evidence in the literature will enhance medical and psychological care for women affected by this disorder.

References

[1] Mathias SD, Kuppermann M, Liberman RF, et al. Chronic pelvic pain: prevalence, health-related quality of life, and economic correlates. Obstet Gynecol 1996;87(3):321–7.
[2] Zondervan KT, Yudkin PL, Vessey MP, et al. Prevalence and incidence of chronic pelvic pain in primary care: evidence from a national general practice database. Br J Obstet Gynaecol 1999;106(11):1149–55.

[3] Howard FM. Chronic pelvic pain. Obstet Gynecol 2003;101(3):594–611.

[4] Brown JS, Vittinghoff E, Wyman JF, et al. Urinary incontinence: does it increase risk for falls and fractures? Study of osteoporotic fractures research group. J Am Geriatr Soc 2000;48: 721–5.

[5] Ackerman MJ. "Fact sheet: the visible human project". National library of medicine. Proceedings of IEEE, Mar 1998;86(3):504–11.

[6] Snell RS. Clinical anatomy for medical students. Boston: Little Brown and Company; 1995.

[7] Vleeming A, Pool-Goudzwaard AL, Hammudoghlu D, et al. The function of the long dorsal sacroiliac ligament. Spine 1996;21:556–62.

[8] Vleeming A, Pool-Goudzwaard AL, Stoeckart R, et al. The posterior layer of the thoracolumbar fascia. Spine 1995;20:753–8.

[9] Vleeming A, Stoeckart R, Snijders C. The sacrotuberous ligament: a conceptual approach to its dynamic role in stabilizing the sacroiliac joint. Clin Biomech (Bristol, Avon) 1989;4: 201–3.

[10] Vleeming A, Stoeckart R, Volkers ACW, et al. Relation between form and function on the sacroiliac joint, part I. Spine 1990;15:133–5.

[11] Vleeming A, Stoeckart R, Volkers ACW, et al. Relation between form and function on the sacroiliac joint, part II. Spine 1990;15:133–5.

[12] Guaderrama NM, Liu J, Nager CW, et al. Evidence for the innervation of pelvic floor muscles by the pudendal nerve. Obstet Gynecol 2005;106(4):774–81.

[13] Wallner C, Maas CP, Dabhoiwala NF, et al. Evidence for the innervation of the puborectalis muscle by the levator ani nerve. Neurogastroenterol Motil 2006;18(12):1121–2.

[14] Wallner C, Maas CP, Dabhoiwala NF, et al. Innervation of the pelvic floor muscles: a reappraisal for the levator ani nerve. Obstet Gynecol 2006;108:529–34.

[15] Barber MD, Bremer RE, Thor KB, et al. Innervation of the female levator ani muscles. Am J Obstet Gynecol 2002;187(1):64–71.

[16] Sampselle CM, DeLancey JO. Anatomy of female continence. J Wound Ostomy Continence Nurs 1998;25(2):63–74.

[17] Ashton-Miller JA, DeLancey JO. Part V., pelvic floor mechanics. Functional anatomy of the female pelvic floor. Ann N Y Acad Sci 2007;1101:266–96.

[18] Bharucha AE. Pelvic floor: anatomy and function. Neurogastroenterol Motil 2006;18(7): 507–19.

[19] Greenman PE. Clinical aspects of sacroiliac function during walking. Journal of Manual Medicine 1990;5:125–30.

[20] Cyphers M. Flexibility. In: Cyphers M, editor. Personal trainer manual-the resource for fitness instructors. San Diego (CA): Council on Exercise; 1991. p. 275–92.

[21] Bache CE, Clegg J, Herron M. Risk factors for developmental dysplasia of the hip: ultrasonographic findings in the neonatal period. J Pediatr Orthop B 2002;11(3):212–8.

[22] Sady SP, Freedson PS. Body composition and structural compositions of female and male athletes. Clin Sports Med 1984;3:755–77.

[23] Cirullo JV. Lower extremity injuries. In: Cirullo JV, editor. The athletic female; American orthopaedic society for sports medicine. Champaign (IL): Human Kinetics; 1993. p. 267–98.

[24] Prather H. Pelvis and hip injuries in the female athlete. In: Swedan N, editor. Women's sports medicine and rehabilitation. Gaithersburg (MD): Aspen Publishers; 2001. p. 35–54.

[25] Laycock J. Pelvic muscle exercises: physiotherapy for the pelvic floor. Urol Nurs 1994;14: 136–40.

[26] Lieber RL. Skeletal muscle structure and function. Baltimore (MD): Williams and Wilkins; 1992.

[27] Laycock J. Incontinence and pelvic floor re-education. Nursing Jul 25–Aug 21, 1991;4(39): 15–7.

[28] Zhu L, Lang JH, Chen J, et al. Morphologic study on levator ani muscle in patients with pelvic organ prolapse and stress urinary incontinence. Int Urogynecol J Pelvic Floor Dysfunct 2005;16(5):401–4.

[29] Sternheim MM, Kane JW. Elastic properties of materials, general physics. Toronoto (Canada): John Wiley & Sons; 1986.

[30] Sahrmann SA. Diagnosis and treatment of movement impairment syndromes. 1st edition. St. Louis (MO): Mosby, Inc; 2002.

[31] DeLancey JOL. Pelvic organ prolapse: clinical management and scientific foundations. Clin Obstet Gynecol 1993;36(4):895–6.

[32] DeLancey JOL. Anatomy and biomechanics of genital prolapse. Clin Obstet Gynecol 1993; 36(4):897–909.

[33] Travell J, Simons D. Myofascial pain and dysfunction: the trigger point manual. Baltimore (MD): Williams & Wilkins; 1992.

[34] Prather H. Pelvis and sacral dysfunction in sports and exercise. Phys Med Rehabil Clin N Am 2000;4:805–36.

[35] Chiarelli PE. Incontinence: the pelvic floor. Aust Fam Physician 1989;18(8):949–57.

[36] Young AW. Burning vulva syndrome: report of the ISSVD task force. J Reprod Med 1984; 29:457–8.

[37] Skene AJ. Treatise on the diseases of women, for the use of students and practitioners. New York: Appleton; 1889.

[38] Moyal-Barracco M, Lynch PJ. 2003 ISSVD terminology and classification of vulvodynia: a historical perspective. J Reprod Med 2004;49:772–7.

[39] Reed BD. Vulvodynia: diagnosis and mangement. Am Fam Physician 2006;73:1231–9.

[40] Metts JF. Vulvodynia and vulvar vestibulitis: challenges in diagnosis and management. Am Fam Physician 1999;59(6):1547–62.

[41] Harris G, Horowitz B, Borgida A. Evaluation of gabapentin in the treatment of generalized vulvodynia, unprovoked. J Reprod Med 2007;52(2):103–6.

[42] Baker PK. Musculoskeletal origins of chronic pelvic pain. Diagnosis and treatment [review]. Obstet Gynecol Clin North Am 1993;20(4):719–42.

[43] Bo K, Stein R. Needle EMG registration of striated urethral wall and pelvic floor muscles activity patterns during cough, valsalva, hip adductor and gluteal muscle contractions in nulliparous healthy females. Neurourol Urodyn 1994;13:35–41.

[44] Bannister L, Berry M, Collins P, et al. Pelvic floor. Gray's anatomy. 38th edition. London: Churhill Livingstone; 1995.

[45] Spitznagle TM. Musculoskeletal chronic pelvic pain. In: Carriere B, Feldt C, editors. Stuttgart (Germany): Georg Thieme Verlag; 2006. p. 35–64.

[46] Markwell SJ. Physical therapy management of pelvic/perineal and perianal pain syndromes. World J Urol 2001;19(3):194–9.

[47] Sinaki M, Merritt JL, Stillwell GK. Tension myalgia of the pelvic floor. Mayo Clin Proc 1977;52:717–22.

[48] Slocumb JC. Neurological factors in chronic pelvic pain: trigger points and the abdominal pelvic pain syndrome. Am J Obstet Gynecol 1984;149(5):536–43.

[49] Maria G, Cadeddu F, Brandara F, et al. Experience with type A botulinum toxin for treatment of outlet-type constipation. Am J Gastroenterol 2006;101(11):2570–5.

[50] Abbott JA, Jarvis SK, Lyons SD, et al. Botulinum toxin type A for chronic pain and pelvic floor spasm in women: a randomized controlled trial. Obstet Gynecol 2006;108(4):915–23.

[51] Brown CS, Glazer HI, Vogt V, et al. Subjective and objective outcomes of botulinum toxin type A treatment in vestibulodynia: pilot data. J Reprod Med 2006;51(8):635–41.

ELSEVIER
SAUNDERS

Phys Med Rehabil Clin N Am
18 (2007) 497–520

PHYSICAL MEDICINE
AND REHABILITATION
CLINICS OF
NORTH AMERICA

Acetabular Labral Tears
of the Hip in Women

Devyani Hunt, MD*, John Clohisy, MD,
Heidi Prather, DO

*Department of Orthopaedic Surgery, Washington University School of Medicine,
Washington University, 4921 Parkview Place, 6th floor, Campus Box 8605,
St. Louis, MO 63110, USA*

The differential diagnosis of anterior hip, groin, and pelvic pain spans many health care specialties from gynecology to general surgery to musculoskeletal medicine and orthopedic surgery. The list of possible causes of pain and dysfunction is extensive. These include causes involving osseous structures and their related soft tissues, as well as pelvic and intraabdominal organs. Structural disorders involving the hip joint itself is a known cause of anterior hip and groin pain. However, many extraarticular structures should also be considered when attempting to elucidate structural and physiological causes of pain. Furthermore, secondary pain and dysfunction may be associated with the complex relationship among the pelvis, spine, and hip, further complicating the diagnostic process and the task of achieving a resolution.

An increasing number of reports suggest acetabular labral tears to be a frequent cause of anterior hip and groin pain. Acetabular labral tears were first described in 1957 [1]. In the last decade, labral disease has been increasingly studied. In addition to hip arthroscopy, better technology related to imaging has been a significant factor in improving the recognition of labral tears. Despite these improvements, patients with labral tears commonly go undiagnosed for several months and patients are often seen by multiple health care providers before obtaining a definitive diagnosis [2,3]. The diagnosis may go unrecognized because the clinical presentation of labral tears varies, especially once secondary changes occur in associated structures, such as the pelvis, the sacroiliac joint, and the related pelvic-floor

---

* Corresponding author. Department of Orthopedics, One Barnes Plaza, West Pavilion Suite 11300, St. Louis, MO 63110.

E-mail address: huntdm@wudosis.wustl.edu (D. Hunt).

1047-9651/07/$ - see front matter © 2007 Elsevier Inc. All rights reserved.
doi:10.1016/j.pmr.2007.05.007 *pmr.theclinics.com*

musculature. A high index of suspicion is necessary to investigate and appropriately treat patients in a timely fashion. The evaluation of patients with anterior hip and groin pain begins with a thorough history, physical examination, radiographic evaluation, and appropriate imaging studies.

The anatomy of the acetabular labrum

The acetabular labrum is a ring of fibrocartilage and dense connective tissue [4] that surrounds the hip joint. It is a continuous, triangular structure that attaches to the boney rim of the acetabulum and is completed at the inferior portion by the transverse acetabular ligament over the acetabular notch (Fig. 1) [5]. The labrum is wider and thinner in the anterior region and thicker in the posterior region. The labrum attaches to the articular side of the acetabulum through a 1- to 2-mm transition zone of calcified cartilage that becomes the hyaline cartilage of the acetabulum. On the nonarticular side, the labrum attaches directly to the acetabular bone (Fig 2) [6,7].

The outer one third of the acetabular base of the acetabular labrum is vascular, while the remaining majority is avascular [4,8]. This is somewhat controversial as McCarthy and colleagues [9] found no areas of relative hypovascularity to the labrum. The vascular supply is provided by the obturator, superior gluteal, and inferior gluteal arteries. These are the

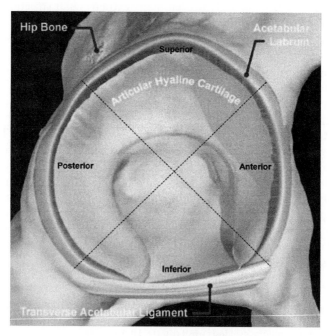

Fig. 1. Acetabular labrum. (*From* Lewis CL, Sahrmann SA. Acetabular labral tears. Phys Ther 2006;86:112. *Adapted from* Primal Pictures, LTD; used with permission.)

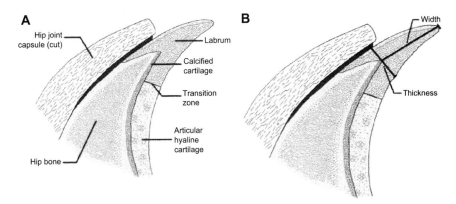

Fig. 2. Cross section of acetabular labrum. (*A*) Labral attachment. (*B*) Labral width and thickness. (*From* Lewis CL, Sahrmann SA. Acetabular labral tears. Phys Ther 2006;86:112; with permission.)

same arteries that supply the bony acetabulum [4,9]. The anterior and superior aspect of the labrum is thought to be the most innervated portions, consisting of free nerve endings and sensory nerve end organs. These structures produce pain, pressure, and deep sensation. As a result, one can conclude that a tear of the labrum could be a source of hip pain [10].

The function of the acetabular labrum remains debatable. It is thought to add stability and protection to the hip joint. The labrum aids in stability by deepening the joint. Some studies show that it deepens the acetabulum by 21% [11]. Additionally, the labrum increases the surface area of the acetabulum by 28% [11], which helps distribute load and therefore decrease contact stress on articular surfaces. The labrum also provides a seal for the joint that helps to maintain the synovial fluid and fluid pressure. This allows some of the load to be transferred to the pressurized joint fluid and off of the femoral and acetabular articular cartilage [12]. Without the labrum, the articular cartilage must withstand significantly increased pressure and a compromise of this system could lead to early joint deterioration. A study testing a labrum-free model of the hip showed that, without the labrum, contact stress may increase by as much as 92% [13].

Etiology

Tears of the acetabular labrum are increasingly recognized as a source of hip pain and dysfunction, especially in young adult and middle aged patients [2,14–17]. Historically, labral tears were associated with slipped capital epiphyses, [18] Legg-Calve-Perthes disease, major structural abnormalities of the hip, or high-velocity trauma, such as motor vehicle accidents or falls [19]. Athletic activities that involve repetitive pivoting motions on a loaded femur have also been associated with damage to the acetabular labrum

[1,20]. Specific sporting activities, such as soccer, hockey, golf, and ballet, have been linked to labral abnormalities [9,18,21]. The end-range motion in positions of hyperabduction, hyperextension, and external rotation is thought to contribute to the higher incidence of labral tears seen in this population of active individuals [9,18,21]. However, most labral tears have recently been reported to be insidious in onset, without a specific inciting event [2]. In these cases, the underlying inciting event is thought to be repetitive microtrauma [9,18].

Hip dysplasia and femoroacetabular impingement are widely accepted as major initiators of early hip disease and secondary osteoarthritis and are now also thought to contribute to acetabular labral tears [2,9,14,15,18,22,23]. Both of these structural abnormalities predispose the hip to abnormal articular loading. This results in progressive labral and chondral injury, and can lead to the development of acetabular labral tears, articular cartilage delamination, and eventual secondary osteoarthritis.

Recent literature correlates subtle bony changes of the acetabulum and femur to acetabular labral and chondral abnormalities [2,14,21,23]. These abnormalities include mild or subclinical hip dysplasia and femoroacetabular impingement. Peelle and colleagues [24] studied the radiographs of 78 patients treated arthroscopically for labral tears. Forty-nine percent of patients with symptomatic labral tears were found to have at least one radiographic abnormality: 17% occurred at the acetabulum, 14% at the femur, and 18% at both anatomic sites. These changes contribute to joint incongruency and are postulated to increase stress on the acetabular labrum. These data emphasize the common association of intraarticular hip disease and structural abnormalities.

Some researchers believe that labral fraying and tears represent the natural history of the aging hip joint. In cadaver studies, labral tears and abnormalities were found in 93% of hips with the average age of 78 and range of 48 to 102 years [9]. Labral abnormalities have also been found in patients without hip pain with the incidence increasing with age [25].

Demographics

Most studies report that symptomatic labral tears occur more frequently in women than in men [2,9,15–17,26]. This may partly be due to the increased incidence of hip dysplasia in women [27], especially between the ages of 15 to 41 years (Table 1) [2,9,15–17,26,28–30]. It is unknown if women with increased joint laxity are predisposed to labral injuries.

Presentation

More than 90% of patients diagnosed with acetabular labral tears complain of anterior hip or groin pain [2,17,21,31–33]. Burnett and colleagues [2]

Table 1
Characteristics of patients with labral tears across studies

Study	N	Population	Male	Female	Dysplasia	Age range (y)	Average age (y)
Suzuki and colleagues [30]	5	Patients with hip pain of unknown origin; labral tear, undiagnosed by arthrography, noted at arthroscopy	60%	40%	0%	13–16	15
Ikedo and colleagues [29]	7	Patients with hip pain and normal radiographs	42.8%	57.1%	14.3%	13–26	16.7
Hase and Ueo [28]	10	Patients with arthroscopically diagnosed and treated labral tears	30%	70%	10%	13–67	28.7
Dorrell and Catterall [15]	11	Patients in which acetabular dysplasia was associated with labral tears	0%	100%	100%	13–47	32.6
Farjo and colleagues [16]	28	Patients who underwent hip arthroscopy and were found to have labral tears	53.6%	46.4%	50% had arthritis or dysplasia	14–70	41
Fitzgerald [17]	55	Patients with a diagnosis of labral tears	45.5%	54.5%	Not reported	18–75	36.5
Sanlori and Villar [26]	58	Patients with labral tears that were arthroscopically detected and treated with partial resection of the labrum	43.1%	56.9%	Not reported	8–70	36.7
Burnett and colleagues [2]	66	Patients with labral tears that were confirmed by hip arthroscopy	29%	71%	22.7%	15–64	38
McCarthy and colleagues [21]	241	Patients with labral tears and mechanical hip symptoms	45.6%	54.4%	Not reported	14–72	39.9

Abbreviation: N, number of patients in study.
Data from Lewis CL, Sahrmann SA. Acetabular labral tears. Phys Ther 2006;86:115.

studied 66 patients found to have labral tears by arthroscopy and reported 92% had predominant localized groin pain, 52% had associated anterior thigh pain, and 59% described lateral hip pain. Fewer patients, 38%, reported associated buttock pain. No patient presented with isolated buttock pain.

The onset of symptoms was described as insidious in 61% of patients. Many patients with labral tears describe a constant dull pain with intermittent episodes of sharp pain that worsens with activity. Walking, pivoting, prolonged sitting, and impact activities, such as running, often aggravate symptoms. Seventy-one percent of patients describe night pain, 53% report mechanical symptoms of popping or snapping, while 41% report true locking or catching (Table 2). The data on functional limitations of patients with acetabular labral tears is scarce. Burnett and colleagues [2] found 89% of patients with labral tears reported limping, 67% required the use of banister with stairs, 36% reported limited walking to six blocks, and 32% reported difficulty donning and doffing socks (Table 3).

Table 2
Summary of hip symptoms associated with labral tears

Clinical parameter	Number of patients
Onset of symptoms	
Insidious	40 (61%)
Acute	20 (30%)
Trauma	6 (9%)
Moderate or severe symptoms	57 (86%)
Location of Pain	
Groin	61 (92%)
Anterior thigh or knee	34 (52%)
Lateral hip	39 (59%)
Buttock	25 (38%)
Quality of pain	
Sharp pain	57 (86%)
Dull pain	53 (80%)
Combination of sharp and dull pain	46 (70%)
Activity-related pain	60 (91%)
Constant pain	36 (55%)
Intermittent pain	30 (45%)
Night pain	47 (71%)
Mechanical snapping, popping, or locking	35 (53%)
Mechanical locking	27 (77%)
Painful mechanical locking	24 (89%)
Pain during walking	46 (70%)
Pain during pivoting	46 (70%)
Pain during impact activities	41 (62%)
Pain during sitting	40 (61%)

Data from Burnett S, Della Rocca G, Prather H, et al. Clinical presentation of patients with tears of the acetabular labrum. J Bone Joint Surg Am 2006;88(7):1450.

Table 3
Functional limitations associated with labral tears

Limitation	Number of Hips (N = 66)
Limp at any time during symptoms	59 (89%)
Severity of limp	
Slight or mild	51 (77%)
Moderate	5 (8%)
Severe	3 (5%)
Use of cane, crutches, or assistive device at any time during symptoms	6 (9%)
Limitation in walking distance	24 (36%)
Limited to six blocks	10 (15%)
Limited to two blocks	11 (17%)
Limited to household	3 (5%)
Stairs	
Requires use of banister	44 (67%)
Unable	1 (2%)
Sitting	
<30 min	17 (26%)
Unable or short duration	3 (5%)
Donning shoes and socks	
Difficult	21 (32%)
Unable	3 (5%)
Unable to use public transportation	6 (9%)

Data from Burnett S, Della Rocca G, Prather H, et al. Clinical presentation of patients with tears of the acetabular labrum. J Bone Joint Surg Am 2006;88(7):1451.

Unique in women is the possible concomitant pelvic-floor pain that may occur in association with labral tears, hip impingement, dysplasia, and early and late arthritis. Because these hip disorders are more common in women, a thorough history should include the discussion of pelvic-floor symptoms. The obturator internus is considered one of the primary musculature sources of pelvic-floor pain that often presents with the complaint of deep vaginal pain. Because the obturator internus is a primary hip rotator, a hip-related cause of pelvic pain should be considered in the differential diagnosis when the pain is determined to be originating from this muscle and when other causes have been excluded.

In an unpublished case series (Prather H, Hunt D. Unpublished data, 2006.), the investigators found that an acetabular labral tear was the source of pain in five women with groin and vaginal pain after a vaginal hysterectomy or attempted vaginal hysterectomy. It is unknown if these women had the labral tears before surgery and became symptomatic after surgery or if the tears occurred during surgery. Regardless, the investigators speculate that hip positioning in flexion and external rotation required to perform a vaginal hysterectomy may have exacerbated or caused the symptoms related to the labral disease.

In the article by Dugan and Prather specifically on pelvic-floor pain elsewhere in this issue, a more in-depth discussion includes information regarding the presentation and evaluation of pelvic-floor disorders.

Diagnosis and physical examination

The diagnosis of a labral tear relies on a high index of suspicion based on recognition of a specific pattern of presentation as well as a thorough physical examination. Determining that a labral tear is the cause of the patient's symptoms can be difficult and many patients experience a delay in diagnosis due to the elusive nature of the signs and symptoms. Fig. 3 presents an algorithm helpful in assessing the structural causes of hip and groin pain.

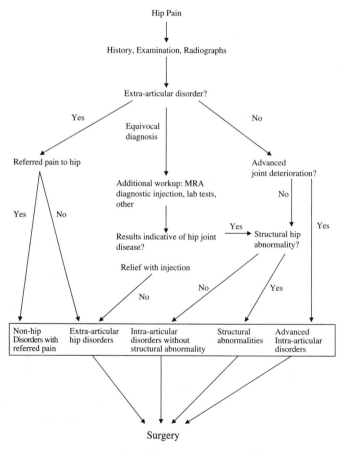

Fig. 3. Algorithm for assessing and treating hip pain. (*Data from* Clohisy JC, Keeney JA, Schoenecker P. Preliminary assessment and treatment guidelines for hip disorders in young adults. Clin Orthop Relat Res 2005;441:168–79; with permission.)

The first step is to discern between an intra- and extraarticular problem, which can be challenging because dysfunction in extraarticular structures coexist or are secondary to intraarticular disorders. An assessment of spine motion and positions of provocation of symptoms is important in determining if a spine issue is contributing to the patient's pain. A thorough neurological examination with neural tension provocative maneuvers in the lower extremity can help discern a neurological component. Evaluation of muscle length and strength, particularly in the core muscles, including the hip and abdominal musculature, is key to identifying areas of system breakdown that may contribute or cause the dysfunction and pain. Extraarticular muscle imbalances between posterior hip abductors and external rotators in combination with shortened hip flexors and iliotibial band can lead to groin and lateral hip pain. Hip range-of-motion parameters are variable in the literature and are described in normal asymptomatic volunteers. For young adults with early hip disorder, range-of-motion parameters have not been developed. The evidence regarding evaluation and management of early intraarticular hip disorders is emerging. For this reason, reliable values for range of motion of the hips in asymptomatic individuals are needed. The influence of age, gender, position, and active or passive movement on range of motion of the hip has not been adequately documented [34–41]. Simoneau and colleagues [41] found that measurements of active hip internal rotation were not significantly affected when subjects were in the prone, rather than seated, position. However, prone positioning significantly affected external rotation. Women also had statistically greater active hip internal and external rotation than men had. More studies are needed to establish the factors that influence range of motion in healthy individuals.

Though the normal ranges for range of motion of the hip are wide, assessing for asymmetries in motion of the hip from side to side is important. Passive range of motion can be measured with specific degrees of motion for comparison.

Hip disorders, especially in their early presentation, are often most symptomatic during weight-bearing activities. Gray [42] proposed and popularized motion testing of the linked musculoskeletal system with the use of a matrix to help measure motion in weight-bearing throughout different planes of motion. The three planes are frontal, sagittal, and transverse (Figs. 4–6). Though these parameters proposed by Gray have not been validated, researchers have looked at similar parameters for lower-extremity function and stability. Star excursion balance tests (SEBTs) have been found to be reliable in assessing dynamic stability [43–45]. SEBTs quantify lower-extremity reach while challenging the individual's stability. The test involves assessing balance on one lower extremity while the other extremity is reaching in one of eight directions of the matrix. SEBTs have been found to be effective for determining reach deficits in persons with unilateral chronic ankle instability [45]. The end point on this method of testing was a reach distance while maintaining single-leg balance on the opposite leg. The

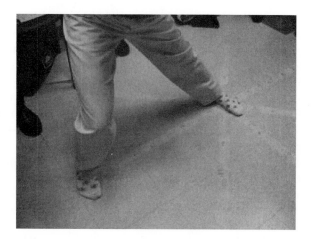

Fig. 4. Frontal plane lunge.

examiners did not record pain complaints in subjects studied. To date, SEBTs have been primarily used in studies to assess distal lower-extremity reach and balance [43,45–48]. In a recent study by Lanning and colleagues [49,50] the SEBTs were a part of a battery of tests to assess trunk endurance and strength in college athletes. Pain limitations were not a part of the assessment and the study was performed in asymptomatic athletes. Though weight-bearing measures have not been consistently validated, some form of weight-bearing is important to assess because it best represents true function of the hip.

A limited number of physical examination provocative tests can be helpful. The most consistent physical examination finding in patients with

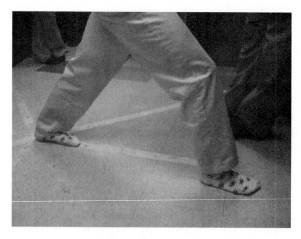

Fig. 5. Sagittal plane lunge.

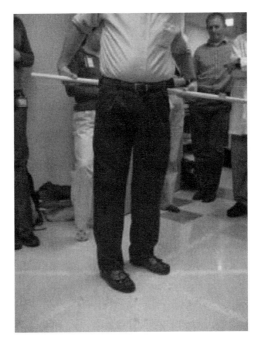

Fig. 6. Transverse plane.

acetabular labral tears is a positive hip-impingement test [2,51]. This is performed with the patient supine with the hip and knee at 90° of flexion. The hip is internally rotated while an adduction force is applied. A positive test results in pain provocation in the anterolateral hip or groin. Other provocative tests that can be helpful to elicit intraarticular pathology have been described, but are not specific to labral tears (Table 4). These include tests that help isolate pathology specific to the hip joint versus other related structures, such as the sacroiliac joint, pelvis, and spine. However, physical examination findings remain inconsistent. This is thought to be secondary to the variable locations of labral tears (Table 5). Most tears reported in the United States occurred in the anterior portion of the labrum [9,13,16,26,28–30]. Studies from Japan found the majority of tears occurring in the posterior aspect of the labrum [28–30]. This is most likely explained by the frequent practice in Japan of squatting or sitting on the ground or floor [28]. As a result, no universal test includes or excludes labral tears in the differential diagnosis because the tears occur in different locations.

Diagnostic imaging

Diagnostic imaging usually begins with a radiographic evaluation with special attention to subtle structural abnormalities of the hip and pelvis.

Table 4
Special tests of the hip

Name of test	Purpose of test	Description of test
Anterior hip impingement test	To assess hip pathology, impingement, or anterior superior labral tear	Patient lies prone. Examiner passively flexes hip and knee, internally rotates and adducts hip. A positive test reproduces anterior or lateral hip pain.
Patrick's test or flexion abduction external rotation (FAbER) test	To discern between hip and sacroiliac joint or low back pathology	Patient lies supine. Examiner places the ankle of the test leg just above the opposite knee in a figure-4 position. The opposite ASIS is stabilized with one hand and over pressure applied to the test leg's knee toward the table. A positive test for hip pathology reproduces groin pain. A positive test for sacroiliac joint or low back pathology reproduces posterior pelvic pain.
Resisted straight leg raise test or Stitchield test	To assess hip pathology	Patient lies supine and actively flexes hip with knee extended to 30° against resistance. A positive test reproduces anterior or lateral hip pain.
Log-roll test	To assess hip pathology	Patient lies supine with hips and knees extended. Examiner passively internally and externally rotates test leg while stabilizing knee and ankle so that motion occurs at the hip. A positive test reproduces anterior or lateral hip pain.
Apprehension test	To assess hip pathology, labral tear	Patient lies prone with hip and knee extended. Examiner passively extends, adducts, and externally rotates hip. A positive test reproduces apprehension or anterior hip pain.
Posterior hip impingement	To assess hip pathology, posterior labral tear	Patient lies prone with hip and knee extended. Examiner passively extends, adducts, and externally rotates hip. A positive test reproduces anterior hip or posterior pelvic pain.

(*continued on next page*)

Table 4 (*continued*)

Name of test	Purpose of test	Description of test
Ober's test	To assess iliotibial band posterior fiber length	Patient lies on side. Lower leg flexed at the hip and knee. Examiner passively extends the patient's upper leg with the knee flexed at 90°. While supporting the knee, the examiner slowly lowers the leg. If the iliotibial band is shortened, the leg remains abducted and does not fall to the table.
	Assess iliotibial band anterior fiber length	Patient lies on side. Lower leg flexed at the hip and knee. Examiner passively flexes the patient's upper limb hip with the knee flexed at 90°. While supporting the knee, the examiner slowly lowers the leg. If the iliotibial band is shortened, the leg remains abducted and does not fall to the table.
Thomas test	Assess hip flexor contracture	Patient sits at edge of table. Patient flexes one knee to chest and rolls on to back while allowing test leg to remain extended at the hip off the edge of the table. If the hip does not fully extend, this indicates a hip flexion contracture. If the leg abducts, this indicates iliotibial band tightness.

Screening radiographs helps detect obvious sources of disease, such as advanced arthritis, tumor, developmental dysplasia of the hip (DDH), or femoroacetabular impingement (FAI). A complete evaluation includes an anteroposterior view of the pelvis; a cross-table lateral view, a frog lateral view, or both [52]; and a false profile [53] view. These projections allow for specific measurements of the acetabulum and femoral head to improve recognition of subtle DDH or FAI. Lateral uncovering of the femoral head and superior lateral inclination of the acetabulum are seen in hip dysplasia (Fig. 7). FAI results from excessive acetabular coverage of the femoral head, an aspherical femoral head, or head–neck offset. These structural abnormalities can result in repetitive abutment of the acetabular-labral-femoral articulation. Cam type of impingement occurs more commonly in young active male patients and is more frequently due to

Table 5
Locations of acetabular labral tears across studies

Study	Number of patients undergoing surgical treatment	Country of study	Anterior	Posterior	Superior or lateral	Other
Suzuki and colleagues [30]	5	Japan	0%	60%	0%	
Ikedo and colleagues [29]	7	Japan	14% anterosuperior	86% posterosuperior	0%	
Hase and Ueo [28]	10	Japan	20%	50%	10%	20% posterior and anterior
Farjo and colleagues [16]	28	United States	61%	25%	15%	
Fitzgerald [17]	49	United States	92%	8%	0%	
Sanlori and Villar [26]	58	England	67%	28%	5%	
Burnett and colleagues [2]	66	United States	64%	7%	14%	15% anterosuperolateral
McCarthy and colleagues [21]	241	United States	86%	11%	3%	

Data from Lewis CL, Sahrmann SA. Acetabular labral tears. Phys Ther 2006;86:115.

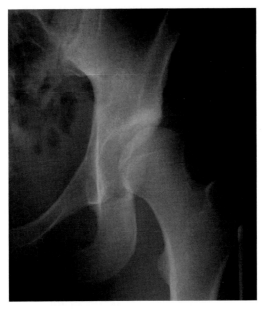

Fig. 7. Anterioposterior radiographs of the hip demonstrating lateral uncovering of the femoral head.

a decreased head–neck offset. Pincer type of impingement occurs more commonly in women and is due to excessive femoral head coverage. Cam and pincer impingement abnormalities also occur concurrently in many hips (Fig. 8) [54]. An association between subtle structural abnormalities of the hip and labral tears has been elucidated [24,55]. The more common structural risk factors found include a shallow acetabulum, acetabular retroversion (Fig. 9), and decreased head–neck offset (Fig. 10).

Once an acetabular labral tear is suspected, a magnetic resonance arthrogram (MRA) can be helpful to further clarify the diagnosis. An MRA is also helpful to rule out other abnormalities within the differential, which include but are not limited to stress fractures, neoplasm, avascular necrosis, osteitis pubis, synovitis, ligamentum teres rupture, and other extraarticular soft tissue abnormalities, such as sports hernias and tendon avulsions. MRI alone is inadequate for visualizing the acetabular labrum [56]. The intraarticular or systemic infusion of gadolinium is required to obtain the detail necessary to study the labrum (Fig. 11) [56]. MRA can also be helpful to assess structural abnormalities. Despite these benefits, MRA has its limitations in regards to sensitivity for diagnosis of acetabular labral and articular cartilage abnormalities. A recent study [46] showed a 71% sensitivity and 44% specificity with a positive predictive value of 93% for acetabular labral pathology as compared with arthroscopic visualization. Other studies that compared MRA to surgical findings show a range of sensitivity from 60%

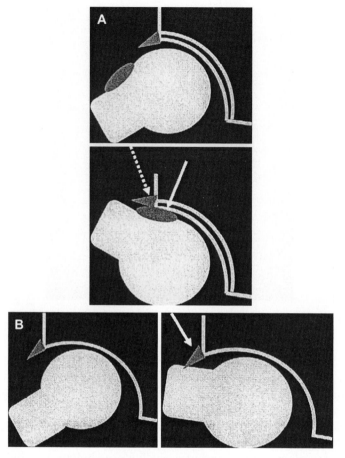

Fig. 8. (*A*) Cam type of femoroacetabular impingement. (*B*) Pincer type of femoroacetabular impingement. (*Reprinted from* Manaster BJ, Zakel S. Imaging of Femoral Acetabular Impingement Syndrome. Clin Sports Med 2006;25:637, 639; with permission from Elsevier.)

to 91% [57–61]. These studies demonstrate that a negative scan does not fully rule out a labral tear and that hip arthroscopy remains the gold standard.

Diagnostic-image–guided intraarticular hip injections can also be helpful in the diagnosis of labral tears. Prior studies have shown that fluoroscopically guided diagnostic hip injections have 88% sensitivity and 100% specificity for localizing groin pain to an intraarticular location [62]. Other studies have shown 90% accuracy of diagnostic hip injections to detect the presence of intraarticular abnormality when compared with hip arthroscopy.

Information from the clinical history, physical examination, diagnostic hip injection, radiographic evaluation, and MRA findings must be considered when contemplating a diagnosis of a labral tear. Any one of these components alone is usually inadequate.

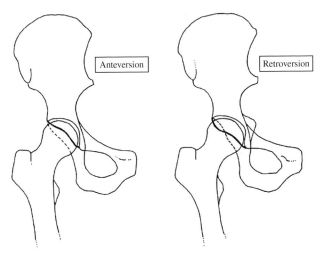

Fig. 9. Acetabular Version. (*From* Espinosa N, Rothenfluh DA, Beck M, et al. Treatment of femoro-acetabular impingement: preliminary results of Labral refixation. J Bone Joint Surg Am 2006 May;88(5):927. Reprinted with permission from The Journal of Bone and Joint Surgery, Inc.)

Treatment

The most important goals of evaluation are to determine the specific cause of symptoms, characterize associated structural abnormalities, and select an optimal treatment plan. Once the diagnosis has been determined, available treatment options are diverse and continue to evolve. These include medications, modalities, therapeutic exercise, image-guided

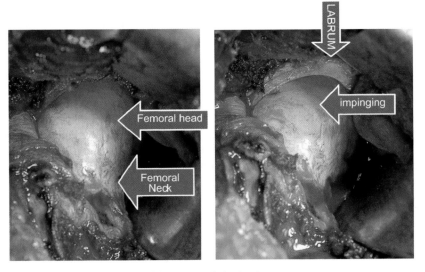

Fig. 10. CAM type of femoroacetabular impingement seen at surgery.

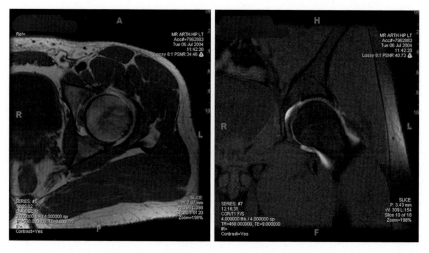

Fig. 11. Labral tear seen on MR Arthrogram.

intraarticular hip injections with or without steroid, and an array of surgical techniques. Many of these options have not been rigorously evaluated with respect to clinical outcomes.

Conservative treatment

Specific methodology regarding therapeutic exercise for labral tears, FAI, DDH, or early arthritic hip disorders has not been formally studied. Labral tears, FAI, and DDH are considered precursors to arthritis and can be associated with early arthritis often noted only at hip arthroscopy. This article discusses the conservative treatment of this group of disorders, which, if left untreated, can lead to moderate and severe hip arthritis. The conservative approach to labral tears of the hip often involves a program to combine several options toward the goal of pain reduction and functional improvement. However, no description provides guidance about when to shift treatment from one option to another. Furthermore, no one has precisely identified which specific therapeutic exercises are most beneficial [63]. The choice of which therapeutic exercises to employ depends on the judgement of the independent examiner and the individual providing treatment. Timing as to when to initiate surgical referral is unclear. All things considered, conservative management and its clinical efficacy have not been well defined.

Typically, a trial of conservative management, including relative rest, anti-inflammatory medications, and pain medications as necessary, combined with a focused physical therapy protocol for 10 to 12 weeks is recommended initially. Occasionally, it is necessary to restrict weight-bearing in patients with acute or traumatic onset of symptoms. A fluoroscopically guided intraarticular injection with or without steroid can also be used to quiet an acute flare. The decision to add a long-acting steroid to the injectate should be based on the degree of associated degenerative changes seen on radiographic evaluation. In a young patient with no degenerative changes, intraarticular steroids may damage chondral surfaces and are not recommended.

The physical therapy protocol should be individualized and based on a thorough musculoskeletal evaluation that includes examination of related structures (spine, pelvis, and lower extremities) and their dynamic functioning. Lewis and Sahrmann [63] recently described a physical therapy protocol for acetabular labral tears with the goal of optimizing the alignment of the hip joint and the precision of joint motion by reducing anteriorly directed forces on the hip and addressing abnormal patterns of recruitment of muscles that control the hip. Limiting pivoting motions and other movement patterns that increase forces across the labrum is of utmost importance because the acetabulum rotates on a loaded femur. Much of the focus is on strengthening muscles found to be inhibited, analyzing gait, and retraining as indicated. Assessing foot motion, especially through the subtalar joint, and correcting stiffness or adding support to the medial arch through taping or orthotics are crucial in making corrections to gait patterns. Progressing the strengthening pattern over time is important in maintaining long-term success in treatment. This can be done through increasing the lever arm length of a particular exercise, adding weight-bearing exercises, and enhancing proprioception and balance through the use of uneven surfaces, balance boards, or force challenges. Ultimately, some of the exercises should resemble the functional activities the patient is trying to return to or accomplish.

Surgical treatment

When conservative measures do not control the patient's symptoms or when functional limitations remain unsatisfactory, a surgical referral is appropriate. Table 6 provides an outline of the specific surgical treatment options based on disease categories as determined by history, physical exam, and imaging studies [14]. In regards to treatment, the literature to date has focused on arthroscopic debridement of labral tears and surgical repair of associated structural problems [2,14,17,18,21,33,64]. Results after arthroscopic debridement are promising. Burnett and colleagues [2] reported 89% of patients with continued "improved" status at an average of 16.5 months after arthroscopic debridement of a labral tear. Similar results are seen across the literature [2,14–17,21]. However, when patients are classified by degree of labral tear [21] and extent of secondary osteoarthritic changes [16], success rates are lower. McCarthy and colleagues [21] reported on patients with stage 3 labral tears (diffuse tears that involve more that one anatomic region and are associated with more pronounced degenerative changes) having 40% good to excellent results compared with 91% good

Table 6
Surgical treatment options for selected disorders

Disease category	Examples	Treatment options
Nonhip disorders with referred pain	Lumbar spine disease	Patient-specific or disease-specific treatment
Extraarticular hip disorder	Snapping psoas	Psoas lengthening
	Piriformis syndrome	Piriformis release
Intraarticular disorders without structural abnormality	Labral tear, chondral flap, chondral defect, loose body, synovitis	Hip arthroscopy
Structural abnormalities	Classic DDH	Reconstructive acetabular osteotomy (periacetabular osteotomy) (arthrotomy, femoral osteotomy, head–neck osteoplasty as needed)
	Cam impingement	(1) Hip arthroscopy with osteoplasty; (2) hip arthroscopy and combined open osteoplasty, (3) surgical dislocation and osteoplasty
	Pincer impingement	(1) Reconstructive acetabular osteotomy (periacetabular osteotomy) (acetabular retroversion); (2) surgical dislocation with rim osteoplasty (coax profunda); (3) (for focal impingement) hip arthroscopy with rim osteoplasty; (4) (for focal impingement) hip arthroscopy and combined open osteoplasty
	Perthes-like deformity	(1) Reconstructive acetabular osteotomy (periacetabular osteotomy); (2) surgical dislocation with osteoplasty (proximal femoral osteotomy, trochanteric advancement, head–neck osteoplasty as needed)
	Slipped capital femoral epiphysis	(1) Cam impingement procedures (above) for mild deformity; (2) intertrochanteric femoral osteotomy and heat–neck osteotomy
	Osteonecrosis	(1) Core decompression; (2) nonvascularized grafting; (3) vascular grafting; (4) proximal femoral osteotomy
Advanced intraarticular disorder	Secondary Osteoarthritis, posttraumatic osteoarthritis, osteonecrosis, chondrolysis, inflammatory arthritis	(1) Prosthetic replacement procedures (2) Arthrodesis

From Clohisy JC, Keeney JA, Schoenecker P. Preliminary assessment and treatment guidelines for hip disorders in young adults. Clin Orthop Relat Res 2005;441:169; with permission.

to excellent results in patients with stage 1 labral lesions (localized to one anatomic region with mild degenerative changes). Farjo and colleagues [16] reported associated arthritic changes as a poor prognostic indicator to arthroscopic repair of labral tears. Clohisy [14,64] and O'Leary and colleagues [33] reproduced similar results.

Arthroscopy also allows visualization of related intraarticular structures, such as the articular cartilage and ligamentum teres. McCarthy and colleagues [21] found 63% of hips scoped for labral tears were found to have articular cartilage abnormalities. In 80% of these patients, labral and articular lesions were found in the same zone of the acetabulum as the labral tear, with most lesions in the anterior quadrant of the acetabulum.

In patients with significant associated structural abnormalities, arthroscopic debridement alone is commonly inadequate. Depending on the underlying type of structural abnormality, other joint-preserving procedures may be indicated. Patients with FAI may benefit from a femoral and/or acetabular osteoplasty procedure. This can be achieved with various techniques, including hip arthroscopy, limited open osteoplasty [64], or open hip procedures. Likewise, those patients with associated developmental dysplasia may benefit most from acetabular reorientation for correction of the dysplasia [65,66].

Summary

Acetabular labral tears are a major cause of hip dysfunction in young patients and are now recognized as a primary precursor to hip osteoarthritis. In addition, labral disease more commonly occurs in women and can present with nonspecific symptoms. With improved imaging and advances in the understanding of structural hip disorders and their relation to labral and chondral pathology, it is now possible to diagnose, quantify, and treat labral tears before the onset of secondary joint deterioration [9,14,23]. The diagnosis requires a high index of suspicion, special attention to subtle patterns of presentation, and timely consideration for imaging studies. Treatment options are still evolving and include a wide array of nonsurgical and surgical techniques. Treatment should also address secondary dysfunction that can be associated with hip pathology, such as pelvic, spine and lower-extremity abnormalities. An initial trial of conservative management is recommended and failure to progress is an indication for surgical consultation.

References

[1] Paterson I. The torn acetabular labrum; a block to reduction of a dislocated hip. J Bone Joint Surg Br 1957;39:306–9.
[2] Burnett S, Della Rocca G, Prather H, et al. Clinical presentation of patients with tears of the acetabular labrum. J Bone Joint Surg Am 2006;88(7):1448–57.

[3] Byrd JW, Jones KS. Hip arthroscopy in the presence of dysplasia. Arthroscopy 2003;19: 1055–60.

[4] Petersen W, Petersen F, Tillmann B. Structure and vascularization of the acetabular labrum with regard to the pathogenesis and healing of labral lesions. Arch Orthop Trauma Surg 2003;11:403–8.

[5] Seldes RM, Tan V, Hunt J, et al. Anatomy, histologic features, and vascularity of the adult acetabular labrum. Clin Orthop Relat Res 2001;382:232–40.

[6] Keene GS, Villar RN. Arthroscopic anatomy of the hip: an in vivo study. Arthroscopy 1994; 10(4):392–9.

[7] Keeney JA, Peelle MW, et al. Magnetic resonance arthrography versus arthroscopy in the evaluation of articular hip pathology. Clin Orthop Relat Res 2004;429:163–9.

[8] Kelly BT, Shapiro GS, Digiovanni CW, et al. Vascularity of the hip labrum: a cadaveric investigation. Arthroscopy 2005;21(1):3–11.

[9] McCarthy JC, Noble PC, Schuck MR, et al. The Otto E Aufranc Award: the role of labral lesions to development of early degenerative hip disease. Clin Orthop 2001;393:25–37.

[10] Kim YT, Azuma H. The nerve endings of the acetabular labrum. Clin Orthop Relat Res 1995;320:176–81.

[11] Tan V, Seldes RM, Katz MA, et al. Contribution of acetabular labrum to articulating surface area and femoral head coverage in adult hip joints: an anatomic study in cadavera. Am J Orthop 2001;30(11):809–12.

[12] Hlavacek M. The influence of the acetabular labrum seal, intact articular superficial zone and synovial fluid thizotropy on squeeze-film lubrication of a spherical synovial joint. J Biomech 2002;35(10):1325–35.

[13] Ferguson SJ, Bryant JT, Ganz R, et al. The influence of the acetabular labrum on hip joint cartilage consolidation: a poroelastic finite element model. J Biomech 2000;33(8):953–60.

[14] Clohisy JC, Keeney JA, Schoenecker PL. Preliminary assessment and treatment guidelines for hip disorders in young adults. Clin Orthop Relat Res 2005;441:168–79.

[15] Dorrell JH, Catterall A. The torn acetabular labrum. J Bone Joint Surg Br 1986;68:400–3.

[16] Farjo LA, Glick JM, Sampson TG. Hip arthroscopy for acetabular labral tears. Arthroscopy 1999;15:132–7.

[17] Fitzgerald RH. Acetabular labrum tears: diagnosis and treatment. Clin Orthop 1995;311: 60–8.

[18] Mason JB. Acetabular labrum tears. Diagnosis and treatment. Clin Sports Med 2001;20: 779–90.

[19] Leunig M, Casillas MM, Hamlet M, et al. Slipped capital femoral epiphysis: early mechanical damage to the acetabular cartilage by a prominent femoral metaphysic. Acta Orthop Scand 2000;71:370–4.

[20] Depaulis F, Cacchio A, Michelini O, et al. Sports injuries in the pelvis and hip: diagnostic imaging. Eur J Radiol 1998;27(Suppl 1):S49–59.

[21] McCarthy J, Nable P, Alusio FV, et al. Anatomy, pathologic features and treatment of acetabular labral tears. Clin Orthop Relat Res 2003;38–47.

[22] Clohisy JC, McClure T. Treatment of anterior femoracetabular impingement with combined hip arthroscopy and limited anterior decompression. Iowa Orthop J 2005;25:164–71.

[23] Ganz R, Parvizi J, Beck M, et al. Femoroacetabular impingement: a cause for osteoarthritis of the hip. Clin Orthop Relat Res 2003;417:112–20.

[24] Peelle MW, Della Rocca GJ, Maloney WJ, et al. Acetabular and femoral radiographic abnormalities associated with labral tears. Clin Orthop Relat Res 2005;441:327–33.

[25] Abe I, Haranda Y, Oinuma K, et al. Acetabular labrum: abnormal findings at MR imaging in asymptomatic hips. Radiology 2000;216(2):576–81.

[26] Santori N, Villar RN. Acetabular labral tears: results of arthroscopic partial limbectomy. Arthroscopy 2000;16(1):11–5.

[27] Bache CE, Clegg J, Herron M. Risk factors for developmental dysplasia of the hip: ultrasonographic findings in the neonatal period. J Pediatr Orthop B 2002;11(3):212–8.

[28] Hase T, Ueo T. Acetabular labral tear: arthroscopic diagnosis and treatment. Arthroscopy 1999;15(2):138–41.

[29] Ikeda T, Awaya G, Suzuki S, et al. Torn acetabular labrum in young patients. Arthroscopic diagnosis and management. J Bone Joint Surg Br 1988;70:13–6.

[30] Suzuki S, Away G, Okada Y, et al. Arthroscopic diagnosis of ruptured acetabular labrum. Acta Orthop Scand 1986;57:513–5.

[31] Binningsley D. Tear of the acetabular labrum in an elite athlete. Br J Sports Med 2003;37(1): 84–8.

[32] Klaue K, Durnin CW, Ganz R. The acetabular rim syndrome. A clinical presentation of dysplasia of the hip. J Bone Joint Surg Br 1991;73(3):423–9.

[33] O'Leary JA, Berend K, Vail TP. The relationship between diagnosis and outcome in arthroscopy of the hip. Arthroscopy 2001;17(2):181–8.

[34] Aalto TJ, Airasinen O, Harkonen TM. Effect of passive stretch on reproducibility of hip range of motion measurements. Arch Phys Med Rehabil 2005;86(3):549–57.

[35] Bierma-Zeinstra SM, Bohnen AM, Ramlal R, et al. Comparison between two devices for measuring hip joint motions. Clin Rehabil 1998;12(6):497–505.

[36] Evans RC. Illustrated orthopedic physical assessment. Mosby; 2001.

[37] Godges JJ, MacRae PG, Engelke KA. Effects of exercise on hip range of motion, trunk muscle performance, and gait economy. Phys Ther 1993;73(7):468–77.

[38] Hoppenfeld S. Physical examination of the spine and extremities. Prentice Hall; 1976.

[39] Kendall FP, McCreary EK, Provance PG, et al. Muscles testing and function with posture and pain. Lippincott Williams and Wilkins, 5th Edition; 2005.

[40] Magee DJ. Orthopedic physical assessment. WB Saunders Co., 4th Edition; 2002.

[41] Simoneau GG, Hoenig KJ, Lepley JE, et al. Influence of hip position and gender on active hip internal and external rotation. J Orthop Sports Phys Ther 1998;28(3):158–64.

[42] Gray GW. Lower extremity functional profile. Adrian (MI): Wynn Marketing Inc; 1995.

[43] Hertel J, Braham RA, Hale SA, et al. Simplifying the star excursion balance test: analyses of subjects with and without chronic ankle instability. J Orthop Sports Phys Ther 2006;36(3): 131–7.

[44] Kinzey SJ, Armstrong CW. The reliability of the star-excursion test in assessing dynamic balance. J Orthop Sports Phys Ther 1998;27:356–60.

[45] Olmsted LC, Carcia CR, Hertel J, et al. Efficacy of the star excursion balance tests in detecting reach deficits in subjects with chronic ankle instability. J Athl Train 2002;37(4):501–6.

[46] Cote KP, Brunet ME, Gansneder BM, et al. Effects of pronated and supinated foot postures on static and dynamic postural stability. J Athl Train 2005;40(1):40–6.

[47] Gribble PA, Hertel J, Denegar CR, et al. The effects of fatigue and chronic ankle instability on dynamic postural control. J Athl Train 2004;39(4):321–9.

[48] Plisky PJ, Rauh MJ, Kaminski TW, et al. Star excursion balance test as a predictor of lower extremity injury in high school basketball players. J Orthop Sports Phys Ther 2006;36(12): 911–9.

[49] Lanning CL, Uhl TL, Ingram CL, et al. Baseline values of trunk endurance and hip strength in collegiate athletes. J Athl Train 2006;41(4):427–34.

[50] Lecouvet FE, Vande Berg BC, Malghem J, et al. MR imaging of the acetabular labrum: variations in 200 asymptomatic hips. AJR Am J Roentgenol 1996;167(4):1025–8.

[51] Saw T, Villar R. Footballer's hip: a report of six cases. J Bone Joint Surg Br 2004;86(5): 655–8.

[52] Eijer H, Myers SR, Ganz R. Anterior femoroacetabular impingement after femoral neck fractures. J Orthop Trauma 2001;15(7):475–81.

[53] Garbuz DS, Masri BA, Haddad F, et al. Clinical and radiographic assessment of the young adult with symptomatic hip dysplasia. Clin Orthop Relat Res 2004;418:18–22.

[54] Beck M, Kalhor M, Leunig M, et al. Hip morphology influences the pattern of damage to the acetabular cartilage: femoroacetabular impingement as a cause of early osteoarthritis of the hip. J Bone Joint Surg Br 2005;87(7):1012–8.

[55] Wenger DE, Kendell KR, Miner MR, et al. Acetabular labral tears rarely occur in the absence of bony abnormalities. Clin Orthop Relat Res 2004;426:145–50.

[56] Byrd JWT, Jones K. Diagnostic accuracy of clinical assessment, magnetic resonance imaging, magnetic resonance arthrography, and intra-articular injection in hip arthroscopy patients. Am J Sports Med 2004;32(7):1668–74.

[57] Czerny C, Hofmann S, Urban M, et al. MR arthrography of the adult acetabular capsular-labral complex: correlation with surgery and anatomy. AJR Am J Roetgenol 1999;173: 345–9.

[58] Czerny C, Hoffman S, Neuhold A, et al. Lesions of the acetabular labrum: accuracy of MR imaging and MR arthrography in detection and staging. Radiology 1996;200:225–30.

[59] Petersilge CA, Haque MA, Petersilge WJ, et al. Acetabular labral tears: evaluation with MR arthrography. Radiology 1996;200:231–5.

[60] Plotz GMJ, Brossmann J, Schunke M, et al. Magnetic resonance arthrography of the acetabular labrum: Macroscopic and histological correlation in 20 cadavers. J Bone Joint Surg 2000;82:426–32.

[61] Schmid MR, Notzli HP, Zanetti M, et al. Cartilage lesions in the hip: diagnostic effectiveness of MR arthrography. Radiology 2003;226:382–6.

[62] Faraj AA, Kumaraguru P, Kosygan K. Intra-articular bupivacaine hip injection in differentiation of co-arthrosis from referred thigh pain: a 10 year study. Acta Orthop Belg 2003; 69(6):518–621.

[63] Lewis CL, Sahrmann SA. Acetabular labral tears. Phys Ther 2006;86:110–21.

[64] Clohisy JC, McClure T, Robison J, et al. Treatment of anterior femoroacetabular impingement with combined hip arthroscopy and limited open osteoplasty. Iowa Orthop J 2005;25: 164–71.

[65] Siebenrock KA, Schoeniger R, Gans R. Anterior femoro-acetabular impingement due to acetabular retroversion: treatment with periacetabular osteotomy. J Bone Joint Surg Am 2003;85:278–86.

[66] Trousdale RT, Ekkernkamp A, Ganz R, et al. Periacetabular and intertrochanteric osteotomy for the treatment of osteoarthrosis in dysplastic hips. J Bone Joint Surg Am 1995;77(1): 73–85.

ELSEVIER
SAUNDERS

Phys Med Rehabil Clin N Am
18 (2007) 521–537

PHYSICAL MEDICINE
AND REHABILITATION
CLINICS OF
NORTH AMERICA

Rehabilitation in Women with Breast Cancer

Julie K. Silver, MD

*Department of Physical Medicine and Rehabilitation, Harvard Medical School,
Countway Library, 10 Shattuck Street, 2nd Floor, Boston, MA 02115, USA*

A historical perspective

Around 2650 BC, early Egyptians documented breast cancer and the treatment, which was cautery of the tumors [1]. Later, in 460 BC, Hippocrates described a case report of breast cancer. He was responsible for naming cancer *karkinos*, which is the Greek word for crab and described the way tumors seem to have tentacles resembling crabs' legs [2]. For hundreds of years, despite trying various other treatments, surgery was the only therapy with a chance of being effective. Therefore, according to historian Olson [2], by the beginning of the 20th century operations for breast cancer outnumbered all other caner surgeries by four to one and the "Halstead mastectomy became the most common major surgical procedure in the world." Doctors tried many different remedies to save women. However, essentially no effective therapeutic options were available other than severely disfiguring and disabling surgery.

Cancer treatment dramatically improved when chemotherapy and radiation therapy came into use during the middle of the 20th century. However, these therapies also resulted in significant toxicity to healthy tissues and disability in women who survived the disease and the treatments. Nearly all cancer survivors, even now, share the experience of having to recover from not only cancer but also the toxic treatments. Sheed [3] wrote of his experience with radiation treatment for oral cancer in his memoir, *In Love with Daylight: A Memoir of Recovery*. Sheed noted,

> As the radiologist [radiation oncologist] reads off the list of possible side- and after-effects, to run concurrently and forever, it's awfully hard to remember that this guy is supposed to be on your side. There he is, about to kill off thousands of your favorite cells, adding up to a large tract of the body that brought you this far, and they call this man a healer! Talk

E-mail address: jksilver@bics.bwh.harvard.edu

about bombing villages to liberate them; talk about napalming whole forests on suspicion. For all anyone knew, I might not even *have* cancer at this stage. But bomb we must. One can't be too careful [3].

Cancer has challenged physicians to save lives without unnecessarily causing pain and disability. This challenge is ongoing, and women who have breast cancer often experience dramatic negative physical effects that may linger for years or even a lifetime. Esophageal cancer survivor, French [4], wrote about this challenge in her book, *A Season in Hell*. French succinctly stated the obvious about oncologists, "Simply to treat cancer means they must violate the primary tenet of their code: First, do no harm."

Another challenge in the cancer community has been the historical secrecy and shame associated with the diagnosis. According to the book *Crusade: The Official History of the American Cancer Society:*

> If the Society would succeed, it first had to take cancer out the closet. In 1913 the disease was not named in polite society. Patients were routinely shielded from knowing that they had a malignancy. The patient's family might be told, but they were unlikely to discuss this even with their closest friends; it was shameful to have a relative with cancer. The seventh leading cause of death in the United States at that time, responsible for some 75,000 deaths per year, cancer was not mentioned in newspaper obituaries. The standard euphemism was "a long illness." It ranked in shame with syphilis and other unmentionable afflictions [5].

Two seminal events happened in 1979, in what the author refers to as "The Tale of Two Bettys." First Lady Betty Ford and news correspondent Betty Rollin shared with the world their diagnoses of breast cancer and subsequent mastectomies. These admissions and the ensuing media coverage helped pave the way for other women to come forward and tell their stories, and a huge national movement, symbolized by pink ribbons, followed.

Epidemiology

Today breast cancer is the third leading cause of cancer in the world (after lung and gastric cancer) and the most common malignancy in women, accounting for 23% of cancers in women worldwide. In the United States, the numbers are higher, with breast cancer accounting for 32% of all new cancer cases, and just more than 200,000 cases of invasive breast cancer and approximately 60,000 cases of in situ breast cancer diagnosed annually [6]. Worldwide among women from all ethnic classes, and in the United States among women who are of African-American and Hispanic descent, it is the leading cause of cancer mortality. Overall in the United States, it is the second leading cause of cancer deaths (after lung cancer) in women [1].

The incidence of breast cancer in the United States has been increasing at the rate of 1% to 2% per year. Although it is the most common cause of cancer death in young women, a decrease in mortality in this age group seems to be "attributable to the combination of patient education, earlier diagnosis with mammogram screening, and increased use of systemic adjuvant therapy" [1]. Nevertheless, breast cancer remains a very real threat to women of all ages, with one in nine women developing this disease.

Although mortality statistics are readily available, morbidity statistics associated with breast cancer treatments have not been studied as extensively. Lymphedema of the upper extremity after breast cancer treatment has probably been studied more than any other complication, and yet the statistics on the incidence of this vary from 10% to 30% [7]. However, other physical impairments and disability in breast cancer survivors have also been studied. In a prospective study, Karki and colleagues [8] surveyed 96 breast cancer patients at 6 months and 12 months postsurgery and found that "Impairments and their impact on activities were frequent and constant." At 6 months, more than half of the respondents experienced limitations in lifting, carry, and reaching, with the most common impairments being axillary scar tightness, axillary edema, and neck–shoulder pain [8]. Another study by Rietman and colleagues [9] retrospectively evaluated 55 women who underwent a modified radical mastectomy or a segmental mastectomy with axillary lymph node dissection. The mean follow-up was 2.7 years after treatment and impairments included pain (60%) and reduced grip-strength (40%). Fehlauer and colleagues [10] evaluated long-term quality of life status in breast cancer survivors related to age at diagnosis and found that physical functioning, role functioning, and sexual functioning were decreased in patients older than 65 years at therapy.

In another study entitled "Functional Limitations in Elderly Female Cancer Survivors," the researchers found that women who had a history of cancer experienced a decline in physical functioning compared with age-matched peers. For example, 42% of the 1068 5-year survivors in this study reported that they were unable to do heavy household work compared with 31% of the 23,501 participants who never had cancer [11]. Finally, a study examining the impact of rehabilitation services on breast cancer survivors found that only the group that received an early home-based physical therapy intervention experienced a significant benefit in reduced arm morbidity and upper-body disability and improved functional well-being, compared with two other groups studied—women who participated in a group-based exercise and psychosocial intervention and a non-intervention group [12].

Cancer rehabilitation, like all rehabilitation, involves focusing on physical function while concurrently maximizing psychosocial and vocational function. To best understand the potential morbidity and subsequent disability in women who have a history of breast cancer, reviewing the current treatment regimens and their potential physical side effects is helpful.

Treatment options and their impact on women's health

Surgery

Surgery, whether it is a localized excision of the malignant cells or tumor (frequently termed *breast conservation surgery*) or a partial or complete mastectomy, is often the first treatment. Some women may undergo chemotherapy first and then surgery or, if evidence of distant metastasis (stage IV) is present, they may not undergo surgery at all. If a mastectomy is planned, women may opt to undergo reconstruction at mastectomy, at a later date, or not at all. Several types of reconstructive procedures are available and each influences healing after surgery. Chemotherapy and radiation therapy can also slow healing after surgery. Whether women undergo axillary lymph node dissection or sentinel lymph node biopsy also influences subsequent disability. Women who have a history of breast cancer may also decide to undergo prophylactic mastectomy or oophorectomy, the latter of which is beyond the scope of this article.

Seromas are a frequent complication of breast cancer surgery, with an incidence of 25% to 50% after mastectomy and up to 25% after axillary dissection [13]. In one retrospective analysis of 359 consecutive patients (94% of whom were Hispanic), Gonzalez and colleagues [14] found that seromas occurred in 19.9% of patients who underwent modified radical mastectomy and in 9.2% of patients who underwent breast-conserving surgery.

Axillary lymph node dissection (ALND) is becoming less common because of the advent of sentinel lymph node biopsy (SLNB), which has been shown to reduce postoperative morbidity in the arm and shoulder region in women who have early-stage breast cancer [15–19]. The presence of metastatic disease in axillary lymph nodes is known to predict recurrence and has important negative prognostic import [20,21]. Therefore, investigation is ongoing to determine the overall efficacy of SLNB compared with ALND and weighing this against the potential for subsequent arm and shoulder symptoms from SLNB versus ALND. In a recent study in the *Journal of Surgical Oncology*, Schulze and colleagues [20] evaluated the long-term morbidity of 134 patients with early-stage breast cancer and found that 31 had SLNB only and 103 had SLNB followed by ALND. Participants were followed up from November 1995 through January 2001. In this study, only one patient from each group experienced a local recurrence (3.2% in the SLNB group and 1.0% in the ALND group). The incidence of lymphedema was 15.8% and 19.7% in the SLNB and ALND groups, respectively. No statistically significant differences were seen in arm range of motion between the groups. The measurement of arm strength showed that significantly fewer patients experienced reduced arm strength in the SLNB group. In another study, Rietman and colleagues [17] evaluated 204 patients who had stage I/II breast cancer and a mean age of 55.6 years, finding that patients who underwent SLNB experienced less treatment-related upper extremity morbidity, less perceived disability in activities of daily living, and a better reported quality of life.

Many women choose to undergo breast reconstruction after mastectomy. Implants are considered a less-invasive reconstructive technique and are performed by inserting a silicone or saline implant behind or in front of the pectoral muscle. In some cases the surgeon will use a balloon expander, which is inserted beneath the skin and chest muscle, and will inject a salt-water solution through a valve mechanism to gradually fill the expander over weeks to months. When the skin is sufficiently stretched, saline is let out until the reconstructed breast and natural breast are equal sizes [22].

Breast reconstruction with the transverse rectus abdominus musculocutaneous (TRAM) flap may need more follow-up surgical procedures than implants or latissimus dorsi flaps [23]. Complications may arise at the donor site level or in the region of the reconstructed breast. Secondary procedures can include liposculpturing, fat necrosis excision, scar revision, and hernia repair. TRAM flaps are similar to deep inferior epigastric perforator (DIEP) flaps; however, theoretically, no muscle is harvested with a DIEP flap. In a retrospective study, Futter and colleagues [24] examined abdominal and back extensor muscle strength, comparing 50 women (23 who had a DIEP flap and 27 who had a free TRAM flap) and 32 nonoperated controls. This study found no statistical difference between the DIEP flap group and controls but that the DIEP group was weaker. They noted a statistical difference between the TRAM and DIEP flap groups, with the former having more significant weakness. In a 2-year analysis of trunk function after TRAM flap, Alderman and colleagues [25] found that breast cancer patients who underwent TRAM reconstructions experienced a less-than-20% long-term deficit in trunk flexion, and no significant difference was seen in patients who receive pedicle versus free TRAM reconstructions.

Chemotherapy

Chemotherapy-related disability may be short-term or long-term, depending on the drugs used and individual patient susceptibility. Neutropenia and gastrointestinal complaints, especially nausea and fatigue, are common during active therapy. Long-term disability (which can vary depending on the regimen used, dosing, interval timing, and individual susceptibility) may include cardiomyopathy and neuropathy. Neuropathy is particularly common with the taxane class of drugs, including paclitaxel and docetaxel. Grade 2 to 3 peripheral neuropathy incidence is believed to be approximately 6% to 10% [26]. For women who have metastatic disease, the taxanes are commonly used for prolonged periods, which may increase their toxicity [27].

The specific drugs used to treat breast cancer and their potential side effects are beyond the scope of this article. However, currently a trend is occurring toward more aggressive chemotherapy regimens, including dose-dense regimens that seek to reduce the interval between the administration of each dose. The cumulative drug dose remains constant, and essentially the same amount of medication is given over a shorter period. Whether dose densification will ultimately be the optimal way to treat some women who have breast cancer is currently unclear [28].

Radiation

Radiation therapy combined with other treatments, including surgery and sometimes chemotherapy, can cause significant disability in women who have undergone breast cancer treatment [29–35]. Long-term disability can be caused by cardiac or pulmonary sequelae, lymphedema, brachial plexopathy, impaired arm/shoulder range of motion, and second malignancies [36]. Blomqvist and colleagues [32] examined range of motion and strength of the arm and shoulder after modified radical mastectomy and radiation therapy and found that of 75 participants, the 30 who underwent radiation experienced significantly reduced range of motion and strength. These authors concluded, "The present analysis indicates that the adjuvant radiotherapy is responsible for most of the reduction of [range of motion] and strength of the shoulder joint in patients operated with mastectomy and axillary dissection" [33].

Another study examining long-term complications associated with breast conservation surgery followed by radiation found that approximately 10% of the participants experienced a grade 2 or higher late complication, including edema, fat necrosis, skin fibrosis, decreased arm/shoulder range of motion, neuropathy, pneumonitis, and rib fracture [31].

Endocrine treatment

The decision to use adjuvant therapy for several years after breast cancer treatment depends on many factors, including whether a woman is pre- or postmenopausal and whether her tumor was estrogen receptor–positive or –negative. Traditionally, tamoxifen was the preferred drug, but recent results from randomized controlled trials indicate that aromatase inhibitors (eg, letrozole, anastrozole) have better anticancer efficacy and toxicity profiles for treating breast cancer in women who are postmenopausal, node-negative, and hormone receptor–positive [36].

The decision to use adjuvant therapy and, if so, what kind is made by the medical oncologist and the patient. However, many women who have breast cancer who present with rehabilitation issues will either take tamoxifen or one of the aromatase inhibitors. Thus, understanding the, listed in Box 1, is important.

Rehabilitation interventions

Undoubtedly many patients who have cancer are much healthier in the beginning of treatment than at the end. Of course, this doesn't minimize the lethal progress of a malignancy that is not treated, but rather acknowledges that the rehabilitation process in cancer treatment is essential for optimal recovery. In the Institute of Medicine report, *From Cancer Patient*

Box 1. Side-effect profiles of adjuvant therapy

Tamoxifen
Changes in appetite/weight
Changes in menstruation
Decreased libido
Dizziness
Dyspareunia
Fatigue
Headache
Hot flashes
Increased risk for ophthalmologic problems
Increased risk for secondary cancer
Increased risk for thromboembolic events, including stroke
Increased triglycerides
Mood disturbance
Nausea/vomiting
Rash
Vaginal discharge

Aromatase inhibitors
Bone loss
Dizziness
Dyspareunia
Fatigue
Headache
Hot flashes
Loss of libido
Mood disturbance
Myalgias and arthralgias
Nausea/vomiting
Vaginal dryness

This is not a complete list of side effects and ongoing investigations may reveal other issues (eg, cardiovascular side effects are currently unclear).

to Cancer Survivor: Lost in Transition [37], one of the key recommendations was to make survivorship a distinct phase of treatment. The focus on physical and emotional healing is key during this phase and health care professionals can do much to intervene in a positive manner.

Therapeutic exercise

Exercise can certainly help healing in women who have a history of breast cancer, and may in fact assist in preventing cancer recurrence [38–40]. These factors have led to national media attention and speculation on the value of exercise in cancer. Many studies suggest that exercise is extremely valuable in the survivorship phase of treatment and that it can enhance physiologic outcomes and function [41,42] and alleviate many disabling symptoms, such as fatigue [43–45]. These factors also have important quality of life implications [46,47]. For example, in a cross-sectional study of 40 early-stage breast cancer survivors who reported regular exercise compared with 79 who were sedentary, those who exercised regularly reported higher body esteem and mood than their sedentary counterparts [48]. Additionally, the women who exercised experienced significantly less confusion, fatigue, and depression. In women who have a history of cancer, exercise can affect long-term complications from treatment, such as osteoporosis [49]. Exercise also seems to have a positive benefit in incurable cancer and is one treatment option in palliative care [50].

Therefore, exercise may affect the quality and quantity of a breast cancer survivor's life, making it an extremely important part of the survivorship phase of oncology care. In fact, all women should be encouraged to exercise, unless it is contraindicated. However, women tend to exercise less during treatment [50,51] and may not return to prediagnosis levels of physical activity [51]. To facilitate continuation of exercise, having them use a pedometer and count how many steps a day they are taking may be helpful. Then, using short-term goals to increase the number of steps will help their progress. Ultimately, the number of steps for active, healthy adults should be approximately 10,000 steps per day.

This technique is a simple way for women to begin exercising, but it doesn't address the specific cardiovascular, strength training, and flexibility exercises that may be particularly beneficial for breast cancer survivors, depending on their specific treatment and physical condition. In a study evaluating 61 patients who had various types of cancer, Midtgaard and colleagues [52,53] reported that a supervised exercise program encouraged participation and that rates dropped significantly once the program ended. However, participants reported a higher level of exercise after the program ended than their baseline. This study suggests that ongoing supervision for exercise may be necessary to encourage participation, but that even short-term intervention may have some lasting effects. In another study focusing on the effects of a cardiovascular and strength training program, Herrero and colleagues [54] found that this combined program "improves the [quality of life] and the overall physical fitness of breast cancer survivors following even a brief (8-week) exercise program."

Exercise in women who have undergone breast cancer treatment should be initiated with caution and as much adherence to the current level of research as possible. However, many gaps exist in what experts know and can safely and authoritatively recommend. For example, the ideal time for women to begin upper extremity exercises and how aggressive to be with upper body strength training are unclear. In a review of randomized clinical trials examining this issue, Shamley and colleagues [55] concluded, "This review has identified support for delaying exercises to reduce seroma formation. However, incomplete reporting of trials and faults in study designs resulting in poor internal and external validity have been identified." In one randomized controlled study evaluating the effect of upper and lower body weight training on the incidence of lymphedema in 45 women who were 4 to 36 months post-treatment, 13 of whom had prevalent lymphedema at baseline, found that the 6-month intervention of exercise did not increase the risk for, or exacerbate the symptoms of, lymphedema [56].

In the rehabilitation setting, exercise may be important in reducing upper extremity pathology after breast cancer treatment. Physical and occupational therapy can help increase shoulder range of motion, promote upper extremity strength, decrease pain, and reduce swelling, including lymphedema, if that is an issue. Prescribing medications, such as anti-inflammatories, to reduce pain and inflammation, may facilitate therapeutic exercise [57].

In one randomized controlled study examining the timing of physical therapy after breast cancer surgery, Lauridsen and colleagues [58] found that the optimal time for treatment was 6 to 8 weeks postoperatively. They also noted that physical therapy treatment can be initiated up to 6 months after surgery with similarly good results.

Timing of exercise and how best to perform the exercises are important issues. In a unique study that attempted to evaluate the latter issue, Ferreira de Rezende and colleagues [59] found that the patients who had a very directed physical therapy program consisting of 19 specific exercises were better rehabilitated than the free group who also exercised but did not have such a structured regimen. Although the best way to exercise after breast cancer treatment is extremely important to consider, very few studies have examined this aspect of care, and evidence-based guidelines do not exist.

Reduce pain

The impact of pain on quality of life can be profound. Although the definition of *quality of life* varies, certain measures are used in research protocols, such as those listed in Box 2 [60–70].

The World Health Organization promotes the definition of health as a state of complete physical, mental, and social well-being and not merely the absence of disease or infirmity. Essentially, that quality of life is important in restoring health. Some of the ways that pain can affect quality of life in cancer patients are listed in Box 3.

In rehabilitation medicine, physicians spend much time focusing on how best to alleviate pain and restore function. In all patients, pain can lead to increased disability and poor function; however, the added concern for cancer survivors is that pain may be heralding recurrent or worsening malignancy. However, in women who have a history of breast cancer, much of

---

Box 2. Measures of quality of life

Functional Assessment of Cancer Treatment (FACT)
Cancer Rehabilitation Evaluation System (CARES)
Visual Analog Scale Global Quality of Life (VASQOL)
Sickness Impact Profile (SIP)
Nottingham Health Profile (NHR)
Medical Outcomes Study Short Form 36 (SF-36)
European Organization for Research and Treatment of Cancer
    (EORTC) modular questionnaire
Rotterdam Symptom Checklist (RSCL)

---

the pain they experience is musculoskeletal because of the invasive nature of the treatments. In a study assessing upper extremity decline in women who have a history of breast cancer, Westrup and colleagues [71] followed up 644 early-stage breast cancer patients for up to 51 months post-surgery. This study found that breast cancer survivors had a fivefold increase in upper body decline compared with age-matched controls. Thus, alleviating pain in a woman who has breast cancer not only can help make her more comfortable and improve her ability to function but can also help sideline a major source of anxiety.

Possible sources of musculoskeletal pain in women who have a history of breast cancer are listed in Box 4. Postmastectomy pain is a unique chronic neuropathic pain syndrome that can affect women postoperatively and does not necessarily correlate with a specific surgical procedure or set of risk factors [72]. The prevalence of postmastectomy pain ranges from 4% to 27% [73–75] and is believed to be underidentified and undertreated. In a study of 95 women with a history of breast cancer, of the 19 women identified

---

Box 3. Pain interfering with quality of life

Interference with appetite, sleep, and other physical functions
Reduced memory and concentration
Decreased ability to work
Loss of interest or other barriers to physical intimacy
Difficulty participating in home activities (eg, household chores,
    caring for children)
Limited social activity and engagements
Decline in financial resources
Change in spiritual connections (eg, fear of dying)
Loss of autonomy and marginalized at home, at work, and in
    social contexts

Box 4. Possible upper extremity pain disorders in women who have a history of breast cancer

Adhesive capsulitis
Arthritis
Brachial plexopathy
Cervical radiculopathy
Cervical sprain/strain
Cellulitis
Complex regional pain syndrome
Deep vein thrombosis
Edema
Epicondylitis
Lymphedema
Median, radial, or ulnar mononeuropathy
Metastases
Neuroma
Phantom breast pain
Postmastectomy pain syndrome
Tendinitis

---

with postmastectomy pain, 75% reported taking no analgesics for their pain [59]. Lymphedema, though classically reported as nonpainful, can cause discomfort in some women. To effectively treat pain, it's important to identify the cause if possible. For example, neuropathic pain can result from taxane-based chemotherapy induced sensory neuropathy. Phantom breast pain is also a source of pain in some women (refer to Box 4).

There are few randomized controlled studies that have evaluated the treatment of pain after breast cancer therapy. As with all types of chronic, disabling pain conditions, a multi-disciplinary approach is ideal. This approach should take into account the physical and emotional aspects of pain management and can include a cognitive behavioral program as well [76]. Box 5 lists possible pain treatment options in women with a history of breast cancer, but again appropriate therapy depends primarily on the underlying diagnosis. Table 1 lists classes of pain medications and their common uses in a rehabilitation setting.

Physical modalities have not been well studied in cancer or more specifically in women with a history of breast cancer. Their safety and efficacy, therefore, is not certain. However, those modalities that are generally believed to be safe include cryotherapy, biofeedback, iontophoresis, transcutaneous electrical nerve stimulation (TENS), and massage [60,77]. Caution is used for most modalities directly over tumor sites. Deep heat such as ultrasound or phonophoresis is usually contraindicated in cancer patients [60].

Box 5. Potential treatment options for pain in women who have a history of breast cancer

Acupuncture
Injected medications
Massage
Oral medications
Physical/occupational therapy
Topical medications

Spinal traction is avoided in patients with spinal bony metastasis or with significant osteoporosis.

Lessen fatigue

Fatigue is the most common and problematic complaint of women who have breast cancer [78–82]. Self-reported fatigue in patients who have cancer correlates with a decline in function [83]. The reasons for fatigue can be multifactorial because of chemotherapy side effects that are physiologically based and may persist for many years after treatment [84]. Associated cognitive symptoms of memory dysfunction and decreased concentration (*chemo brain*), although still somewhat controversial, seem to have a physiologic basis and may contribute to fatigue [85,86]. The triad of fatigue, mood disorders, and cognitive complaints is not uncommon in female breast cancer survivors [74].

Other causes of fatigue may be treatment-induced menopause, wherein the accompanying hot flashes interfere with sleep, as can pain and anxiety

Table 1
Classes of pain medications and their uses

Class	Uses	Examples
Opioids	Visceral, soft tissue, bone, neuropathic	Fentanyl, hydromorphone, methadone, morphine, oxycodone
NSAIDs	Soft tissue, bone	Celecoxib (COX-2), ibuprofen, nabumetone, naproxen
TCAs	Neuropathic, myofascial	Amitriptyline, desipramine, nortriptyline, cyclobenzaprine
SSRIs	Neuropathic, depressive component	Duloxetine, tramadol[a]
Anticonvulsants	Neuropathic	Carbamazepine, clonazepam, gabapentin, pregabalin
Antispasmodics	Spasticity	Baclofen, dantrolene, tizanidine
Benzodiazepines	Muscle spasm, anxious component	Alprazolam, diazepam, lorazepam

Abbreviations: NSAID, nonsteroidal anti-inflammatory drug; SSRI, selective serotonin reuptake inhibitor; TCA, tricyclic anti-depressant.
[a] Has properties of SSRI and opioid receptor agonist.

Box 6. Potential treatment options for fatigue in women who have a history of breast cancer

Address pain
Consultation with a dietitian
Consultation with a mental health professional
Counsel on naps and the effect they may have on sleep at night
Reduce hot flashes
Therapeutic exercise

---

[87]. Fatigue may have a physical and/or an emotional component. For example, physical deconditioning and clinical depression can both contribute to symptoms of fatigue.

Exercise has been shown to be effective in treating fatigue in women who have a history of breast cancer [88,89]. Cancer-related fatigue seems to respond to exercise in many different types of cancer. In a study evaluating 72 survivors who had different diagnoses, a 15-week rehabilitation intervention program improved fatigue and physical parameters [84]. Treating hot flashes with antidepressant medications and other nonhormonal agents is currently favored [90–92]. In a double-blind study of 420 women who were having two or more hot flashes per day, Pandya and colleagues [93] found that gabapentin effectively controlled this symptom at a dose of 900 mg/d but not at a lower dose.

Similar to pain, the treatment of fatigue should focus on the underlying cause and account for the multiple factors that can influence this symptom and the physical and emotional underlying components. Rehabilitation strategies are therefore multidisciplinary and focus on appropriate strategies that are summarized in Box 6.

The management and rehabilitation of women who have a history of breast cancer should certainly be a distinct phase of oncology care and are invaluable in improving quality of life and potentially affecting long-term survival. Because this area has recently been the focus of academic research, many things are still unknown. Where a lack of evidence-based medicine exists, knowledgeable practitioners will have to rely on what seems reasonable and appropriate given a particular woman's medical status. Undoubtedly, the future will offer much more to in terms of evidence-based clinical guidelines.

References

[1] Silva OE, Zurrida S, editors. Breast cancer: a practical guide. 3rd edition. New York: Elsevier Saunders; 2005. p. 15, 21–3, 24.
[2] Olson JS. Bathsheba's breast. Baltimore (MD): Johns Hopkins University Press; 2002. p. 13, 68–9.

[3] Sheed W. In love with daylight: a memoir of recovery. Pleasantville: Akadine Press; 1999. p. 234.

[4] French M. A season in hell. New York: Ballantine; 2000. p. 60.

[5] Ross W. Crusade: the official history of the American Cancer Society®. New York: Arbor House; 1987. p. 18.

[6] Jemal A, Murray T, Ward E, et al. Cancer statistics, 2005. CA Cancer J Clin 2005;55:10–30.

[7] Kligman L, Wong RKS, Johnston M, et al. The treatment of lymphedema related to breast cancer: a systematic review and evidence summary. Support Cancer Care 2004;12:421–31.

[8] Karki A, Simonen R, Malkia E, et al. Impairments, activity limitations and participation restrictions 6 and 12 months after breast cancer operation. J Rehabil Med 2005;37:180–8.

[9] Rietman JS, Dijkstra PU, Debreczeni R, et al. Impairments, disabilities and health related quality of life after treatment for breast cancer: a follow-up study 2.7 years after surgery. Disabil Rehabil 2004;26:78–84.

[10] Fehlauer F, Tribius S, Mehnert A, et al. Health-related quality of life in long term cancer survivors treated with breast conserving therapy: impact of age at therapy. Breast Cancer Res Treat 2005;92:217–22.

[11] Sweeny C, Schmitz KH, Lazovich D, et al. Functional limitations in elderly female cancer survivors. J Natl Cancer Inst 2006;98:521–9.

[12] Gordon LG, Battistutta D, Scuffham P, et al. The impact of rehabilitation support services on health-related quality of life for women with breast cancer. Breast Cancer Res Treat 2005; 93:217–26.

[13] Chilson T, Chan F, Lonser F, et al. Seroma prevention after modified radical mastectomy. Am Surg 1992;58:750–4.

[14] Gonzalez EA, Saltzstein EC, Riedner CS, et al. Seroma formation following breast cancer surgery. Breast J 2003;9:385–8.

[15] Haid A, Koberle-Wuhrer R, Knauer M, et al. Morbidity of breast cancer patients following complete axillary dissection or sentinel node biopsy only: a comparative evaluation. Breast Cancer Res Treat 2002;73:31–6.

[16] Rietman JS, Dijkstra PU, Geertzent JHB, et al. Treatment-related upper limb morbidity 1 year after sentinel lymph node biopsy or axillary lymph node dissection for stage I or II breast cancer. Ann Surg Oncol 2004;11:1018–24.

[17] Rietman JS, Geertzen JHB, Hoekstra HJ, et al. Long term treatment related upper limb morbidity and quality of life after sentinel lymph node biopsy for stage I and II breast cancer. Eur J Surg Oncol 2006;32:148–52.

[18] Ronka R, von Smitten K, Tasmuth T, et al. One-year morbidity after sentinel node biopsy and breast surgery. Breast 2005;14:28–36.

[19] Schulze T, Mucke J, Markwardt J, et al. Long-term morbidity of patients with early breast cancer after sentinel lymph node biopsy compared to axillary lymph node dissection. J Surg Oncol 2006;93:109–19.

[20] Canavese G, Catturich A, Vecchio C, et al. Prognostic role of lymph-node level involvement in patients undergoing axillary dissection for breast cancer. Eur J Surg Oncol 1998;24: 104–9.

[21] Jatoi I, Hilsenbeck SG, Clark GM, et al. Significance of axillary lymph node metastasis in primary breast cancer. J Clin Oncol 1999;17:2334–40.

[22] Crompvoets S. Comfort, control, or conformity: women who choose breast reconstruction following mastectomy. Health Care Women Int 2006;27:75–93.

[23] Losken A, Carlson GW, Schoemann MB, et al. Factors that influence the completion of breast reconstruction. Ann Plast Surg 2004;52:258–62.

[24] Futter CM, Webster MHC, Hagen S, et al. A retrospective comparison of abdominal muscle strength following breast reconstruction with a free TRAM and DIEP flap. Br J Plast Surg 2000;53:578–83.

[25] Alderman AK, Kuzon WM, Wilkins EG. A two-year prospective analysis of trunk function in TRAM breast reconstructions. Plast Reconstr Surg 20006;117:2131–8.

[26] Gianni L, Capri G. New chemotherapy drugs. In: Bonadonna G, Hortobagyi GN, Gianni AM, editors. Textbook of breast cancer—a clinical guide to therapy. London: Martin Dunitz Ltd; 1997. p. 253–80.

[27] Makino H. Treatment and care of neurotoxicity from taxane anticancer agents. Breast Cancer 2004;11:100–4.

[28] Orzano JA, Swain SA. Concepts and clinical trials of dose-dense chemotherapy for breast cancer. Clin Breast Cancer 2005;6:402–11.

[29] Deutsch M, Flickinger JC. Shoulder and arm problems after radiotherapy for primary breast cancer. Am J Clin Oncol 2001;24:172–6.

[30] Meric F, Bucholz TA, Mirza NQ, et al. Long-term complications associated with breast-conservation surgery and radiotherapy. Ann Surg Oncol 2002;9:543–9.

[31] Beenken SW, Bland KI. Long-term complications of breast-conservation therapy: can the incidence be reduced? Ann Surg Oncol 2002;9:524–5.

[32] Blomqvist L, Stark B, Engler N, et al. Evaluation of arm and shoulder mobility and strength after modified radical mastectomy and radiotherapy. Acta Oncol 2004;43: 280–3.

[33] Gaya AM, Ashford RFU. Cardiac complications of radiation therapy. Clin Oncol 2005;17: 153–9.

[34] Pierce LJ. The use of radiotherapy after mastectomy: a review of the literature. J Clin Oncol 2005;23:1706–17.

[35] Senkus-Konefka E, Jassem J. Complications of breast-cancer radiotherapy. Clin Oncol 2006;18:229–35.

[36] Ranger GS. Current concepts in the endocrine therapy of breast cancer: tamoxifen and aromatase inhibitors. J Clin Pharm Ther 2005;30:313–7.

[37] Hewitt M, Greenfield S, Stovall E, editors. From cancer patient to cancer survivor: lost in transition. Washington, DC: The National Academies Press; 2006.

[38] Holmes MD, Chen WY, Feskanich D, et al. Physical activity and survival after breast cancer. JAMA 2005;293:2479–86.

[39] McNeely ML, Campbell KL, Rowe BH, et al. Effects of exercise on breast cancer patients and survivors: a systematic review and meta-analysis. CMAJ 2006;175:34–41.

[40] Dallal CM, Sullivan-Halley J, Ross RK, et al. Long-term recreational physical activity and risk of invasive and in situ breast cancer. Arch Intern Med 2007;167:408–15.

[41] MacVicar MG, Winningham ML, Nickel JL. Effects of aerobic interval training on cancer patients' functional capacity. Nurs Res 1989;38:348–51.

[42] MacVicar MG, Winningham ML. Promoting functional capacity of cancer patients. Cancer Bull 1986;38:235–9.

[43] Mock V, Dow KH, Meares CJ, et al. Effects of exercise on fatigue, physical functioning, and emotional distress during radiation therapy for breast cancer. Oncol Nurs Forum 1997;24: 991–1000.

[44] Mock V, Pickett M, Ropka ME, et al. Fatigue and quality of life outcomes of exercise during cancer treatment. Cancer Pract 2001;9:119–27.

[45] Schwartz AL, Mori M, Gao R, et al. Exercise reduces daily fatigue in women with breast cancer receiving chemotherapy. Med Sci Sports Exerc 2001;33:718–23.

[46] Segal R, Evans W, Johnson D, et al. Structured exercise improves physical functioning in women with Stage I and II breast cancer: results of a randomized controlled trial. J Clin Oncol 2001;19:657–65.

[47] Couneya KS, Mackey JR, Bell GJ, et al. Randomized controlled trial of exercise in postmenopausal breast cancer survivors: cardiopulmonary and quality of life outcomes. J Clin Oncol 2003;21:1660–8.

[48] Pinto BM, Trunzo JJ. Body esteem and mood among sedentary and active breast cancer survivors. Mayo Clin Proc 2004;79:181–6.

[49] Hoff AO, Gagel RF. Osteoporosis in breast and prostate cancer survivors. Oncol 2005;19: 651–8.

[50] Oldervoll LM, Loge JH, Paltiel H, et al. The effect of a physical exercise program in palliative care: a Phase II study. J Pain Symptom Manage 2006;31:421–30.

[51] Courneya KS, Friedenreich CM. Relationship between exercise pattern across the cancer experience and quality of life in colorectal cancer survivors. J Altern Complement Med 1997;3:215–26.

[52] Denmark-Wahnefried W, Hars V, Conaway MR, et al. Reduced rates of metabolism and decreased physical activity in breast cancer patients receiving adjuvant therapy. Am J Clin Nutr 1997;65:1495–501.

[53] Midtgaard J, Tveteras A, Rorth M, et al. The impact of supervised exercise intervention on short-term postprogram leisure time physical activity level in cancer patients undergoing chemotherapy: 1- and 3-month follow-up on the body & cancer project. Palliat Support Care 2006;4:25–35.

[54] Herrero F, San Juan AF, Fleck SJ, et al. Combined aerobic and resistance training in breast cancer survivors: a randomized, controlled pilot trial. Int J Sports Med 2006;27: 573–80.

[55] Shamley DR, Barker K, Simonite V, et al. Delayed versus immediate exercises following surgery for breast cancer: a systematic review. Breast Cancer Res Treat 2005;90:263–71.

[56] Ahmed RL, Thomas W, Yee D, et al. Randomized controlled trial of weight training and lymphedema in breast cancer survivors. J Clin Oncol 2006;24:2765–72.

[57] Hase K, Kamisako M, Fujiwara T, et al. The effect of zaltoprofen on physiotherapy for limited shoulder movement in breast cancer patients: a single-blinded before-after trial. Arch Phys Med Rehabil 2006;87:1618–22.

[58] Lauridesen MC, Christiansen P, Hessov IB. The effects of physiotherapy on shoulder function in patients surgically treated for breast cancer: a randomized study. Acta Oncol 2005;44: 449–57.

[59] Ferreira de Rezende L, Franco RL, Ferreira de Rezende M, et al. Two exercise schemes in postoperative breast cancer: comparison of effects on shoulder movement and lymphatic disturbance. Tumori 2006;92:55–61.

[60] Silver J, Mayer RS. Barriers to pain management in the rehabilitation of the surgical oncology patient. J Surg Oncol 2007;95:427–35.

[61] Cella DF, Tulsky DS, Gray G, et al. The functional assessment of cancer therapy scale: development and validation of the general measure. J Clin Oncol 1993;11(3):570–9.

[62] Coscarelli Schag CA, Heinrich RL. Development of a comprehensive quality of life measurement tool: CARES. Oncology 1990;4(5):135–8.

[63] Coscarelli Schag CA, Ganz PA, Heinrich RL. Cancer rehabilitation evaluation system—short form (CARES-SF). Cancer 1991;68:1406–13.

[64] Spitzer WO, Dobson AJ, Hall J, et al. Measuring the quality of life of cancer patients: a concise QL index for use by physicians. J Chronic Dis 1981;34:585–97.

[65] Watt-Watson JH, Graydon JE. Sickness impact profile: a measure of dysfunction with chronic pain patients. J Pain Symptom Manage 1989;4:152–6.

[66] Bardsley MJ, Astell S, McCallum A, et al. The performance of three measures of health status in an outpatient diabetes population. Diabet Med 1993;10:619–26.

[67] Hays RD, Sherbourne CD, Mazel RM. The RAND 36-item health survey 1.0. Health Econ 1993;2(3):217–27.

[68] Aaronson NK, Bullinger M, Ahmedzai S. A modular approach to quality of life assessment in cancer clinical trials. Recent Results Cancer Res 1988;111:231–49.

[69] Aaronson NK, Ahmedzai S, Bergman B, et al. The European organisation for research and treatment of cancer QLQ-C30: a quality-of-life instrument for use in international clinical trials in oncology. J Natl Cancer Inst 1993;85(5):365–76.

[70] Watson M, Law M, Maguire GP, et al. Further development of a quality of life measure for cancer patients: the Rotterdam symptom checklist (revised). Psychooncology 1992;1:35–44.

[71] Westrup JL, Lash TL, Thwin SS, et al. Risk of decline in upper-body function and symptoms among older breast cancer patients. J Gen Intern Med 2006;21:327–33.

[72] Carpenter JS, Sloan P, Andrykowski MA, et al. Risk factors for pain after mastectomy/lumpectomy. Cancer Pract 1999;7:66–70.

[73] Stevens PE, Dibble SL, Miaskowski C. Prevalence, characteristics, and impact of postmastectomy pain syndrome: an investigation of women's experiences. Pain 1995;61:61–8.

[74] Carpenter JS, Andrykowski MA, Sloan P, et al. Postmastectomy/postlumpectomy pain in breast cancer survivors. J Clin Epidemiol 1998;51:1285–92.

[75] Foley KM. Pain syndromes in patients with cancer. Med Clin North Am 1987;71:169–84.

[76] Robb KA, Williams JE, Duvivier V, et al. A pain management program for chronic cancer-treatment-related pain: a preliminary study. J Pain 2006;7:82–90.

[77] Watkins T, Maxeiner A. Musculoskeletal effects of ovarian cancer and treatment: a physical therapy perspective. Rehabil Oncol 2003;21(2):12–7.

[78] Servaes P, Verhagen C, Bleijenberg G. Fatigue in cancer patients and after treatment: prevalence, correlates and interventions. Eur J Cancer 2002;38:27–43.

[79] Broeckel JA, Jacobsen PB, Horton J, et al. Characteristics and correlates of fatigue after adjuvant chemotherapy for breast cancer. J Clin Oncol 1998;16:1689–96.

[80] Loge J, Abrahamsen A, Ekeberg C, et al. Fatigue and psychiatric morbidity among Hodgkin's disease survivors. J Pain Symptom Manage 2000;19:91–9.

[81] Servaes P, van-der-Werf S, Prins J, et al. Fatigue in disease-free cancer patients compared with fatigue in patients with chronic fatigue syndrome. Support Care Cancer 2001;9:11–7.

[82] Longman AJ, Braden CJ, Mishel MH. Side effects burden, psychological adjustment, and life quality in women with breast cancer: pattern of association over time. Oncol Nurs Forum 1999;26:909–15.

[83] Mallinson T, Cella D, Cashy J, et al. Giving meaning to measure: linking self-reported fatigue and function to performance of everyday activities. J Pain Symptom Manage 2006;31:229–41.

[84] Van Weert E, Hoekstra-Weebers J, Otter R, et al. Cancer-related fatigue: predictors and effects of rehabilitation. Oncologist 2006;11:184–96.

[85] Matsuda T, Takamaya T, Tashiro M, et al. Mild cognitive impairment after adjuvant chemotherapy in breast cancer patients—evaluation of appropriate research design and methodology to measure symptoms. Breast Cancer 2005;12:279–87.

[86] Bender CM, Ergun FS, Rosensweig MQ, et al. Symptom clusters in breast cancer across 3 phases of the disease. Cancer Nurs 2005;28:219–25.

[87] Hickey M, Saunders CM, Stuckey BGA. Management of menopausal symptoms in patients with breast cancer: an evidence-based approach. Lancet Oncol 2005;6:687–95.

[88] Mock V, Frangakis C, Davidson NE, et al. Exercise manages fatigue during breast cancer treatment: a randomized controlled trial. Psychooncology 2005;14:464–77.

[89] Hewitt JA, Mokbel K, van Someren KA, et al. Exercise for breast cancer survival: the effect on cancer risk and cancer-related fatigue. Int J Fertil 2005;50:231–9.

[90] Carroll DG. Nonhormonal therapies for hot flashes in menopause. Am Fam Physician 2006; 73:457–64, 467.

[91] Perez DG, Loprinzi CL. Newer antidepressants and other nonhormonal agents for the treatment of hot flashes. Compr Ther 2005;31:224–36.

[92] Stearns V, Loprinzi CL. New therapeutic approaches for hot flashes in women. J Support Oncol 2003;1:11–21.

[93] Pandya KJ, Morrow GR, Roscoe JA, et al. Lancet 2005;366:818–24.

ELSEVIER
SAUNDERS

Phys Med Rehabil Clin N Am
18 (2007) 539–553

PHYSICAL MEDICINE
AND REHABILITATION
CLINICS OF
NORTH AMERICA

Current and Future Trends in Lymphedema Management: Implications for Women's Health

Andrea L. Cheville, MD, MSCE

*Department of Physical Medicine and Rehabilitation, Mayo Clinic,
200 First Street SW, Rochester, MN 55905, USA*

This article presents a comprehensive overview of cancer-related lymphedema in women. However, its secondary agenda is to increase the reader's awareness of changing trends in lymphedema incidence and practice patterns that may have important future public health implications. Breast cancer unquestionably brought lymphedema to national awareness and will remain an important lymphedema-related focus. However, it is time that we broadened our vision and recognized the growing problem of lymphedema in other populations. The forces that placed lymphedema at the forefront of cancer survivorship concerns are shifting.

Understanding lymphedema requires an examination of past, current, and future practice patterns. In the early 1990s lymphedema was seldom mentioned, and then solely to advise patients that a compression pump or sleeve might be helpful [1]. The dramatic expansion in the availability and caliber of lymphedema care over the past 17 years can be attributed to breast-cancer–related political advocacy, high-quality epidemiological and quality-of-life research, growing emphasis on cancer survivorship, and the introduction of a truly effective treatment modality. In concert, these factors have made lymphedema screening and prevention an integral part of comprehensive cancer care. Consciousness has been dramatically raised among oncologic clinicians and more patients than ever are being appropriately referred for lymphedema treatment.

The progress achieved through breast cancer lymphedema advocacy is extremely welcome as shifting epidemiological trends increase the proportion of medically complex patients presenting to lymphedema clinics. Images of the typical lymphedema patient as a middle-aged breast cancer

E-mail address: cheville.andrea@mayo.edu

1047-9651/07/$ - see front matter © 2007 Elsevier Inc. All rights reserved.
doi:10.1016/j.pmr.2007.06.001

pmr.theclinics.com

survivor with a swollen arm are inappropriate if not frankly inaccurate. With the alarming rise in obesity, lymphedema clinics are grappling with an influx of morbidly obese patients with lower-extremity lymphedema. Recurrent cellulitis, unhealing wounds, and mycotic infestation are common among this cohort [2]. Many of these patients come from lower socio-economic strata and, consequently, have limited resources to devote to lymphedema treatment [3]. Shifting population demographics have led to an increase in elderly lymphedema patients, many of whom have medical comorbidities and limited capacity to perform the maintenance activities required for long-term lymphedema control [4].

The epidemiology of cancer-related lymphedema is also changing. Innovations in primary breast cancer treatment designed to spare lymphatics (discussed below) have reduced lymphedema incidence in early-stage breast cancer patients. As a consequence, patients with high-risk breast cancer (eg, large tumors, lympho-vascular invasion, positive lymph nodes), whose breast cancers are is most likely to recur, constitute an increasing proportion of lymphedema patients. Cancer recurs in 30% to 35% of these patients [5,6]. Thanks to improved antihormonal and antineoplastic agents, they live considerably longer with stage IV disease. Hence, a greater proportion of breast-cancer–related lymphedema develops in patients with stage IV disease or in those at high risk of recurrence. The clinical demands of caring for these patients can be substantial.

Similar trends are affecting other female cancer cohorts and resulting in more cases of lymphedema. Patients with gynecological, colon, and bladder malignancies, as well as pelvic sarcomas, are generally living longer with stage IV disease [7,8]. Increasing numbers of patients with ovarian cancer are living to develop lymphedema. Lymphedema awareness has fortunately extended beyond breast cancer and more patients with lymphedema secondary to other malignancies are finding their way to lymphedema clinics. Many of these patients have been aggressively treated with combined modality therapies. Such treatments not only can cause lymphedema but also can trigger a host of other complications that must be addressed for treatment to succeed. The forces that are extending cancer 5-year survival rates—principally, better screening techniques, a wider range of anticancer drugs, and greater sophistication in combined modality therapy—will continue in the foreseeable future. We can therefore expect that increasing numbers of cancer patients will live to develop lymphedema.

Is lymphedema a gender issue?

Lymphedema unrelated to cancer occurs more often in women than in men. Eighty-three percent of primary lymphedema (lymphedema that develops in the absence of iatrogenic or other sources of lymphatic compromise) patients are female [9]. This estimate must be interpreted as imprecise because definitive epidemiological work is lacking. However, anecdotal clinical experience corroborates the preponderance of women among lymphedema patients. This phenomenon may be partially explained by the higher prevalence of obesity in women [3]. As suggested above, an elevated body mass index is a risk factor for lymphedema [10]. Obese women without histories of lymphatic compromise are frequent lymphedema patients. Recent projections anticipate a continued rise in the prevalence of female obesity, which will undoubtedly have an impact on the future composition of lymphedema patients [3].

Assessing lymphedema risk

All patients who have undergone lymph node resection or irradiation are at some risk of developing lymphedema. Generally, lymphedema risk increases directly as treatments become more aggressive and anatomically disruptive [10,11]. Each patient's "at risk" territory depends on the lymphotome or lymphotomes affected by their treatment. A lymphotome is the territory drained by a superficial lymph node bed. Fig. 1 shows the body's six superficial lymph node beds (ie, a pair of cervical/supraclavicular beds, a pair of axillary beds, and a pair of inguinal beds) and their associated lymphotomes. Breast cancer patients are solely at risk in the axillary lymphotome on their affected side. The axillary lymphotome encompasses the ipsilateral arm, breast, and upper truncal quadrant. Patients treated for gynecological cancers potentially have much more extensive territory at risk. Their pelvic and peri-aortic lymph nodes may have been resected and irradiated. These deep nodes receive lymph from both superficial inguinal beds, which drain the lower extremities, lower truncal quadrants, and external genitalia. Due to extensive compromise of these deep lymph nodes, treatment of gynecological cancers places the entire lower half of the body at risk for lymphedema. Despite the potential for widespread lymphedema, patients generally present with lower-extremity swelling.

Many factors have been studied with regard to lymphedema risk. The contribution of obesity and weight gain to lymphedema development has been previously mentioned. Of note, obesity increases risk of lymphedema progression and refractoriness to conventional therapy [10,12]. Venous insufficiency and recurrent soft tissue infections may harm the lymphatic system and undermine lymph drainage [13]. The underlying mechanisms are imperfectly understood. Medical comorbidities, including diabetes, hypertension, congestive heart failure, and autoimmune conditions, have not been implicated in lymphedema despite considerable epidemiological scrutiny. Vocational and avocational pursuits that require vigorous and repetitive upper-extremity use do not appear to increase lymphedema risk in breast cancer patients [12,14]. Similar studies have yet to be conducted with patients who have developed or are at risk of lower-extremity

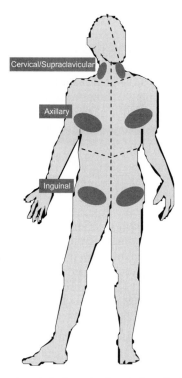

Fig. 1. Three pairs of lymph node beds receive lymph from the body's six lymphotomes.

lymphedema. It has been suggested that postoperative complications, such as infection, axillary web syndrome, and seroma or hematoma formation, increase lymphedema risk. Prospective cohorts of sufficient size have not been followed to definitively address these concerns.

Primary prevention

The success of researchers and breast cancer patient advocates in bringing lymphedema to popular attention has spurred surgical innovations that reduce axillary lymph node compromise. Sentinel lymph node biopsy (SLNB) represents the most recent and significant step forward in this effort. In brief, SLNB involves the injection of radioactive tracer and blue dye into the soft tissue surrounding a breast tumor. When the axillary lymph node bed is surgically exposed, visual inspection and a hand-held gamma probe allow identification of lymph nodes that have taken up both tracer and dye. These "sentinel lymph nodes" are then resected. Sentinel lymph nodes are subjected to rigorous pathological scrutiny. If metastases are not detected, no additional lymph nodes are removed. The absence of cancer cells in the sentinel lymph nodes supports the inference that cancer has not spread beyond the primary tumor. Further anticancer treatments are planned accordingly.

SLNB has become the standard approach to the initial axillary surgical sampling. SLNB represents a dramatic advance in that it reflects prioritization of patients' long-term functional status and morbidity among surgical outcomes. SLNB apparently has significantly reduced the incidence and severity of lymphedema among breast cancer survivors. Initial reports of zero incidence have emerged as overly optimistic [15]. Even so, the current best estimate of a 7% incidence at 6 months postoperation is an improvement over prevalence rates as high as 68% after full axillary lymph node dissection and irradiation [16].

One of the most challenging aspects of lymphedema is that by the time swelling becomes clinically obvious, significant changes have already occurred in the lymphatic system and interstitium. Anecdotal evidence suggests that these changes may be irreversible and, once established, preclude restoration of normal lymphatic homeostasis [17]. Several technologies show promise of detecting lymphedema in its preclinical phase. These are bioimpedance and high-frequency ultrasound [18,19]. However, these remain largely experimental and current evidence does not support their integration into clinical practice.

An additional impediment to primary prevention is the lack of empirically based models of lymphedema pathogenesis. Many primary-risk–reducing strategies have been rigorously endorsed [20]. Some make good theoretical sense and are aligned with general health recommendations (eg, avoiding sunburns and trauma to the at-risk body part). Other strategies, such as avoidance of exercise and repetitive upper-extremity use (in the case of breast cancer), have potentially adverse consequences for patients' quality of life and general well-being. Evidence suggests that exercise may reduce patients' risk of breast cancer recurrence by as much as 50% [21]. Further, well-designed trials increasingly suggest that exercise, when properly performed, may protect against lymphedema [22,23]. Thus, advice against exercise or other activities with quality-of-life implications must be carefully weighed in light of each patient's overall clinical picture and the shifting evidence base.

Additional common risk-reduction approaches include prophylactic use of a compression sleeve, avoidance of needle sticks and blood-pressure cuffs, avoidance of manicures, and use of protective clothing (eg, gloves) while engaging in tasks that may compromise skin integrity [24]. Endorsement of any approach to risk reduction, given the tenuous evidence base, should depend on a number of factors. These include patients' lymphedema risks, activity profiles (eg, frequency and duration of air travel), and anxiety levels regarding lymphedema. Given the previously mentioned challenges to accurate lymphedema-risk prediction, estimates are inevitably imprecise. However, patients who have undergone extensive surgical nodal clearing and irradiation are unquestionably at higher risk.

Thanks to expanded cancer survivorship services and the abundance of Web-based information, patients have ever-increasing awareness of their lymphedema risk. Inaccurate and sensational portrayals of lymphedema and lymphedema risk represent a down side to this generally desirable trend. Confronted by photos of advanced elephantiasis (stage III lymphedema), patients may experience understandably high levels of anxiety and inadvertently cause harm in their zeal to prevent lymphedema. Providing patients with accurate lymphedema-risk prevention information may, by relieving their anxiety, do much to improve their quality of life while potentially reducing their lymphedema risk very little [25].

The following paragraph offers a few pointers about the pros and cons of prophylactic compression garments. Many patients are instructed to obtain and wear compression garments during provocative circumstances (eg, air travel) [26]. Far from being a global recommendation, unmonitored garment use can cause significant problems. Garments should always be provided by a formally trained and experienced fitter. Poorly fit sleeves can trigger lymphedema. Constriction at the proximal band and the flexed elbow may severely impede lymph flow. Sleeves should always be dispensed with a glove or gauntlet. Compressing the arm may interrupt lymph drainage from the hand and potentially create a gradient that favors fluid accumulation in the hand. The author has managed patients whose hand lymphedema was unfortunately triggered by sole use of an overly tight sleeve without hand compression.

Though less problematic, proper fit remains a concern with lower-extremity garments. The issue of tight proximal bands is similar, compounded by the tendency of excessively long stockings to be rolled up or bunched and form a tourniquet. Patients should never fold over the proximal portion to reduce length. Additionally, most off-the-shelf stockings are designed for use in venous stasis disease, which generally spares the feet. Compression in most off-the-shelf stockings, therefore, begins at the distal calf and leaves the feet relatively uncompressed. A gradient may be established that favors fluid accumulation over the dorsal feet. Compressive footwear may offset the tendency for dorsal swelling, yet patients should remain vigilant.

Diagnosis

Timely diagnosis remains a barrier to optimal lymphedema treatment for many patients. The reasons for this are complex and aggravated by lymphedema's frequently insidious onset. While some patients develop dramatic acute swelling, more commonly initial swelling is transient without obvious precipitants. Patients, hopeful that the episode will be brief and isolated, do not recognize the incipient stage of lymphedema. Lymphedema generally progresses in the absence of treatment [27]. In light of mounting evidence that progression can be prevented through early treatment, failure of timely lymphedema referrals represents an important target for future improvement in lymphedema management [28].

A diagnosis of lymphedema should be entertained in any cancer patient that develops swelling or sensations of heaviness, tingling, fatigue, or aching within "at risk" territory, regardless of complicating vascular, cardiac, or endocrine factors [29]. Information should be sought regarding tightness of jewelry, clothing, or footwear. Careful inspection of all "at risk" territories should be made on clinical examination with vigilance for loss of anatomic architecture (eg, bony prominences, veins, tendons, skin creases) [30]. Subtle asymmetry should be sought in limb contour, recalling that while most lower-extremity lymphedema is bilateral, one limb is generally more involved. Rapidly progressive edema, particularly with associated pain or neurological deficits, should raise concern about recurrent cancer.

Lymphoscintigraphy may be diagnostically helpful in cases of etiologic uncertainty, but is not generally required. Lymphoscintigraphy involves intradermal injection of technetium-labeled sulfur colloid, generally into the interdigital webspaces of the dorsal foot or hand [31]. A gamma camera records tracer movement in serial images obtained at 1-hour intervals for 4 to 6 hours. Lymphedema may cause reduced tracer movement, sluggish or failed arrival of tracer in draining lymph nodes, and a "dermal pattern" of tracer distribution indicating retrograde flow and lymphatic incompetence. Lymphoscintigraphy results are qualitative and therefore subject to inconsistent interpretation. Prognostication must be exceedingly conservative as long-term follow-up of a sufficiently large cohort has never been reported. Precise sensitivity and specificity estimates are also lacking. Anecdotally, lymphoscintigraphy has a high false-negative rate.

Treatment

Complex or complete decongestive therapy (CDT) represents the current international standard of care for lymphedema management as formalized in a white paper by the International Society of Lymphology in 2001 [32]. CDT, an intensive integration of manual approaches, achieves and maintains substantial volume reduction in most lymphedema patients. Surgical, dietary, and pharmacological approaches offer equivocal benefit at best, but can be considered when appropriate manual and compression therapy fails to achieve adequate reduction [13].

CDT is a multimodal, two-phase system that incorporates manual lymphatic drainage (MLD), multilayer short-stretch compressive bandaging, skin care, therapeutic exercise, and compression garments. The initial "reductive" phase, sometimes designated with a Roman numeral I, is primarily focused on reducing limb volume [33]. Typically, phase I CDT sessions include 45 minutes of MLD followed by the application of compression bandages and performance of remedial exercises. Treatment should ideally be performed 7 days per week. The 5-day workweek is accommodated by instructing patients and caregivers to rebandage over weekends. Compressive bandages must be left in place 21 to 24 hours per day for optimal volume reduction. The efficacy of treatment delivered at this intensity has been demonstrated in numerous case series [34–36]. Figs. 2 through 4 show pre- and post-CDT images in a patient with bilateral stage III lymphedema of the lower extremities.

Following maximal volume reduction, patients are gradually transitioned to phase II, a long-term maintenance program. During phase II, compressive garments are used during the day, and compressive bandages are applied overnight. Patients perform remedial exercises on a daily basis while bandaged, and receive MLD as needed. Phase II continues indefinitely and consistent adherence is required for long-term lymphedema control.

Compression forms the basis of virtually all successful lymphedema therapy. During CDT phases I and II, compression is achieved through the use of short-stretch bandages (Fig. 5). Short-stretch bandages have a high "working pressure" and compressive forces are maximal when the underlying muscles contract [37,38]. Bandages exert low "resting pressure" when muscles relax. A distal-to-proximal compression gradient is achieved by applying more layers of bandages distally, rather than increasing tension when bandages are applied. Foam may be used under bandages to increase patients' pressure tolerance, to apply focal pressure for restoration of normal anatomic contour, and to break down fibrosis. Caution must be exercised to ensure that overzealous use of foam does not compromise skin integrity.

Compression garments are essential during phase II CDT. Their use achieves multiple goals, including (1) improved lymphatic flow, (2) reduction of accumulated proteinaceous debris, (3) enhanced venous return, (4) proper shaping of the limb, (5) sustained volume control, (6) maintenance of skin integrity, and (7) protection of the limb from potential trauma.

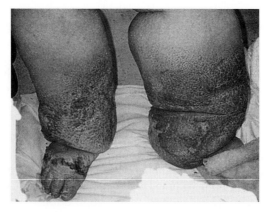

Fig. 2. Patient with primary stage III lymphedema.

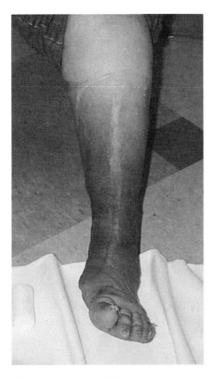

Fig. 3. Patient in Fig. 2 after dramatic lymphedema volume reduction and tissue softening achieved through phase I CDT.

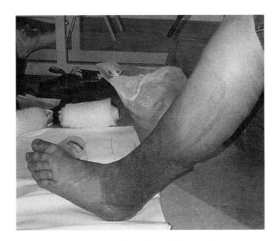

Fig. 4. Patient in Figs. 2 and 3, lateral view.

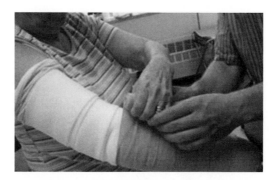

Fig. 5. Multilayer short-stretch bandages are applied with a distal-to-proximal compression gradient.

Garments may be prefabricated (off-the-shelf) or custom fitted, with the latter being either sewn or knitted (Fig. 6). Custom-knitted garments offer greater support and are recommended in advanced lymphedema. The need for custom garments must be determined on a case-by-case basis. General indications include irregular limb contour, compression requirements greater than or equal to 45 mm Hg, extensive fibrosis, and lymphedema progression with prefabricated garments. Prefabricated and custom garments can be combined, enabling patients to reap the significant cost savings afforded by prefabricated garments. For example, a custom sleeve might be combined with an off-the-shelf glove or vice versa. Garments should be replaced every 6 to 9 months.

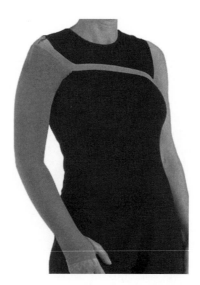

Fig. 6. One-piece compression sleeve and gauntlet.

MLD or "lymphatic massage" is a highly specialized technique that facilitates lymph sequestration and transport. Specific stroke duration, orientation, pressure, and sequence characterize MLD. MLD stimulates smooth muscle contraction in the lymph vessel walls, which underlies their inherent pumping action [37]. Through gentle, rhythmic skin distension, congested lymph is directed through intact lymph vessels into functioning lymphotomes with preserved drainage. MLD is administered with light finger or hand pressures of 30 mm Hg. Treatments begin with stimulation of intact lymph node beds and "clearing" of intact lymphotomes. Treatment of congested lymphotomes begins proximally, adjacent to the cleared territory, and gradually progresses "backwards" (distally and away from functioning lymphotomes) into congested territory. In this manner, lymphedematous areas are sequentially decongested. Hand strokes are constantly oriented toward functioning lymphotomes. The treatment ultimately moves far distally and generally terminates in the hands or feet.

"Remedial" lymphedema exercises are a very specific group of repetitive movements designed to encourage repeated muscle contractions within the lymphedematous territory. Remedial exercises are always performed with some form of external compression, most commonly garments or bandages. Rhythmic muscle contraction and relaxation gently compresses the lymph vessels, triggering smooth muscle contraction within the lymph vessel walls [17]. When external compression is adequate, an internal pumping mechanism is established that encourages lymph to flow along a compression gradient [37].

Skin care is an integral part of CDT and most important in advanced lymphedema when recurrent cellulitis is most common. The goals of skin care include controlling bacterial and fungal colonization, eliminating microbial overgrowth in skin crevices, and hydrating the skin to control dryness and fissuring. Daily cleansing with mineral-oil–based soap removes desquamated skin and bacteria while ensuring adequate skin moisture [37]. Topical antimicrobials, such as Batroban and Nystatin, may be required for patients troubled by recurrent infection.

Patients frequently inquire about the potential benefits of pumps and other compression devices. Current recommendations advise against the isolated use of external pumps to treat lymphedema. A single under-powered and unreplicated study suggests that pumps may be useful adjuncts to CDT [39]. More recently, the Flexitouch, a novel pumping device designed to mimic MLD, was introduced. Current evidence is insufficient to warrant endorsing the Flexitouch and its cost at $10,000 is prohibitive. More widely used, though admittedly also lacking a robust evidence base, are "alternative" compression devices. Recognizing that many lymphedema patients are unable or unwilling to bandage the recommended 7 nights per week, various manufacturers have developed "alternative" devices to substitute for nighttime bandaging. All conform to one of two basic designs. The simpler design is a long foam mitt or boot over which an elastic outer sleeve or stocking can be placed for greater compression. The Solaris Tribute, Jovi-Pak, Peninsula Medical Opera, and CircAid Silhouette garments conform to this design. The second design adds an outer canvas shell over the inner foam sleeve. Attached straps are cinched to create a compression gradient. The Peninsula Medical Reid Sleeve, CircAid Graduate (Fig. 7), and Leg-/Arm-Assist are examples of the second design. In the author's experience, patient tolerance of these devices varies dramatically. It is critical that patients appreciate the bulk and potentially cumbersome nature of these devices before substantial resources are invested in their purchase.

The current shortage of adequately trained lymphedema therapists in the United States is a frequent impediment to successful lymphedema decongestion. The Lymphology Association of North America (LANA) has developed a certification examination to accredit therapists with the knowledge base and manual skills required for successful lymphedema treatment. A list of certified therapists is available through the LANA Web site, www.cltlana.org. To sit for the LANA exam, therapists must have completed a training course of 135 hours or more offered by a variety of lymphedema schools. All schools have Web sites through which therapists in specific geographic regions can be located (www.nortonschool.com, www.acols.com, www.klosetraining.com, www.vodderschool.com). The National

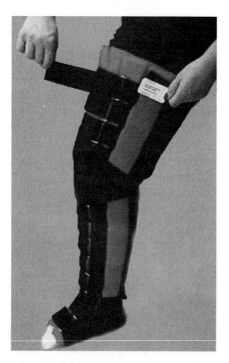

Fig. 7. CircAid Graduate nocturnal compression device. (*Courtesy of* CircAid Medical Products Inc., San Diego, CA; with permission.)

Lymphedema Network (www.lymphnet.org) also offers an extensive list of lymphedema-related resources. Patients with lymphedema complicated by recurrent cancer, dermal metastases, chemotherapeutic neuropathies, or pain may require specialized care generally only available through lymphedema specialists at tertiary centers.

Financial issues

Decongestive lymphedema therapy has been subject to inconsistent insurance coverage since its introduction to the United States in the early 1990s. The twice daily, 7-day-per-week treatment regimen, considered standard of care in Europe, is only available at self-pay clinics within the United States. Most care providers attempt to reproduce European success rates by treating patients 5 days per week with a heavy emphasis on patient self-care over the intervening weekends. The compromise in success rates with this adulterated regimen has yet to be rigorously quantified.

Lymphedema is a chronic condition and the associated costs mount indefinitely. Many lymphedema-related costs are not covered by conventional insurance. Medicare does not cover compression garments. Even basic off-the-shelf varieties can be expensive, at $100 to $150 for a sleeve and glove. If patients are to replace two sets every 6 months, the costs can become prohibitive. The expense of custom garments can be significant. Custom panty hose may cost as much as $500 to $700 per pair. Presenting a compelling case for custom garments to uninformed insurers requires physicians' limited time and energy. Many practitioners must confront the reality that it is untenable to make a case for all affected patients.

Future trends

The only down side of the progress that has been achieved in lymphedema prevention and management is the potential that clinicians, patients, and funding agencies will erroneously assume that lymphedema is a thing of the past. This could not be further from the truth. Relative to lymphedema from other causes, breast-cancer–related lymphedema will comprise a smaller proportion of future lymphedema cases. Nonetheless, breast-cancer–related lymphedema will remain problematic in the foreseeable future. In addition to the 7% or more of SLNB patients who develop lymphedema, lymphedema will affect up to 68% of the 30% to 35% of patients who present with node-positive breast cancer. This cohort is not only at highest risk of developing lymphedema, but also for developing severe, treatment-refractory lymphedema. The aging of the population, increasing prevalence of obesity, and extended cancer-survival rates will collectively ensure that lymphedema clinics will remain busy and challenged in the foreseeable future.

References

[1] Runowicz CD. Lymphedema: patient and provider education: current status and future trends. Cancer 1998;83(12 Suppl American):2874–6.

[2] Scheinfeld NS. Obesity and dermatology. Clin Dermatol 2004;22(4):303–9.

[3] Wang Y, Beydoun MA. The obesity epidemic in the United States—gender, age, socioeconomic, racial/ethnic, and geographic characteristics: a systematic review and meta-regression analysis. Epidemiol Rev 2007.

[4] Cesari M, Onder G, Russo A, et al. Comorbidity and physical function: results from the aging and longevity study in the Sirente geographic area (ilSIRENTE study). Gerontology 2006;52(1):24–32.

[5] Cady B. Case against axillary lymphadenectomy for most patients with infiltrating breast cancer. J Surg Oncol 1997;66(1):7–10.

[6] Bland KI, Menck HR, Scott-Conner CE, et al. The National cancer data base 10-year survey of breast carcinoma treatment at hospitals in the United States. Cancer 1998;83(6):1262–73.

[7] Institute NC. Surveillance epidemiology and end results database. Available at: http://seer.cancer.gov/.

[8] Society AC. Cancer facts & figures. Available at: http://www.cancer.org/docroot/STT/content/STT_1x_Cancer_Facts__Figures_2007.asp.

[9] Weissleder H. Lymphedema: diagnosis and treatment. Cologne (Germany): Viavital Verlag GmbH; 2001.

[10] Soran A, D'Angelo G, Begovic M, et al. Breast cancer-related lymphedema—what are the significant predictors and how they affect the severity of lymphedema? Breast J 2006;12(6):536–43.

[11] Goltner E. Das postmastektomie-lymphodem. In: Berens von Rautenfeld D, editor. Lymphologica. Bonn: Hannover: Kagerer Kommunikation; 1991.

[12] Johansson K, Ohlsson K, Ingvar C, et al. Factors associated with the development of arm lymphedema following breast cancer treatment: a match pair case-control study. Lymphology 2002;35(2):59–71.

[13] Szuba A, Rockson SG. Lymphedema: classification, diagnosis and therapy. Vasc Med 1998;3(2):145–56.

[14] Petrek JA, Senie RT, Peters M, et al. Lymphedema in a cohort of breast carcinoma survivors 20 years after diagnosis. Cancer 2001;92(6):1368–77.

[15] Erickson V, Pearson M, Ganz P, et al. Arm edema in breast cancer patients. J Natl Cancer Inst 2001;93:96–111.

[16] Wilke LG, McCall LM, Posther KE, et al. Surgical complications associated with sentinel lymph node biopsy: results from a prospective international cooperative group trial. Ann Surg Oncol 2006;13(4):491–500.

[17] Olszewski WL. Contractility patterns of normal and pathologically changed human lymphatics. Ann N Y Acad Sci 2002;979:52–63.

[18] Cornish BH, Chapman M, Hirst C, et al. Early diagnosis of lymphedema using multiple frequency bioimpedance. Lymphology 2001;34(1):2–11.

[19] Gniadecka M, Quistorff B. Assessment of dermal water by high-frequency ultrasound: comparative studies with nuclear magnetic resonance. Br J Dermatol 1996;135(2):218–24.

[20] Ridner SH. Breast cancer lymphedema: pathophysiology and risk reduction guidelines. Oncol Nurs Forum 2002;29(9):1285–93.

[21] Holmes MD, Chen WY, Feskanich D, et al. Physical activity and survival after breast cancer diagnosis. JAMA 2005;293(20):2479–86.

[22] Ahmed RL, Thomas W, Yee D, et al. Randomized controlled trial of weight training and lymphedema in breast cancer survivors. J Clin Oncol 2006;24(18):2765–72.

[23] McKenzie DC, Kalda AL. Effect of upper extremity exercise on secondary lymphedema in breast cancer patients: a pilot study. J Clin Oncol 2003;21(3):463–6.

[24] Network NL. Risk reduction position paper. Available at: http://www.lymphnet.org/pdfDocs/nlnriskreduction.pdf.

[25] Thomas-MacLean R, Miedema B, Tatemichi SR. Breast cancer-related lymphedema: women's experiences with an underestimated condition. Can Fam Physician 2005;51:246–7.

[26] Network NL. Air travel position paper. Available at: http://www.lymphnet.org/pdfDocs/nlnairtravel.pdf.

[27] Casley-Smith JR. Alterations of untreated lymphedema and it's grades over time. Lymphology 1995;28(4):174–85.

[28] Gergich N. Lymphedema secondary prevention. Paper presented at the National Lymphedema Network 7th International Conference. Nashville (TN), November 2–5, 2006.

[29] Armer JM, Radina ME, Porock D, et al. Predicting breast cancer-related lymphedema using self-reported symptoms. Nurs Res 2003;52(6):370–9.

[30] Society AC. Lymphedema: understanding and managing lymphedema after cancer treatment. 2005.

[31] Szuba A, Shin WS, Strauss HW, et al. The third circulation: radionuclide lymphoscintigraphy in the evaluation of lymphedema. J Nucl Med 2003;44(1):43–57.

[32] Bernas MJ, Witte CL, Witte MH. The diagnosis and treatment of peripheral lymphedema: draft revision of the 1995 Consensus Document of the International Society of Lymphology Executive Committee for discussion at the September 3-7, 2001, XVIII International Congress of Lymphology in Genoa, Italy. Lymphology 2001;34(2):84–91.

[33] Foldi E, Foldi M, Weissleder H. Conservative treatment of lymphoedema of the limbs. Angiology 1985;36(3):171–80.

[34] Foldi M. [Lymphostatic diseases and their treatment. Pathological aspects. consequences for treatment]. Sem Hop Ther 1975;51(9):483–6 [in French].

[35] Ko DS, Lerner R, Klose G, et al. Effective treatment of lymphedema of the extremities. Arch Surg 1998;133(4):452–8.

[36] Morgan RG, Casley-Smith JR, Mason MR. Complex physical therapy for the lymphoedematous arm. J Hand Surg [Br] 1992;17(4):437–41.

[37] Cheville AL, McGarvey CL, Petrek JA, et al. Lymphedema management. Semin Radiat Oncol 2003;13(3):290–301.

[38] Partsch H, Mostbeck A. [Pathogenesis of phlebopathic and lymphogenous edemas]. MMW Munch Med Wochenschr 1980;122(22):821–2 [in French].

[39] Szuba A, Achalu R, Rockson SG. Decongestive lymphatic therapy for patients with breast carcinoma-associated lymphedema. A randomized, prospective study of a role for adjunctive intermittent pneumatic compression. Cancer 2002;95(11):2260–7.

ELSEVIER
SAUNDERS

Phys Med Rehabil Clin N Am
18 (2007) 555–575

PHYSICAL MEDICINE
AND REHABILITATION
CLINICS OF
NORTH AMERICA

Exercise for Health and Wellness at Midlife and Beyond: Balancing Benefits and Risks

Sheila A. Dugan, MD[1]

*Rush Medical College, Rush University Medical Center, 1725 W. Harrison Street,
Suite 970, Chicago, IL 60612, USA*

The health-promotion aspects of exercise and physical activity have been clearly documented and substantiated in the medical literature [1–3]. Many individuals turn to exercise to manage or prevent chronic medical conditions, control or reduce body weight, and reduce stress [4–6]. It has been shown that exercise can reduce the risk of breast cancer in women [7–9]. Exercise is positively correlated with cognitive function in older persons [10]. Moreover, exercise is an effective means of rehabilitation and is thought to contribute to injury prevention and functional ability in older persons [11–14].

Functional limitations

Identifying and managing functional limitations is an ever-increasing task for health care practitioners, especially those caring for aging females. Fifty-two million Americans are estimated to be living with physical limitation and disability secondary to injury, disease, birth defects, and the aging process [15]. Several researchers have identified a gender difference in reporting disability. Women are more likely to self-report disability than men [16,17]. A recent cross-sectional study of women of multiple races in an age range of 40 to 55 years found that approximately 20% self-reported limitations in physical functioning [18]. Clarification is needed regarding the role of age-related musculoskeletal changes, injuries, and diseases in causing these

---
[1] Department of Physical Medicine & Rehabilitation, Rush University Medical Center, 1725. W Harrison Street, Suite 970, Chicago, IL 60612, USA.
E-mail address: sheila_dugan@rush.edu

1047-9651/07/$ - see front matter © 2007 Elsevier Inc. All rights reserved.
doi:10.1016/j.pmr.2007.05.006
pmr.theclinics.com

limitations. Further, exercise is an important component of the functional restoration program and must be prescribed in a safe and efficient manner. Over the past two decades, women with a wide variety of medical conditions and physical disabilities have been counseled to partake in regular exercise programs. For some women who missed the boom in women's athletics after the early 1970s and Title IX, this may be their initial foray into exercise. Others have been active in sports all their lives or just later in life, perhaps following in the footsteps of their daughters. As in other age groups, exercise novices may be at risk of different musculoskeletal injuries than those common to women experienced in regular exercise. Sports-specific mechanisms of injury should be considered. Understanding the exercise, physical-activity, and previous-injury history of one's patient is important for diagnosing and managing her musculoskeletal injury. Remember too that injuries in older females impact a system with shrinking physiological reserves. Lifestyle issues and changes associated with aging must be considered when evaluating women and exercise. For example, postpartum pelvic floor weakness can be the precursor to urinary incontinence, pelvic pain, and lumber pain later in life. Soft tissue atrophy and bone density loss in the setting of declining estrogen levels cause changes in strength and posture that may predispose a woman to injury in the perimenopause and postmenopause period. In a system with reduced estrogen, pain related to the musculoskeletal system may be more symptomatic [19]. Master athletes have degenerative changes of the spine and extremities that may limit joint mobility, leading to altered movement patterns and increased injury risk.

Midlife and cardiovascular disease risk profile

Women in midlife tend to gain weight and develop a variety of risk factors for cardiovascular disease. It has been shown that women who are physically active tend to be leaner and have a better lipid profile (higher high-density lipoprotein and lower low-density lipoprotein, triglycerides, and glucose) than women who are not physically active. The impact of physical activity on health outcomes is beneficial. In cross-sectional studies, physical activity was significantly predictive of body mass index [20]. In a longitudinal study, an increase in sports participation or exercise was associated with decreases in weight and in waist circumference [21]. An Australian study of an intervention involving diet and exercise showed significant improvements in weight, body mass index, waist circumference, and diastolic blood pressure [22]. In a clinical trial in the United States, physical activity and diet together were successful in preventing weight gain from pre-, to peri-, to postmenopause and reduced rises in low-density lipoprotein cholesterol, triglycerides, and glucose [23]. The same study reported later that the progression in intima-media thickness, a measure of atherosclerosis, was slowed in the intervention group [24]. In the Nurses' Health Study, obesity (whether measured by body mass index or waist girth) and physical inactivity independently contributed to the development of coronary heart disease in women followed over 20 years [25].

Menopause itself, rather than age alone, brings an increase in cardiovascular disease risk. Physical activity may be able to ameliorate this risk. A cross-sectional study of a biracial sample of women at midlife demonstrated that physical activity negatively correlated with intraabdominal fat independent of multiple covariates as measured by CT [26] (Fig. 1). Intraabdominal fat is associated with higher risk of cardiovascular disease. The study shows that motivating white and black women to increase their physical activity during their middle years can positively modify age-related increases in intraabdominal fat, which in turn may improve cardiovascular disease risk profiles. In addition, mood has been shown to have an independent effect on cardiovascular disease. Depression and depressive symptoms were significantly associated with cardiovascular disease morbidity and mortality [27]. The same researchers found that the associations between depressive symptoms and insulin resistance and risk for diabetes in a sample of middle-aged women were largely mediated by central adiposity, as assessed by waist circumference [28]. Exercise and physical activity can improve mood, providing another means to improve one's cardiovascular disease risk profile in midlife.

Goals of article

This article addresses musculoskeletal disorders that can present in women at midlife and later. Beyond understanding the disorders and their

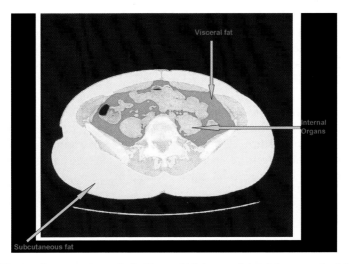

Fig. 1. CT scan demonstrating a single 10-mm thick image of the abdomen at the L4-L5 vertebral space to quantify amount of visceral fat area, subcutaneous fat area, and total abdominal fat area.

management, individuals caring for women must recognize that rehabilitation goals may differ across a woman's life span. For some women, returning to competition as soon as possible, without risking ongoing injury, is their challenge. For others, returning to independent performance of activities of daily living may suffice. In moving forward with both basic science and clinical issues, clinicians must continue to examine how activity modifies the musculoskeletal system, both negatively and positively, thus making the best use of exercise for promoting health, preventing injury, and fostering rehabilitation. The task for health care practitioners and exercise scientists is to identify the appropriate "dosing" of exercise to achieve desired goals and avoid undesirable side effects. Nowhere is this more relevant than with the aging female. For example, clinicians must develop exercise programs that limit joint injuries and decrease the force of impacts and the size of torsional loads in high-impact activities. Such exercise programs would diminish the risk of osteoarthritis while delivering site-specific loading of bone to enhance osteogenesis and limit postmenopausal osteoporosis. Thankfully, first-rate research continues on these challenging fronts.

The aging process

As the body ages, it loses its capacity to adapt because of structural change and loss of reserve in multiple-organ systems. As early as the fourth decade of life, a decline in capacity begins, involving the cardiovascular, pulmonary, hormonal, thermoregulatory, and nervous systems. This decline contributes to a decline in health and function. Changes particular to the musculoskeletal system can lead directly to painful and disabling conditions in the aging female and are discussed below. When considering a current musculoskeletal condition, clinicians should keep in mind that concurrent medical conditions, the effects of previous illnesses and injuries, and the side effects of medical treatments may be implicated. Certain behaviors earlier in life, in particular those related to physical activity, may be implicated in a real-time musculoskeletal condition but are not modifiable later in life. For instance, strong evidence indicates that physical activity as a youth contributes to peak bone density [29–31]. Previous injury to a joint has been associated with osteoarthritis [32,33]. However, it is important to consider the contemporaneous effects of such behaviors for current and future health concerns when dealing with an older population.

Musculoskeletal changes associated with aging

Bone resorption is age-related with bone density decreasing after the age of 50. This is likely related more to loss of bone volume than mineralization, the latter being largely unaffected by the aging process alone. Osteoporotic vertebral fractures are a more common cause of morbidity in elderly women than in elderly men. Bone density, mineral content, and bone strength losses can be ameliorated through more physical activity. This can be affected regionally. For instance, study participants performing calisthenics and low-impact aerobics increased their lumbar spine bone density [34]. A recent review article reported that progressive-resistance training has been shown to have a more potent impact on bone density than cardiovascular exercise [31]. Refer to the chapter on osteoporosis by Sinaki in this issue for a more comprehensive review of this subject.

The joint capsules become stiffer with age, which leads to a loss of active and passive range of motion. Articular cartilage degeneration is related to age, as well as to joint geometry, sex, injury, activity history, and genetics. Age-related proteoglycan structural changes have been identified and are more fully discussed in the osteoarthritis section below. Functional limitations frequently become the final common pathway of loss of range of motion, strength, and endurance. Radiographic studies have demonstrated that disc degeneration is found uniformly by the eighth decade of life [35]. This is associated with spondylosis, including osteophytes at the vertebral endplates and zygoaphophyseal joints. Degenerative changes in collagen are also in part age-related and occur at the cellular and morphological level. Most studies of age-related changes in tendons and ligaments have focused on the peripheral joints, with the anterior cruciate ligament most commonly studied. Decline in the proprioceptive function of these tissues has been documented [36]. Muscle demonstrates the most evident changes with aging. These changes include loss of muscle mass and decline in the number of motor units, especially type II fibers [37]. This results in a reduced ability to generate force, which can impact functional activity. Muscle mass is a major determinant of age- and gender-related differences in strength. Once function is impaired, a downward spiral of deconditioning or injury can bring significant morbidity. Globally, the reaction time of elders is reduced due to multiple peripheral and central factors. An example of the former is the age-related slowing of motor and sensory nerve conduction velocities. Motor unit recruitment declines centrally. Comorbid factors in the elderly include chronic disease processes and medications directly or indirectly impacting the nervous system. Sensory changes affecting the visual, vestibular, and proprioceptive systems can be age-related or illness-related. Any decline in sensory processing affects the motor responsiveness. Postural control is impaired and can lead to loss of balance. Falling and the fear of falling can be debilitating. Health care practitioners for women must recognize how these physiological and biomechanical changes affect health and function. Functional loss leads to safety concerns and further deconditioning, causing a vicious downward spiral, at times with high morbidity and mortality. This can be a precipitous decline, such as that following a hip fracture in a frail, debilitated elderly female, or a more gradual decline, such as when an elderly female with osteoarthritis becomes isolated in her home as her pain increases and she loses strength, endurance, and balance.

Osteoarthritis: a global musculoskeletal disorder

Osteoarthritis, the most common joint disorder, affects over 25 million Americans, leading to a large economic and functional burden on individuals and society [38–40]. Disability attributable to knee osteoarthritis is equal to that for cardiac disease and greater than that for any other medical condition in the elderly [41–43]. It is also important to consider the impact of osteoarthritis in younger women. A recent cross-sectional study identified radiographic evidence of hand and knee osteoarthritis in women under age 40, with a higher prevalence of knee osteoarthritis in African-American women (23.1%) compared with that in Caucasian women (8.5%) [44].

Osteoarthritis is a chronic, degenerative joint disease characterized by focal articular cartilage loss with variable amounts of subchondral bone reaction. It is a disease of the cartilage of weight-bearing joints primarily with "wear and tear" as a presumptive etiology. The articular or hyaline cartilage is composed of collagen (providing strength), chondrocytes (providing viscous synovial fluid for lubrication), and proteoglycans (providing distensibility and hydration). As loads are placed across the joint, cartilage and subchondral bone can be damaged, especially if the joint has an abnormal alignment. This damage leads to loss of adequate proteoglycan synthesis and release of lysosomal proteases that cause further cell death.

The association between physical activity and osteoarthritis has been studied primarily in areas of (1) level of activity, especially sports participation; (2) postinjury osteoarthritis (secondary osteoarthritis); and (3) exercise in managing osteoarthritis. There have been few well-controlled prospective longitudinal studies in these areas. The strongest evidence correlates previous injury with developing osteoarthritis [45–47]. Studies looking at exercise as treatment for osteoarthritis have shown that exercise can limit the disability associated with osteoarthritis in elderly individuals [48].

Animal research shows that normal repetitive weight-bearing use of a joint preserves the structure and function of the joint [49]. In vitro studies of chondrocytes have shown that loading in the physiologic range stimulated proteoglycan synthesis and improved flow of nutrients [50]. The articular surfaces of joints demonstrated degeneration when loading was prohibited [51]. Prolonged joint disuse results in structural degeneration of cartilage. Despite these findings, a recent review article evaluating the relationship between physical activity and osteoarthritis prevention concluded that no studies demonstrate direct preventive effects of physical activity on the development of osteoarthritis [52]. A more salient concept for rehabilitation providers is the risk to cartilage if immobilization is prescribed.

Studies have been contradictory in associating level of activity and developing osteoarthritis. Framingham study data were used to evaluate the level of current physical activity and the risk of radiographic, symptomatic knee osteoarthritis in older individuals (mean age: 70.1 years; SD: 4.5 years) and demonstrated that current heavy weight-bearing exercise in elderly men and women may increase the risk [53]. Researchers loosely defined heavy weight-bearing exercise as lifting greater than 5 lb, outdoor work with heavy tools, and "other strenuous sports or recreational activity." The researchers concluded that elderly men and women engaging in greater than 3 h/d of heavy physical activity for many years have an increased risk of knee osteoarthritis. The risk was greatest in subjects with the highest body mass index, demonstrating the link between obesity and osteoarthritis found in other studies [54]. Another study using Framingham data found no increased risk of symptomatic knee osteoarthritis in men or women who engaged in regular physical activity in their middle years [55]. A prospective study of adults correlated self-reported physician diagnosis of osteoarthritis with running greater than 20 miles/wk in men under 50 years old but found no such relationship among older men or women under or over 50 years of age [56]. The general consensus is that runners without underlying lower-extremity biomechanical abnormalities are at no additional risk of developing osteoarthritis [57].

There has been limited success with defining a dose-response curve between physical activity and osteoarthritis. In addition to time of exposure, factors such as torsional loading and speed of force application are relevant, with slowly applied loads considered better tolerated, perhaps due to damping by muscles [52]. Increased development of osteoarthritis may be associated with sports that involve tortional impacts or apply torsional loads over time, but this has not been specifically defined.

Several risk factors have been identified for osteoarthritis. Osteoarthritis of the knee, the hand, and possibly the hip is more prevalent in women, especially postmenopausal women, than in men, suggesting that hormonal changes play a role [58]. Researchers concluded that postmenopausal estrogen-replacement therapy might protect against osteoarthritis of the hip in elderly white women [59]. It is difficult to ascertain whether there are gender differences in how physical activity impacts individuals either in the development or treatment of osteoarthritis. Matching men and women by activity to confirm and identify such a difference has been difficult. In addition, other prevailing factors, including genetic predisposition, equipment use, and quality of performance, may play a significant role in physical activity contributing to osteoarthritis. Obesity has repeatedly been correlated with knee osteoarthritis [46,58]. Exercise prescription for obese women presents a rehabilitation challenge. Low-impact aerobic activity without torsional loading is likely the best mode of exercise in this population.

Regional musculoskeletal disorders in midlife and older women

Common spinal disorders

Cervical spondylosis

Spondylosis is the term for progressive bony changes of the spine. Spinal degeneration begins with loss of intervertebral disc height, leading to changes in disc and spinal ligaments. Altered patterns of load-bearing in the spine arise with resultant sclerosis of the vertebral body, uncovertebral joints (cervical spine) and zygoapophyseal joints (z-joints), as described in the lumbar spine [60]. While most older persons do not experience symptoms related to spondylosis, symptomatic patients describe axial neck pain, muscle spasm, stiffness, and loss of motion. Cervical radiculopathy (nerve root injury) or cervical myelopathy (spinal cord injury) can result from narrowing due to progressive cervical sclerosis, loss of disc height, and soft tissue changes (disc herniation, ligament hypertrophy). Cervical myelopathy is the most common spinal cord injury at middle age and older [61]. It presents with gradual loss of motor strength and balance with gait dysfunction and fine motor deficits. Cervical radiculopathy (pathologic process affecting the nerve root) in adults affects most commonly, in order, the C7, C6, C8, and then the C5 nerve root with sensory, motor, and reflex involvement based on severity [62]. Pertinent findings on examination include loss of cervical spine range of motion; loss of accessory gliding at the vertebral segments, uncovertebral joints, and zygoapophyseal joints; and loss of flexibility in the muscles of the neck and thorax. Changes in the neurological examination relate to the root level or spinal cord level, if involved, including deficits on manual muscle testing, sensory testing, coordination testing, and reflex testing. In the setting of myelopathy, hyperreflexia may be demonstrated in the lower limbs due to the upper motor neuron lesion. Provocative maneuvers can be used to augment the physical examination of the neurological system. Spurling's test is done to reproduce discrete radicular symptoms in the lower cervical roots. The examiner places the patient's cervical spine in ipsilateral lateral flexion and extension and asks about radiating symptoms. If negative, an axial load can be applied through the head with the same query for radiating symptomatology.

Diagnostic testing with plain radiographs is not always necessary or useful as osteophytes may be age-related. Radiographs typically demonstrate the spondylosis described above (osteophytic spurs at the vertebral endplates, the uncovertebral joints, and the zygoapophyseal joints) and narrowing of the lateral or central foramina. Flexion and extension films are indicated if instability is a consideration. MRI delineates soft tissues, including disc, spinal cord, nerve root, and ligament (Fig. 2). As noted above, disc degeneration is ubiquitous by the eighth decade and care must be taken to corroborate findings on radiographic studies with the patient's presenting signs and symptoms. CT scan with or without myelography may be clinically useful in individual cases or when other tests are inconclusive. Electrodiagnostic studies (electromyogram, nerve conduction velocity, somatosensory-evoked potentials) can supplement imaging and help to determine acuity of lesions. Laboratory testing is generally normal.

The management of cervical spondylosis is typically nonsurgical. As in other musculoskeletal conditions, pain management is an initial focus. Oral medication, including nonsteroidal anti-inflammatory drugs

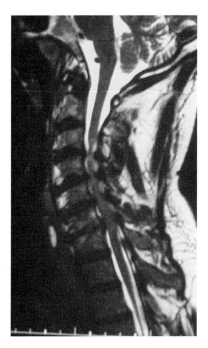

Fig. 2. MRI demonstrating cervical spondylosis with multilevel disc degeneration, ligamentous hypertrophy, osteophytic spurring, and central stenosis with spinal cord narrowing in a patient who presents with signs and symptoms consistent with cervical myelopathy.

(NSAIDS), cyclooxygenase 2 (COX-2) inhibitors, and various analgesics, can be prescribed with close attention to minimizing toxicities, especially in older individuals. Depending on the acuity of symptoms and the patient's preference, ice or heat can be applied topically. Deeper levels of tissue heating are achieved with therapeutic ultrasound. Therapeutic electrical stimulation modalities are used to stimulate local blood flow and reduce associated muscle spasm. Joint mobilization and stretching are employed and advanced as tolerated by the patient, with a goal of maximizing cervical spine range of motion. Long-standing postural abnormalities (eg, forward head) may not be amenable to significant alteration in older women; younger women are counseled regarding normal posture when posture modification is more likely. Manual therapy to evaluate and treat restricted cervical segments is used and requires a skilled practitioner.

The exercise program is tailored to address flexibility, strength, endurance, and motor-control deficits. Many adults have muscle imbalances with chronically shortened phasic musculature (pectoralis, latissimus dorsi, anterior scalene) and lengthened and weak tonic muscles (trapezius, rhomboids, spinal extensors). Once the imbalances are identified, manual resistance techniques are employed to correct the length/tension relationships.

Tactile cueing is frequently necessary to facilitate appropriate co-contraction in the cervicothoracic region. Functional assessment can identify activities of daily living and recreational activity that might be contributing to ongoing abnormal movement patterns. Resting positions and movement patterns can be evaluated ergonomically with recommendations given for adaptation as appropriate.

Interventional procedures, from epidural injections to nucleoplasty, and surgery may be indicated in specific cases, especially in the setting of discogenic or radicular pain. A review of the indications, contraindications, specific procedures, and outcomes of various surgical and interventional procedures are not included in this article.

Thoracic kyphosis

Kyphosis is abnormal curvature in the sagittal plane. Posterior thoracic convexity has been given a normal range of values of 20° to 40° by some investigators, but others have documented a wider range of normal values [63,64]. As one ages, there is a trend, especially in women, toward increased thoracic kyphosis and reduced lumbar lordosis. Kyphotic deformities that are not compensated for in the spinal segments above and below result in anterior spinal decompensation. Conversely, conditions that compromise the anterior structures (vertebral bodies), such as osteoporosis, infection, or tumor, will promote thoracic kyphotic deformity. Postural kyphosis is a term used to describe a flexible curve with poor carriage of the body. It typically corrects with the spine in extension or the subject in prone [65]. If this poor posture continues as one ages, the curve may become more fixed. There are many other etiologies of kyphosis; a review of these is beyond the scope of this article.

Symptomatic patients initially describe an intermittent achy pain that occurs over the apex of the curve. Women with more extensive curvatures may be at risk of disc disease, facet arthropathy, and foraminal and central stenosis and should be carefully questioned and examined to rule out neurological involvement. A history of neuromuscular disease, trauma, infection, surgery, radiation, or bone disease should be queried, as these can be etiologic factors in the development of kyphosis. Impingement of the rotator cuff tendons can occur in conjunction with the thoracic kyphosis because of limitation in scapular mobility on the thoracic wall. This causes abnormal kinematics of the glenohumeral joint leading to impingement of the rotator cuff tendons in the subacromial space. Physical examination includes observation, palpation to localize the pain, range-of-motion testing, and neurological testing. Compensatory hyperlordosis of the cervical and lumbar spine is expected. Evidence shows that kyphotic curves are larger in women older than 40 years than in men older than 40 [63]. During spinal active range of motion, kyphosis in older woman corrects incompletely with extension. Associated flexibility deficits include tight hamstrings and hip flexors. In patients complaining of associated shoulder pain, a complete examination of the shoulder is indicated to assess scapulothoracic rhythm and rule out rotator-cuff tear. Diagnostic testing starts with posteroanterior and lateral radiographs of the spine. Flexion and extension views should be done if instability is a concern. One investigator found an indirect correlation between bone mineral density and thoracic kyphosis [66]. Bone density testing should be considered in the context of the individual woman's medical, menstrual, and family history. MRI, bone scan, and CT scans may also be useful in more complex cases, such as a woman presenting with neurological deficits. For treatment suggestions for symptomatic kyphosis, refer to the preceding section on cervical spondylosis. If the curve corrects with prone lying or extension, there is more opportunity for therapeutic exercise that includes stretching and strengthening to affect posture and symptomatology. In patients with associated rotator cuff impingement, muscular re-education of the scapula can improve scapulothoracic rhythm and should precede rotator cuff strengthening.

Thoracolumbar scoliosis

The incidence of scoliosis, or lateral deviation of the spine, increases with age and affects between 3% and 30% of the population [67]. Scoliosis diagnosed in adults develops before skeletal maturity and is not previously diagnosed or is secondary to bone remodeling issues, such as osteoporosis, osteomalacia, postoperative changes, or degenerative changes [68]. In one review, which found that 3.9% of adults had thoracolumbar or lumbar scoliotic curve that developed in adolescence and progressed in adult life, about 60% of the subjects had spinal pain [69]. Idiopathic scoliosis, the most common type of scoliosis, has a much greater incidence in females. It is difficult to correlate pain symptoms with severity of curve; curves less than 20° are typically asymptomatic while curves greater than 60° lead to impairment in the intraabdominal and thoracic organ systems and neurological structures. As with other spinal lesions, the history includes specific questioning on the location, duration, characteristics, and behavior of the pain. Aggravating and relieving factors can assist in identifying the tissue generating pain. The physical examination includes not only a thorough musculoskeletal assessment, but also a detailed neurological exam to rule out radiculopathy. Right thoracic and left lumbar curvature is the usual presentation. Side to side comparison of shoulder heights, inferior angle of scapula, iliac crest, and leg lengths is important. Long-standing curves can cause abnormalities and asymmetry of the pelvis and hips, which must be evaluated and treated. Manual assessment of the spinal segments and provocative maneuvers of the disc and zygoapophyseal joints are included. The examiner should screen for diseases associated with scoliosis. A joint survey should be completed to assess for Marfan's syndrome. A thorough skin assessment for any stigmata of neurofibromatosis is important. Initial radiographs should include standing posteroanterior and lateral thoracolumbar views [68] (Fig. 3). Serial measurements of the Cobb angle can assess for

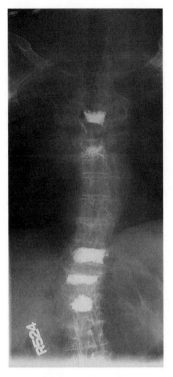

Fig. 3. Posterior anterior radiograph of patient with thoracolumbar scoliosis and with most common presentation of right thoracic and left lumbar curvature.

progression of the curve. MRI can be useful when neurological dysfunction is present. CT scan used in conjunction with myelography can help rule out spinal cord compression. Bone density testing may be indicated in women with risk factors for osteoporosis because women with scoliosis have been shown to have lower bone mass than their peers [70,71].

Because of the inherent inability to correlate curvature measurement and symptoms, the task of making the correct decision on treatment is complex. Nonsurgical management is first-line, except in those patients with progressive neurological impairment. Intractable pain is the most common indication for surgery, but this is an area of controversy. A recent study of patients with idiopathic scoliosis compared surgical fusion patients to nonsurgical patients and to controls [72]. The surgical and nonsurgical groups did not have statistically different pain or functional scores. Both groups had similarly reduced spinal function scores and more complaints of back pain than controls did. Radiographic studies demonstrated similar degenerative changes in both groups of patients, despite surgical intervention. Idiopathic scoliosis patients with or without surgery have been shown to have greater disc degenerative changes [73]. However, these degenerative changes do not necessarily correlate to pain complaints, which concur with the findings of previous studies of scoliotic patients [74].

Rehabilitation practitioners attempt to localize the pain-generating structure to direct treatment. For example, zygoapophyseal joints can generate pain related to abnormal alignment, especially near the apex of the curve. Beyond oral anti-inflammatory and analgesic medications and modalities, possible treatment options include mobilization, manipulation, fluoroscopically guided steroid injections, and medial branch blocks. Interventional procedures can be diagnostic as well as therapeutic. It is beyond the scope of this article to review the indications, contraindications, risks, and benefits of these interventional procedures. They are generally used to control pain and facilitate participation in exercise and functional activities. As already mentioned, exercise protocols are based on reducing pain, restoring flexibility, increasing strength, and enabling the individual with scoliosis. Low-impact aerobics, cycling, and swimming are examples of acceptable forms of cardiovascular exercise. Collaborative research between operative and nonoperative spine physicians is needed to optimize care for scoliosis patients.

Lumbar degeneration and stenosis

While spinal degeneration is ubiquitous, back pain causes disability in about 20% of the elderly [33]. Inactivity may play a significant role in back pain in this age group. Spinal stenosis can result if these degenerative changes cause narrowing of the central canal or lateral foramina. While spinal stenosis is an endpoint of significant spondylosis, it usually progresses slowly and responds to conservative treatment. Symptoms cannot always be correlated with the extent of the stenosis [75–77].

Women with spinal stenosis frequently present with pain that radiates to the lower limbs in a pattern related to the level of stenosis. Aggravating activities include standing, walking, and other activities in which the lumbar spine is in an extended position. Positioning the lumbar spine in flexion typically relieves symptoms and patients will describe a phenomenon of pain reduction or relief upon sitting or forward bending in standing. Due to the variability of symptoms, many individuals do not use pain medications regularly. Diagnostic testing is pursued along the continuum of plain radiographs through MRI. MRIs provide a greater level of detail and are necessary for planning for injections and surgical approaches.

Oral medication, including NSAIDS, muscle relaxants, and analgesics, have increased incidence of adverse effects in older patients; use should be closely monitored. Caudal epidural steroid injections may be effective in reducing or alleviating symptoms at least temporarily [78]. A comprehensive therapy prescription for musculoskeletal back pain should include the following principles: pain control; mobilization; flexibility; strengthening; endurance; functional activity (eg, gait training, occupational- or sports-specific activity, ergonomics); and education, including training in an ongoing exercise program. Modalities, including cold or heat, electrical stimulation, and others, have not proven effective in treating musculoskeletal pain in randomized controlled trials. Modalities may have a role initially in pain management. It is thought that these modalities are not effective for the elderly with spinal degeneration [79]. There may be individual variation in response to modalities and one must be familiar with contraindications in their use, especially in older women with sensory impairments. Patients can be educated in home use of ice and heat if they demonstrate a thorough understanding of safe technique.

While exercise has been shown to be safe and effective in older individuals, there have been no randomized controlled studies examining the use of exercise in low back pain in this age group. In fact, some investigators warn specifically against back strengthening or extension exercises in elderly patients with spinal stenosis or spondylosis [80,81]. However, another investigator demonstrated that exercises over long periods were associated with less back pain in men [82]. In two observational studies without control groups, elderly patients of both sexes with low back pain were shown to tolerate a therapeutic exercise program [76,77]. A recent 10-year follow-up study of 100 individuals with lumbar stenosis concluded that surgical decompression resulted in excellent or fair result in 80% of patients compared with excellent or fair results in 50% of nonsurgical patients at the 4-year follow-up with no significant clinical deterioration over the next 6 years in either group. Patients who initially opted for nonsurgical management had favorable outcome with delayed surgery supporting a decision for initial conservative management [75].

Common appendicular disorders in midlife and older women

Hip and knee osteoarthritis

Women who come to medical attention with hip or knee osteoarthritis describe a history of moderate to severe pain, usually asymmetrical, and associated disability in weight-bearing activities. They may describe progressive limping. Recently, researchers identified a nonrandom pattern in the progression of lower-extremity osteoarthritis, demonstrating that patients who undergo a unilateral total hip replacement for end-stage osteoarthritis are much more likely to require a subsequent contralateral total knee replacement than an ipsilateral total knee replacement [83]. Pertinent physical examination findings include asymmetrical weight-bearing through the lower limbs and genu varum due to disproportionate loss of medial compartment knee joint cartilage. In long-standing cases, the examiner may visualize an enlarged knee joint and palpate nontender osteophytes at the joint line. Joint effusion is present inconsistently and generally associated with an acute inflammatory response. Crepitus may be appreciated with passive and active range of motion of the knee, especially with patellofemoral osteoarthritis. Loss of range of motion is seen in long-standing osteoarthritis. Variable loss of range of motion raises the possibility of a loose body in the joint line. Pain with active and passive range of motion is more likely in the setting of acute inflammation. Joint loading via squatting may elicit pain. The examiner can also load the joint and apply torsional forces with such maneuvers as patellar grinding, hip scouring, or McMurray's testing. McMurray's test is useful in identifying a torn meniscus. Ligamentous testing of the knee may reveal increased excursion, but this may be related to changes in joint congruity rather than pathological ligamentous laxity. The neurological examination is generally normal.

In patients with ongoing symptoms despite treatment or for presurgical planning, radiographs provide insight into the focality and severity of the joint degenerative changes. Weight-bearing films are recommended. Special views of the patellofemoral joint, such as the Merchant's or sunrise view, can be useful. Frog-leg views provide superior visualization of the hip. Disease progression can be elucidated. Treatment planning can be facilitated by more advanced imaging, such as MRI. Laboratory testing is typically normal.

The management of hip and knee osteoarthritis focuses on relieving pain and restoring function. Weight management can be helpful in both of these areas. No medical intervention has been shown conclusively to halt disease progression. In more advanced disease, a reduction in weight bearing through the involved limb with an assistive device may alleviate symptoms. Oral or topical anti-inflammatories and analgesics are used, with close attention to minimizing toxicities. NSAIDS and acetaminophen have been shown to have similar efficacy in reducing pain [84,85]. NSAID use is complicated by gastrointestinal toxicity in a dose-dependent manner. Other risk factors for gastrointestinal complications include advanced patient age and concurrent medical conditions. Selective COX-2 inhibitors were shown to be as valuable as NSAIDS in managing pain [86]. Celecoxib is currently still available in the United Status. Chondroitin sulfate (1200 mg/d) and glucosamine sulfate (1500 mg/d) supplements are taken in divided doses. Glucosamine provided pain relief comparable to NSAIDS in one study [87]. There may be a month-long delay between the start of therapy with glucosamine or chondroitin and the onset of pain reduction. No trials evaluating long-term use of either agent have been completed. Other nonoral medical treatments are prescribed frequently in the setting of osteoarthritis. In a meta-analysis of topical agents, investigators concluded that use of capsaicin (a derivative of cayenne pepper) cream resulted in some clinical improvement [88]. Intraarticular injections of corticosteroids are used for short-term symptom management. There is no consensus in the literature about the absolute number or timing of such injections. Clinical studies of hyaluronic acid intraarticular knee injections have shown clinical improvement but have not defined a specific viscosupplementation protocol [89]. Clinicians typically inject weekly for 3 to 5 weeks. A recent study concluded that the combined use of hyaluronic acid injections with home exercise programs should be considered for management of moderate-to-severe pain in patients with knee osteoarthritis [90].

Patients with symptomatic osteoarthritis are frequently prescribed physical therapy and exercise. A randomized trial of low-intensity (40% heart rate reserve) versus high-intensity (70% heart rate reserve) cycling showed improved function, increased cardiovascular endurance, decreased pain, and improved gait in individuals with knee osteoarthritis performing both protocols [91]. Cycling did not increase acute pain in either group. Physical therapy, including supervised exercise in the setting of known osteoarthritis has been shown to be effective in reducing pain and disability. A review of the literature through the late 1990s demonstrated a modest effect of exercise in patients with knee osteoarthritis [92]. A more recent randomized controlled trial of manual therapy and supervised exercises, including stretching, strengthening, and aerobic exercises for 4 weeks in men and women with knee osteoarthritis showed improvements even at 1 year [93].

Surgical consultation is pursued when conservative management is unsuccessful. Arthroscopy (to debride the joint or remove loose bodies) or osteotomy may be considered earlier in the clinical course while arthroplasty is used in the setting of refractory pain and significant disability. Rehabilitation providers in conjunction with orthopedic surgeons have developed postoperative clinical pathways. It is beyond the scope of this article to review total joint arthroplasty.

Exercise prescription in the older woman

Exercise prescription is an important component of the treatment plan for women with any of a wide variety of medical problems, from heart disease to depression. It is a key tool to combat impairment and disability in aging women with and without musculoskeletal disorders. The prescription is developed in the context of the individual's medical history. For previously sedentary individuals, a complete history and physical examination should be completed before initiating the program. The prescription encompasses the following areas: flexibility, strength, endurance, and functional activity. A 5-minute walk or ride on a stationary bicycle is done for warm-up. Daily stretching of all the major muscle groups includes holding the lengthened position of stretch for 30 seconds and then repeating. Strengthening of the trunk and extremities can be accomplished with resistance training. Light hand weights or household items, weight-training machines, or elastic bands can be used. Choosing a level of resistance that one can lift comfortably and with good form for eight repetitions is a good starting point. When 15 repetitions can be done consistently, one can increase the level of resistance. Weight lifting should be done every other day or 3 days per week. Endurance training includes cardiovascular exercises using low-impact machines, such as the elliptical trainer or stationary bicycle, or walking. The pace is one in which the woman feels she is exerting herself moderately but can continue to count aloud. The goal is 30 minutes preferably 4 to 5 days per week. It may be done in divided sessions (eg, three

10-minute walks). Functional exercises for improving balance can be accomplished through dance, tai chi, or low-impact aerobics classes. Appropriate fluid intake and layering of clothing are keys as older adults are more susceptible to dehydration. Group participation can improve compliance and socialization. The exercise program is progressed slowly to avoid injury. Regular communication with one's health care provider regarding the exercise prescription maximizes effectiveness and compliance.

References

[1] Blair S, Kohl H III, Paffenbarger R Jr, et al. Physical fitness and all-cause mortality: a prospective study of healthy men and women. J Am Med Assoc 1989;262:2395–401.

[2] Buchner D, Wagner EH. Preventing frail health. Clin Geriatr Med 1992;8:1–17.

[3] Pu CT, Johnson MT, Forman DE, et al. Randomized trial of progressive resistance training to counteract the myopathy of chronic heart failure. J Appl Physiol 2001;90:2341–50.

[4] Harris SS, Casperson CJ, DeFriese GH, et al. Physical activity counseling for healthy adults as a primary preventive intervention in the clinical setting: report for the US Preventive Services Task Force. JAMA 1989;261:3588–98.

[5] Pennix BW, Messier SP, Rejeski WJ, et al. Physical exercise and the prevention of disability in activities of daily living in older persons with osteoarthritis. Arch Intern Med 2001;161: 2309–16.

[6] Plona R, Brownstein B. Function in older individuals—orthopedic geriatrics. In: Brownstein B, Bronner S, editors. Evaluation treatment and outcomes functional movement in orthopedic and sports physical therapy. New York: Churchill Livingstone Inc; 1997. p. 311–47.

[7] Bernstein L, Henderson BE, Hanisch R, et al. Physical exercise and reduced risk of breast cancer in young women. J Natl Cancer Inst 1994;86:1403–8.

[8] Carpenter CL, Ross RK, Paganini-Hill A, et al. Lifetime exercise activity and breast cancer risk among post-menopausal women. Br J Cancer 1999;80:1852–8.

[9] Friedenreich CM, Courney KS, Bryant HE. Relation between intensity of physical activity and breast cancer risk reduction. Med Sci Sports Exerc 2001;33(9):1538–45.

[10] Yaffe C, Barnes D, Nevitt M, et al. A prospective study of physical activity and cognitive decline in elderly women; Women who walk. Arch Intern Med 2001;161:1703–8.

[11] Bassey EJ, Fiatarone MA, O'Neill EF, et al. Leg extensor power and functional performance in very old men and women. Clin Sci (Lond) 1992;82(3):321–7.

[12] Fiatarone MA, O'Neill EF, Ryan ND, et al. Exercise training and nutritional supplementation for physical frailty in very elderly people. N Engl J Med 1994;330:1769–75.

[13] Pate RR, Pratt M, Blair SN, et al. Physical activity and public health. A recommendation from the Center for Disease Control and Prevention and the American College of Sports Medicine. JAMA 1995;273(5):402–8.

[14] Pu CT, Nelson ME. Aging, function, and exercise. In: Frontera WR, Dawson DM, Slovik DM, editors. Exercise in rehabilitation medicine. Champaign (IL): Human Kinetics; 1999. p. 391–424.

[15] McNeil JM. Americans with disabilities, 1997. Current population reports, Series P70, No. 73. Washington, DC: US Department of Commerce, Bureau of Census; 2001. p. 1–5.

[16] Maddox GL, Clark DO. Trajectories of functional impairment in later life. J Health Soc Behav 1992;33:114–25.

[17] Public Health Service. Healthy people 2000: national health promotion and disease prevention objectives. Full report, with commentary; 1990. Washington, DC: US Department of Health and Human Services, DHHS Publication #PHS 91–50212.

[18] Sowers MF, Pope S, Welch G, et al. The association of menopause and physical functioning in women at midlife. J Am Geriatr Soc 2001;49:1485–92.

[19] Dugan SA, Powell LH, Kravitz HM, et al. Musculoskeletal pain and menopausal status. Clin J Pain 2006;22(4):325–31.

[20] Matthews KA, Abrams B, Crawford S, et al. Body mass index in mid-life women: relative influence of menopause, hormone use, and ethnicity. Int J Obes 2001;25: 863–73.

[21] Sternfeld B, Wang H, Quesenberry CP Jr, et al. Physical activity and changes in weight and waist circumference in midlife women: findings from the Study of Women's Health Across the Nation. Am J Epidemiol 2004;160:912–22.

[22] Anderson D, Mizzari K, Kain V. The effects of a multimodal intervention trial to promote lifestyle factors associated with the prevention of cardiovascular disease in menopausal and postmenopausal Australian women. Health Care Women Int 2006;27: 238–53.

[23] Kuller LH, Simkin-Silverman LR, Wang RR, et al. Women's Healthy Lifestyle Project: a randomized clinical trial. Circulation 2001;103:32–7.

[24] Wildman RP, Schott LL, Brockwell S, et al. A dietary and exercise intervention slows menopause-associated progression of subclinical atherosclerosis as measured by intima-media thickness of the carotid arteries. J Am Coll Cardiol 2004;44:579–85.

[25] Li TY, Rana JS, Manson JE, et al. Obesity as compared with physical activity in predicting coronary heart disease in women. Circulation 2006;113:499–506.

[26] Dugan SA, Everson-Rose SA, Karavolos K, et al. Physical activity and intra-abdominal fat in a biracial sample of women at midlife. Abstract Presented at theAmerican College of Sports Medicine Annual Meeting. New Orleans (LA), June 1, 2007.

[27] Everson-Rose SA, Lewis TT. Psychosocial factors and cardiovascular diseases. Annu Rev Public Health 2005;26:469–500.

[28] Everson-Rose SA, Meyer PM, Powell LH, et al. Depressive symptoms, insulin resistance, and risk of diabetes in women at midlife. Diabetes Care 2004;27:2856–62.

[29] Chilibeck PD, Sale DG, Webber CE. Exercise and BMD. Sports Med 1995;19:103–22.

[30] Drinkwater BL. Physical activity, fitness, and osteoporosis. In: Bouchard C, Shephard RJ, Stephens T, editors. Physical activity, fitness, and health. International Proceedings and Consensus Statement. Champaign (IL): Human Kinetics; 1994. p. 724–36.

[31] Layne JE, Nelson ME. The effects of progressive resistance training on bone density: a review. Med Sci Sports Exerc 1999;31(1):25–30.

[32] Gelber AD, Hochberg MC, Mead LA, et al. Joint injury in young adults and risk for subsequent knee and hip osteoarthritis. Ann Intern Med 2000;133:321–8.

[33] Rainville J, Ahern DK, Phalen L, et al. The association of pain with physical activities in chronic low back pain. Spine 1992;17:1060–4.

[34] Krolner B, Toft B, Pors Nielsen S, et al. Physical exercise as a prophylaxis against involutional bone loss; a controlled trial. Clin Sci 1983;64:541–6.

[35] Vernon-Roberts B, Pirie CJ. Degenerative changes in the intervertebral disk of the lumbar spine and their sequelae. Rheumatol Rehabil 1977;16:13–21.

[36] Skinner HB, Barrack RL, Cook SD. Age-related decline in proprioception. Clin Orthop Rel Res 1984;184:208–11.

[37] Frontera WR, Hughes VA, Lutz KJ, et al. A cross-sectional study of muscle strength and mass in 45- to 78-year-old men and women. J Appl Physiol 1991;71:644–50.

[38] Cassel CK, Brody JA. Demography, epidemiology, and aging. In: Cassel CK, Riesenberg DE, Sorensen LB, Walsh JR, editors. Geriatric medicine. 2nd edition. New York: Springer-Verlag; 1990. p. 20.

[39] March LM, Bachmeier CJ. Economics of osteoarthritis: a global perspective. Baillieres Clin Rheumatol 1997;11(4):817–34.

[40] Nevitt MC, Lane N. Body weight and osteoarthritis. Am J Med 1999;107(6):632–3.

[41] Guccione AA, Felson DT, Anderson JJ, et al. The effects of specific medical conditions on the functional limitations of elders in the Framingham Study. Am J Public Health 1994; 84(3):351–8.

[42] Kramer JS, Yeltin EH, Epstein WV. Social and economic impacts of four musculoskeletal conditions. A study using national community-based data. Arthritis Rheum 1983;26(7): 901–7.

[43] Hurley MV. The role of muscle weakness in the pathogenesis of osteoarthritis. Rheum Dis Clin North Am 1999;25(2):283–98.

[44] Sowers MF, Lachance L, Hochberg M, et al. Radiographically defined osteoarthritis of the hand and knee in young and middle-aged African American and Caucasian women. Osteoarthritis Cartilage 2000;8(2):69–77.

[45] Cooper C, McAlindon T, Snow S, et al. Mechanical and constitutional risk factors for symptomatic knee osteoarthritis: differences between medial tibiofemoral and patellofemoral disease. J Rheumatol 1994;21:307–13.

[46] Davis MA, Ettinger WH, Neuhaus JM, et al. The association of knee injury and obesity with unilateral and bilateral osteoarthritis of the knee. Am J Epidemiol 1989;130:278–88.

[47] Saxon L, Finch C, Bass S. Sports participation, sports injuries and osteoarthritis. Implications for prevention. Sports Med 1999;28:123–35.

[48] Fisher NM, Greshman GE, Abrams M, et al. Quantitative effects of physical therapy on muscular performance in subjects with osteoarthritis of the knees. Arch Phys Med Rehabil 1993;74:840–7.

[49] Buckwalter JA. Osteoarthritis and articular cartilage use, disuse, and abuse: Experimental studies. J Rheumatol 1995;22(Suppl 43):13–5.

[50] Hall AC, Urban JPG, Gehl KA. The effects of hydrostatic pressure on matrix synthesis in articular cartilage. J Orthop Res 1991;9:1–10.

[51] Engh GA, Chrisman OD. Experimental arthritis in rabbit knees: a study of relief of pressure on one tibial plateau in immature and mature rabbits. Clin Orthop 1997;125:221–6.

[52] Vuori IM. Dose-response of physical activity and low back pain, osteoarthritis, and osteoporosis. Med Sci Sports Exerc 2001;33(6):S551–86.

[53] McAlindon TE, Wilson PW, Aliabadi P, et al. Level of physical activity and the risk of radiographic and symptomatic knee osteoarthritis in the elderly: the Framingham Study. Am J Med 1999;106:151–7.

[54] Felson DT, Zhang Y, Hannan MT, et al. Risk factors for incident radiographic knee osteoarthritis in the elderly. The Framingham Study. Arthritis Rheum 1997;40:728–33.

[55] Hannan MT, Felson DT, Anderson JI, et al. Habitual physical activity is not associated with knee osteoarthritis: the Framingham Study. J Rheumatol 1993;20:704–9.

[56] Cheng Y, Macera CA, Davis DR, et al. Physical activity and self-reported, physician-diagnosed osteoarthritis: is physical activity a risk factor? J Clin Epidemiol 2000;53: 315–22.

[57] Lane NE. Exercise: a cause of osteoarthritis. J Rheumatol 1995;22(Suppl 43):3–6.

[58] Felson DT. The epidemiology of knee osteoarthritis: results from the Framingham Osteoarthritis Study. Semin Arthritis Rheum 1990;20(Suppl 1):42–50.

[59] Nevitt MC, Cummings SR, Lane NE, et al. Association of estrogen replacement therapy with the risk of osteoarthritis of the hip in elderly white women. Study of Osteoporotic Fractures Research Group. Ann Intern Med 1996;156(18):2073–80.

[60] Yong-Hing K, Kirkaldy-Willis WH. The pathophysiology of degenerative disease of the lumbar spine. Orthop Clin North Am 1983;14(3):491–504.

[61] Bohlman HH, Emery S. The pathophysiology of cervical spondylosis and myelopathy. Spine 1988;13:843–6.

[62] Malanga GA. The diagnosis and treatment of cervical radiculopathy. Med Sci Sports Exerc 1997;29(Suppl 7):S236–45.

[63] Fon GT, Pitt MJ, Thies AC. Thoracic kyphosis. Range in normal subjects. AJR Am J Roentgenol 1980;134:979–83.

[64] Stagnara P, DeMauroy JC, Dran G, et al. Reciprocal angulation of vertebral bodies in a sagittal plane. Approach to references for the evaluation of kyphosis and lordosis. Spine 1982;7: 335–42.

[65] Holt RT, Dopf CA, Isaza JE, et al. Adult kyphosis. In: Frymoyer JW (editor-in-chief): The adult spine, principles and practice, 2nd edition, Lippincott-Raven: Philadelphia; 1997. p. 1537–78.

[66] Thevenon A, Pollez B, Cantegrit F, et al. Relationship between kyphosis, scoliosis, and osteoporosis in the elderly. Spine 1987;(12):744–5.

[67] Thomas MA, Wang Y. Scoliosis and kyphosis. In: Frontera WR, Silver JK, editors. Essentials of physical medicine and rehabilitation. Philadelphia: Hanley & Belfus Inc.; 2002. p. 735–42.

[68] Kostuik JP. Adult scoliosis. In: Rothman RH, Simeone FA, editors. The spine. 3rd Edition. Philadelphia: W.B. Saunders; 1992. p. 879–911.

[69] Kostuik JP, Bentivoglio J. The incidence in low back pain in adult scoliosis. Spine 1981;6: 268–73.

[70] Healey JH, Lane JM. Structural scoliosis in osteoporotic women. Clin Orthop 1985;195: 216–23.

[71] Velis KP, Healey JH, Schneider R. Osteoporosis in unstable adult scoliosis. Clin Orthop 1988;237:132–41.

[72] Parsch D, Gaertner V, Brocai DR, et al. The effect of spinal fusion on the long-term outcome of idiopathic scoliosis. A case-control study. J Bone Joint Surg Br 2001;83(8): 1133–6.

[73] Danielsson AJ, Nachemson AL. Radiologic findings and curve progression 22 years after treatment of idiopathic scoliosis: comparison of brace and surgical treatments with matching control group of straight individuals. Spine 1999;24:1693–700.

[74] Weinstein SL, Ponseti IV. Curve progression in idiopathic scoliosis. J Bone Joint Surg Am 1983;65:447–55.

[75] Amundsen T, Weber H, Nordal HJ, et al. Lumbar spinal stenosis: conservative or surgical management? A prospective 10-year study. Spine 2000;25(11):1424–35.

[76] Schaufele MK, Rainville J, Hartigan C, et al. Rehabilitation of senior citizens with chronic low back pain [abstract]. Arch Phys Med Rehabil 1997;78(9):1025.

[77] Simotas AC, Dorey FJ, Hansraj KK, et al. Non-operative treatment for lumbar spinal stenosis; Clinical and outcome results, and a three year survivorship analysis. Spine 2000;25(2): 197–203.

[78] Ciocon JO, Galindo-Ciocon D, Amaranath L, et al. Caudal epidural blocks for elderly patients with lumbar canal stenosis. J Am Geriatics Soc 1994;42(6):593–6.

[79] Wiltse LL, Kirkaldy-Willis WH, McIvor GW. The treatment of spinal stenosis. Clin Orthop 1976;115:83–91.

[80] Jackson CP, Brown M. Analysis of current approaches and a practical guide to prescription of exercise. Clin Orthop Relat Res 1983;179:46–54.

[81] Walker WC, Chiappini RA, Bushbacher RB, et al. Rationale prescription of exercise in managing low back pain. Crit Rev Phys Rehabil Med 1993;5(3):219–26.

[82] Videman T, Sarna S, Battie MC, et al. The long-term effects of physical loading and exercise lifestyles on back-related symptoms, disability, and spine loading pathology among men. Spine 1995;20(6):699–709.

[83] Shakoor N, Block JA, Case JP. The sequence of joint replacements in osteoarthritis is not random. J Investig Med 2001;49(5):304A.

[84] Bradley JD, Brandt KD, Katz BP, et al. Comparison of an anti-inflammatory dose of ibuprofen, an analgesic dose of ibuprofen and acetaminophen in the treatment of osteoarthritis of the knee. N Engl J Med 1991;325:87–91.

[85] Williams HJ, Ward JR, Egger MJ, et al. Comparison of naproxen and acetaminophen in a 2-year study of treatment of osteoarthritis of the knee. Arthritis Rheum 1993;36:1196–206.

[86] Cannon GW, Caldwell JR, Holt P, et al. Rofecoxib, a specific inhibitor of cyclooxygenase 2, with clinical efficacy comparable with that of diclofenac sodium. Arthritis Rheum 2000; 43(5):978–87.

[87] Delafuente JC. Glucosamine in the treatment of osteoarthritis. Rheum Dis Clin North Am 2000;26(1):1–11.

[88] Zhang WY, Po ALW. The effectiveness of topically applied capsaicin: a meta-analysis. Eur J Clin Pharmacol 1994;46:517–22.

[89] Simon LS. Viscosupplementation therapy with intra-articular hyaluronic acid: fact or fantasy. Rheum Dis Clin North Am 1999;25(2):345–57.

[90] Stitik TP, Blacksin MF, Stiskal DM, et al. Efficacy and safety of hyaluronan treatment in combination therapy with home exercise for knee osteoarthritis pain. Arch Phys Med Rehabil 2007;88(2):135–41.

[91] Mangione KK, McCully K, Gloviak A, et al. The effects of high-intensity and low-intensity cycle ergometry in older adults with knee osteoarthritis. J Gerontol A Biol Sci Med Sci 1999; 54:M184–90.

[92] Van Baar ME, Assendeleft WJ, Dekker J, et al. Effectiveness of exercise therapy in patients with osteoarthritis of the hip or knee. A systemic review of randomized clinical trials. Arthritis Rheum 1999;42:1361–9.

[93] Deyle GD, Henderson ME, Matekel RL, et al. Effectiveness of manual physical therapy and exercise in osteoarthritis of the knee. A randomized, controlled trial. Ann Intern Med 2000; 132:173–81.

ELSEVIER
SAUNDERS

Phys Med Rehabil Clin N Am
18 (2007) 577–591

PHYSICAL MEDICINE
AND REHABILITATION
CLINICS OF
NORTH AMERICA

Conservative Care for Patients with Osteoporotic Vertebral Compression Fractures

Heidi Prather, DO[a],*, Devyani Hunt, MD[a],
John O. Watson, MD[a], Louis A. Gilula, MD[b]

[a]Section of Physical Medicine and Rehabilitation, Washington University Orthopedics,
One Barnes-Jewish Hospital Plaza, Suite 11300, Saint Louis, MO 63110, USA
[b]Mallinckrodt Institute of Radiology, Washington University School of Medicine,
510 S. Kingshighway, Box 8131, St. Louis, MO 63110, USA

Epidemiology and natural history

A recent US Census Bureau report shows that in July 2004 there were 36.3 million people in the United States over 65 years of age, accounting for 12% of the total population. It is estimated that in 2050 this number will rise to 86.7 million, comprising 21% of the total population, a 147% increase during half a century [1]. Accompanying this increasing age will be increases in the health risks already affecting the elderly population. The National Osteoporosis Foundation has reported that osteoporosis already affects 10 million people, and another 34 million are at increased risk. The silent disease of osteoporosis will predispose this aging population to fractures. Vertebral fractures will be the most commonly encountered: vertebral fractures account for 700,000 of the 1.5 million annual fractures [1]. Data collected in the 1990s reported that the direct medical cost of vertebral compression fractures in the United States was greater than $746 million. This expense will continue to rise [1]. The physical and emotional consequences that accompany a vertebral compression fracture can be devastating. Many vertebral compression fractures are asymptomatic. As a result, osteoporosis often remains silent, and the incident is attributed to a "back strain."

* Corresponding author. Washington University, 4921 Parkview Place, 6th floor, Campus Box 8605, Saint Louis, MO 63110.
E-mail address: pratherh@wudosis.wustl.edu (H. Prather).

Only 23% to 33% of fractures become clinically evident [2]. In those that are symptomatic, the first symptom usually is back pain, which sometimes can be mistaken for a muscle strain or arthritis. After an acute fracture, the degree of vertebral body height loss can progress and, as a result, so may the spine deformity. Regular surveillance is important to treat current symptoms and prevent future complications. Compression fractures that cause intractable pain cause immobilization. In addition, acute complications, such as transient ileus, urinary retention, and, occasionally, spinal cord compression, can occur [3,4]. Chronic effects include kyphosis with occasional breathing difficulties, deconditioning, insomnia, and depression. Because osteoporosis remains a silent disease process, a painful vertebral compression fracture may be the first time the diagnosis of osteoporosis is confirmed. Every such patient should be referred for evaluation of bone mineral health with appropriate medical intervention for the treatment. Physiatrists may need to function as "watch dogs" to ensure that patients have been evaluated and medical treatment options are offered. Surgical management is reserved for cases of severe spinal instability or neurologic compromise. For all other cases, conservative management should be a structured and ongoing attempt to treat symptoms, monitor for neurologic injury and further vertebral body collapse, and restore function.

Acute fracture management

Diagnostics

The history and physical examination are important in identifying the possibility of the development of a new vertebral compression fracture. Any elderly patient or a patient who has a history of osteoporosis with a new onset of low back pain or trauma associated with pain should be evaluated for a fracture. Obtaining the proper radiographs is the first step in evaluating vertebral compression fracture(s). Radiographs of the lumbar or thoracic spine should include both anteroposterior and lateral views and flexion and extension views if instability is suspected.

The initial plain film evaluation includes properly locating the vertebral body. The level of the fracture can be misidentified when anomalies such as sacralization, lumbarization, or hypoplastic ribs are present. The approximate vertebral loss of body height should be documented and expressed as a percentage. A decrease in height of 20% or more or a decrease of at least 4 mm compared with baseline height has been used to confirm a compression fracture [5]. Definite fractures that have less marked collapse may be confirmed by MRI. Documenting the type of fracture(s) by the height loss of the anterior vertebral body, biconcave, or plana and the estimated amount of height loss is helpful in managing future problems. Reference to previous radiographic hip examinations can help distinguish between progression of a previous fracture and the onset of a new fracture. Evaluating the posterior vertebral line also is very important, because retropulsion can be a devastating complication of vertebral compression fractures.

When retropulsion is suspected, it is essential to obtain either an MRI or CT scan to assess the patency of the spinal column adequately and to evaluate the vertebral discs and nerve roots, which may concurrently be irritated or compressed.

Flexion extension views of the fracture site are important to assess for instability in the setting of a fracture complicated by retropulsion. The health care provider must keep in mind that patients who have a retropulsion associated with the fracture may present with clinical symptoms of spinal stenosis. In this setting, pain may increase with extension, and leg symptoms may be apart of the symptom complex.

It often is difficult to determine the age of a compression fracture, especially when a specific trauma or fall has not occurred. This difficulty becomes an even greater issue when multiple compression fractures are found. A bone scan or MRI will help localize more active compression fractures, but both technologies have limitations. A bone scan may not become positive for up to 10 days after fracture, therefore leading to false-negative findings if a scan is obtained too soon after an acute fracture. With MRI, the compression fracture usually shows decreased signal on T1 sequences and marrow edema on T2 fat-saturation sequences. The physical examination and MRI findings can help determine effective treatment, because not all the patient's pain may be related to an obvious fracture. Pain related to degenerative processes, neurogenic pain, and pain related to deformity may be concomitant or isolated sources in this patient population. One possible scenario is neural foraminal narrowing at the level of the compression fracture, which may refer pain down the dermatomal distribution of the respective nerve root.

Another more recent observation is the dynamic mobility of these compression fractures. McKiernan and colleagues [6] first reported that 35% of the fractures that group evaluated were mobile, as assessed by a supine cross-table lateral radiograph centered on the fractured vertebra. Some patients used a foam bolster to help facilitate this spinal extension, a technique that has led some investigators to try postural reduction of a fracture before performing a vertebral augmentation procedure [7]. The results are encouraging and may offer a valuable new technique for a conservative management plan.

Medications for pain control

Adequate pain control following a vertebral compression fracture is crucial. Narcotics can relieve pain well, but short- and long-acting agents need to be regulated in timing and frequency. Side effects, especially in the elderly population, can be debilitating. Cognitive impairment, nausea, and constipation can be especially problematic. Patient and family education is essential for safe administration. Not all pain responds to narcotic medication. Disorders related to inflammation often respond inadequately to narcotics. Patients who have compression fractures may have pain related to inflammation within the periosteum and soft tissue changes as a result of the fracture that may cause an unrelenting cycle of pain and muscle spasm that is difficult to relieve. As a result, patients who have recent fractures may respond to nonsteroidal anti-inflammatory medications. Again, gastrointestinal side effects such as nausea, gastritis, and ulcers can be problematic. Cyclo-oxygenase 2 inhibitors may help avoid some of these effects. If local inflammatory mediators around the nerve root of a compression fracture are a concern, corticosteroids may be introduced to the area by an epidural injection with a transforaminal approach [8].

Patients who have vertebral fractures can develop radicular pain caused by compression by a retropulsed fragment combined with general inflammation occurring in the region. The exiting nerve root is susceptible to this compression bilaterally as a result of neural foraminal narrowing. On physical examination, a straight leg raise or dural tension test may reveal radicular pain, even when strength and reflex testing are found to be normal. Management of radicular pain should include anti-inflammatory medication, narcotic pain medication if needed, and a fluoroscopically guided contrast-enhanced nerve-root block or transforaminal epidural injection of steroid and an anesthetic. These injections often can minimize patients' radicular pain quickly. If the pain becomes chronic in nature, other medications that address neurogenic pain should be used. The pharmacologic classes that are helpful in addressing neurogenic pain include antidepressants, anticonvulsants, and alpha-2-agonists. The antidepressant medications include tricyclics, selective serotonin-reuptake inhibitors, and monoamine oxidase inhibitors. The tricyclics have been studied most thoroughly for pain. Several studies have demonstrated the analgesic effect of the tricyclics separate from their antidepressant effects [9,10]. Their analgesic effect often is achieved at lower doses than required for an antidepressant effect. Tricyclics reduce pain by modifying the reuptake of norepinephrine and serotonin. Common side effects include anticholinergic symptoms including drowsiness and dry mouth. Other less common adverse reactions are hypotension, cardiac dysrhythmias, and urinary retention. The tertiary amines such as amitriptyline tend to have more side effects that the secondary amines such as desipramine. Patients requiring assistance with sleep regulation might respond best to a tertiary amine, whereas those who complain of hangover symptoms may respond better to a secondary amine. Other antidepressants such as trazodone, citalopram, and the selective serotonin-reuptake inhibitors can help modify pain by their effects on serotonin [11], but few controlled studies have been completed to verify the many anecdotal reports. The initial dosage of a tricyclic medication should be small and increased gradually over several weeks to monitor side effects appropriately. If a selective serotonin-reuptake inhibitor is added to a regimen that already includes a tricyclic, the dose of the tricyclic may need to be halved to maintain the same blood level because of the drug–drug interaction. Discontinuing these medications requires tapering over several weeks to avoid withdrawal phenomena such as mood change or insomnia. Anticonvulsants suppress spontaneous neuronal firing rates through their actions on ion channels and/or neurotransmitters. How anticonvulsants achieve analgesic effect is not entirely clear, but the effect is thought to be related to this modification of the neurons. There are many drugs in this class that act on various sets of receptors. As a result, response to one drug does not predict a response to others in this class. Gabapentin and pregabalin have become commonly used adjunct pain medications with proven analgesic effect on neuropathic pain syndromes [12–14].

Pregabalin reduces pain and improves sleep and mood disturbances in patients who have postherpetic neuralgia and provides pain relief in patients who have painful diabetic neuropathy [15]. Gabapentin and pregabalin have a high degree of safety and are metabolized through renal excretion. The most common side effects include sedation and cognitive clouding. Treatment with gabapentin should be initiated at a low dose (100–300 mg) at night and increased gradually until analgesic benefits are noted. Dosing can be as high as 3600 to 6000 mg/d in three equal doses. Pregabalin should follow the same course of low dosing at 75 mg twice daily increasing to 150 mg twice daily. Both medications should be titrated to the patient's symptoms. Rapidly stopping either medication can lead to seizures, so the patient should be instructed to taper off the medication. Another neuropathic agent to consider is tizanidine, which is a central alpha-2 adrenoreceptor agonist. Tizanidine may help with pain control through a variety of mechanisms, including reducing the release of substance P in polysynaptic pathways, inhibition of the synaptic transmission of nociceptive stimuli to the spinal cord, and postsynaptic reduction in excitatory transmitter activity. Tizanidine is related structurally to clonidine, and therefore cardiovascular side effects such as hypotension and bradycardia must be monitored. Liver function tests also must be monitored regularly, because there have been reports of elevation throughout the treatment episode [16].

As pain lessens and the ability to perform functional activities improves, the treating physician should continue to monitor the patient's need for pain medication and taper the medications as indicated. Removing narcotics and some anticonvulsants rapidly can cause significant morbidity. Gradual tapering adjusted to the patient's symptoms is necessary to ensure a smooth transition.

In summary, it is important to tailor medications to patients' needs based on the level and quality of pain. Taking a careful patient history can assist the physician in prescribing an appropriate pain medication or combination of medications safely. Understanding the indications and side-effect profiles is essential for effective management of pain related to vertebral compression fracture.

Physical therapy

Physical therapy plays a vital role in treating painful vertebral compression fractures. First, education about ways to avoid pain in activities of daily living and mobility is essential for this population of impaired patients who often are elderly. Therapeutic exercise can help reduce pain, build strength and endurance, and prevent future fractures [17]. Aerobic exercise and weight-bearing physical activity are important in maintaining general health and bone health, but resistance training has a more potent impact on bone density [18]. Often, the initial focus of physical therapy is improving posture and body mechanics to reduce compressive loads on the spinal column; therapy then progresses to core-strengthening exercise that facilitates truncal stability and strength [19].

Spinal extensor strengthening can help reduce pain by reducing compressive loads and helping maintain bone mineral density [17,20]. Sinaki and colleagues [17] reported on a prospective study in which postmenopausal women participated in a 2-year back exercise program and were followed for 8 years after completion. Benefits of this program included a reduced risk of compression fractures and improved bone density. In a randomized, controlled trial, Papaioannou and colleges [21] found that women who had vertebral fractures and who complied with a home exercise program improved their quality of life in the domains of symptoms, emotion, and leisure and social activity over a 6-month period [21]. Adding dynamic proprioceptive training can help reduce pain and the risk of falls in patients who have kyphosis related to osteoporotic compression fractures [22]. The physical therapy prescription for patients who have radicular pain should be modified to treat the radicular and back pain. This modification includes avoiding activities involving positions that provoke pain. Strengthening of abdominal, gluteal, and hip muscles is important to support spinal structures with noncompressive forces and can be done by integrating the exercises into a more functional rehabilitation program. Functional exercises that use all planes of motion and simulate activities of daily living may be more beneficial for the patient [19]. Once pain has improved, the patient should be given a home exercise program that facilitates neutral spine posture and improves strength and endurance. Adapting an aerobic conditioning program to the patient's capabilities helps the patient reduce fear of incurring a new vertebral compression fracture or of progression of a current one.

Bracing

For appropriate patients, bracing after a vertebral compression fracture may be an important part of the treatment program. Braces generally are used to facilitate pain control, promote appropriate posture, and provide support for patients who have significant muscular deconditioning. Bracing may facilitate neuromuscular re-education and provide comfort. Although it is not always necessary, bracing for compression fractures can help reduce pain by decreasing postural flexion that causes increased loading on the painful fractured periosteum. There also can be significant relief from lumbar and thoracic paraspinal muscle spasm that develops secondary to the pain and inflammation. The brace must be tailored to fit the patient's need for comfort and function.

Several braces are available. In some patients, bracing can help reduce motion enough to allow the patient to tolerate natural healing and avoid further invasive intervention. After vertebral augmentation, bracing also may facilitate pain reduction and axial support for patients who have poor activity tolerance because of muscle fatigue. Bracing is very helpful for patients who have poor muscular endurance or thoracic kyphosis in which pain might be reduced by facilitating spinal extension. Problems with bracing can include a poor fit in obese patients, patient acceptance, expense, and difficulty in putting on and removing the brace. A brace that fits poorly or is too difficult to use often will end up unused. The type of brace should be directed by the patient's level of activity and comfort. Traditionally, the Jewitt and cruciform anterior spinal extension (CASH) orthoses (Figs. 1 and 2) have been used because the three-point contact facilitates thoracic and lumbar neutral positioning while decreasing flexion. For stable thoracic fractures, the authors often recommended a posture training support (Fig. 3) to facilitate spinal extension and scapular retraction [23]. This brace is easy to put on and remove, can be worn under regular clothing if desired, and is relatively affordable. Most insurance companies and Medicare will pay a portion of the cost. Small weights can be added to this backpack-like device as the patient's strength increases and tolerance improves. A patient should start out with a single 1-pound weight and increase the weight weekly, as tolerated, but not above 3 pounds. If more limitation in motion is required because of pain, a Jewitt (see Fig. 1) or cruciform

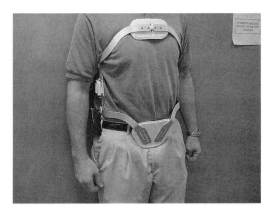

Fig. 1. Jewitt brace used to facilitate thorocolumbar extension and reduce flexion.

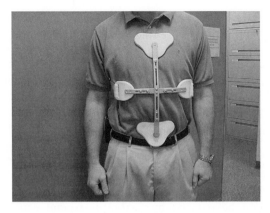

Fig. 2. Cruciform anterior spinal extension (CASH) brace used to facilitate thorocolumbar extension and limit flexion.

anterior spinal extension (CASH) brace (see Fig. 2) can be prescribed. When spine stability is a concern, a custom thoracic lumbar spinal orthosis can be fabricated. For lumbar compression fractures, a simple corset with a moldable plastic posterior shell can be used to facilitate appropriate spine posture and avoid chronic flexion [24]. The purpose and importance of bracing needs to be reviewed with the patient. Not all patients require bracing, however, and not all patients have the body habitus to accommodate available orthoses.

A trial of bracing with the physical therapist working with an orthotist is helpful in determining the appropriate fit while not impeding function. As pain improves, discontinuing the brace usually is easiest when weaned in increments of decreased wearing time. Some patients find that continuing to wear the brace for specific activities after the fracture has healed may help reduce continued pain and facilitate good spine mechanics.

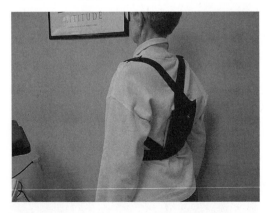

Fig. 3. Posture training support orthosis uses weights to facilitate spinal extension and scapular retraction.

Injections

In addition to the treatment plan outlined previously, some patients may require further intervention to reduce pain and improve function. Patients may present with neurogenic symptoms consistent with radiculopathy. When these symptoms are experienced in combination with motor weakness, spine stability should be confirmed first. Other causes include vertebral body retropulsion as a result of the fracture causing central or lateral recess narrowing (Fig. 4). Disc protrusions may be evident at, below, or above the level involved. These radicular symptoms may be managed with epidural steroid injections directed at the level of the patient's symptoms and correlated with imaging findings. Because of the anatomic variations associated with compression fractures, the authors recommend that these injections be performed under fluoroscopic guidance with contrast enhancement to ensure accurate placement of the medication and to avoid subdural puncture (Fig. 5). In patients who have intractable radicular pain, epidural steroid injections pain often may help the timeliness of the patient's recovery.

Vertebral augmentation

Vertebral augmentation is being used more widely for nonneoplastic vertebral compression fractures [2]. Vertebroplasty, the transpedicular percutaneous infusion of methylmethacrylate into vertebral bodies, has been used in the United States for spinal vertebral compression fractures caused by osteoporosis and cancer (Fig. 6). Prospective [25–32] and retrospective [3,33–39] studies report pain improvement. Kyphoplasty, a procedure that

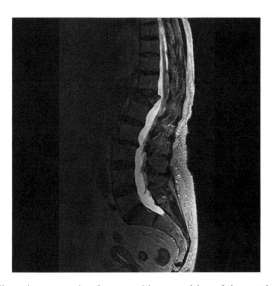

Fig. 4. Thoracic compression fracture with retropulsion of the vertebral body.

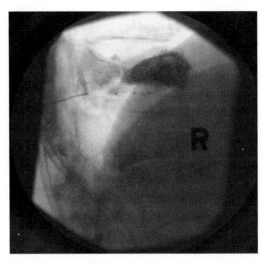

Fig. 5. Sagittal view of a transforaminal epidural steroid injection performed for a patient who experienced radicular pain following vertebroplasty.

involves inflating percutaneously placed balloons within the fractured verte-bra and then infusing cement within the cavities created by the balloon, is another type of vertebral augmentation. The publicized advantage of kyphoplasty over vertebroplasty is the potential restoration of vertebral body height, which ultimately reduces deformity. With less deformity, it can be inferred that subsequent fracture rates would diminish after the

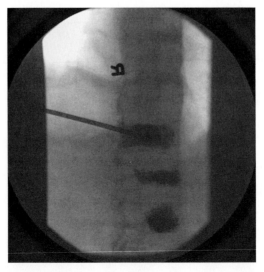

Fig. 6. Sagittal view of vertebroplasty being performed on a painful osteoporotic compression fracture.

procedure. Several studies have shown that this height restoration is measurable, although small in increment [40,41]. Gaitanis and colleagues [40] reported a mean increment of 4.3 mm for anterior wall restoration and a mean increment of 4.88 mm for midvertebral height restoration. This study looked exclusively at pathologic fractures. Although these increments are small, the physiologic and biomechanical advantages still need to be investigated. A recent study by McCann and colleagues [42] found no difference between vertebroplasty and kyphoplasty in restoration of vertebral height in cadaveric vertebral compression fractures. In another study, McKiernan and colleagues [32] treated 46 patients who had a total of 66 painful nonneoplastic vertebral compression fractures with vertebroplasty and measured height restoration after the procedure. At 6 months, there was no difference in pain or quality of life measures in patients who had vertebral height restoration and those who had not. No correlation has been found between pain reduction and the amount of cement infused or vertebral body correction [43,44]. Fribourg and colleagues [45] completed a follow-up study of 38 patients, 13 of whom had received kyphoplasty, and found a higher rate of fracture after the procedure than seen with the natural history of fracture. One study showed that the vertebral body in a cadaver model augmented with kyphoplasty was less stiff than before augmentation, suggesting one possible cause for subsequent fractures [46]. The topic of subsequent fractures after vertebroplasty and kyphoplasty remains controversial [45]. There are many factors involved in subsequent fractures after both procedures, including extent of osteoporosis, kyphosis and scoliosis, motion at the fracture site, posture, activities, and collaborative treatment. Future study of these contributing factors is necessary to decipher risks and prognosticate outcomes better. As with any procedure, patient selection for the procedure and patient management before and after the procedure are mastered with experience. Although known complications of vertebroplasty such as infection, discitis, radiculitis, vertebral fracture, and pulmonary embolism are uncommon, there are fairly straightforward treatment guidelines to follow should they occur [47]. Although uncommon, rib and sternal fractures have been reported with both procedures [3,30,37,48]. The overall incidence of procedural complications with vertebroplasty has been reported to be 2.4% [49], compared with 0.9% with kyphoplasty [50]. Some of this variation involves the recognition of leakage, which some sources call a complication; others, however, find small amounts of leakage commonly present without symptoms [38]. The incidence of transient increases in pain after the procedure has been reported to range from 4% to 23.4% [28,34]. Transient pain increase has been attributed to increased pressure in the fractured vertebral body, inflammatory reaction to polymethylmethacrylate, and osseous ischemia [25].

Vertebral augmentation by means of vertebroplasty or kyphoplasty is a safe and effective treatment option for patients who have intractable pain caused by osteoporotic vertebral compression fractures. In the acute setting, augmentation is preferable to the usual natural course in patients who have intractable pain and marked functional limitations [31,40,51,52]. Another indication for augmentation is to stop further collapse of the rapidly collapsing vertebra. To detect this situation, the authors recommend obtaining a repeat lateral radiographic view of the fractured vertebra after 1 week to be certain that the fractured vertebra is not collapsing rapidly. Ongoing prospective studies comparing standard conservative treatment with vertebroplasty and kyphoplasty should help the treating physician and patient determine which treatment option is best in each individual case. Further studies are also ongoing and necessary to determine the risk factors for developing new fractures after vertebral augmentation. Correlation to extent of bone density is evolving. With improvements in medication such as parathyroid hormone, cotreatment with exercise and vertebral augmentation may help limit further fractures. The answers to management issues such as weight-lifting restrictions, exercise, bracing, and how to treat continued pain after vertebral augmentation are less obvious. Discussing weight-lifting restrictions and avoidance of activities that require repetitive flexion may help reduce the risk of future fracture and pain. Bracing may be advocated for some patients who continue to have axial back pain. The brace may facilitate proprioceptive feedback in proper posture and avoidance of repetitive flexion. Further long-term studies should help determine the best treatment course. For now, careful follow-up is advised, especially a 1-week follow-up lateral radiograph to establish a stable and nonprogressive compressed vertebra.

Summary

Conservative management of osteoporotic vertebral compression fractures is multifaceted and requires a comprehensive approach. For some patients, a painful vertebral fracture may be the first indication of osteoporosis, and a bone mineral health work-up is essential. Fracture care may include relative rest, possibly bracing, medication, and therapeutic exercise. If pain remains intractable, vertebral augmentation may be a good a treatment option to facilitate recovery and reduce or eliminate the risks associated with immobilization.

References

[1] Old JL, Calvert M. Vertebral compression fractures in the elderly. Am Fam Physician 2004; 69(1):111–6.

[2] Rao RD, Singrakhia MD. Painful osteoporotic vertebral fracture. J Bone Joint Surg 2003; 85A(10):2010–22.

[3] Jensen ME, Evans AJ, Mathis JM, et al. Percutaneous polymethylmethacrylate vertebroplasty in the treatment of osteoporotic vertebral body compression fractures: technical aspects. AJNR Am J Neuroradiol 1997;18(10):1897–904.

[4] Bostrom MPG, Lane JM. Augmentation of osteoporotic vertebral bodies. Spine 1997;22: 38S–42S.

[5] Nevitt MC, Ettinger B, Black DM, et al. The association of radiographically detected vertebral fractures with back pain and function: a prospective study. Ann Intern Med 1998; 128(10):793–800.

[6] McKiernan F, Jensen R, Faciszewski T. The dynamic mobility of vertebral compression fractures. J Bone Miner Res 2003;18(1):24–9.

[7] Chin D, Kim Y, Cho Y, et al. Efficacy of postural reduction in osteoporotic vertebral compression fractures followed by percutaneous vertebroplasty. Neurosurgery 2006;58(4): 695–700.

[8] Kim D, Yun Y, Wang J. Nerve root injections for the relief of pain in patients with osteoporotic vertebral fractures. J Bone Joint Surg Br 2003;85(2):250–3.

[9] Max MB, Lynch SA, Muir J, et al. Effects of desipramine, amitriptyline and fluoxetine on pain in diabetic neuropathy. N Engl J Med 1992;326:1250–6.

[10] Max M, Schafer SC, Culnane M. Amitriptyline, but not lorazapam, relieves post-herpetic neuralgia. Neurology 1988;38:1427–32.

[11] Sindrup SH, Gram LF, Brosen K, et al. The selective serotonin reuptake inhibitor paroxetine is effective in the treatment of diabetic neuropathy symptoms. Pain 1990;42:135–44.

[12] Backonja M, Beydoun A, Edwards KR, et al. Gabapentin for the symptomatic treatment of painful neuropathy in patients with diabetes mellitus: a randomized controlled trial. JAMA 1998;280:1831–6.

[13] Rowbotham M, Harden N, Stacey B, et al. Gabapentin for the treatment of postherpetic neuralgia: a randomized controlled trial. JAMA 1998;280(21):1837–42.

[14] Sabatowski R, Galvez R, Cherry D, et al. Pre-gabalin reduces pain and improves sleep and mood disturbances in patients with post-herpetic neuralgia: results of a randomized, placebo-controlled clinical trial. Pain 2004;109(1–2):26–35.

[15] Lesser H, Sharma U, LaMoreaux L, et al. Pregabalin relieves symptoms of painful diabetic neuropathy: a randomized controlled trial. Neurology 2004;63(11):2104–10.

[16] Semenchuk MR, Sherman S. Effectiveness of tizanidine in neuropathic pain: an open-label study. Clin J Pain 2000;1(4):285–92.

[17] Sinaki M, Itoi E, Wahner HW, et al. Stronger back muscles reduce the incidence of vertebral fractures: a prospective 10 year follow-up of postmenopausal women. Bone 2002;30(6): 836–41.

[18] Layne JE, Nelson ME. The effects of progressive resistance training on bone density: a review. Med Sci Sports Exerc 1999;31(1):25–30.

[19] Akuthota V, Nadler SF. Core strengthening. Arch Phys Med Rehabil 2004;85(3 Suppl 1): S86–92.

[20] Bonner FJ Jr, Sinaki M, Grabios M, et al. Health professional's guide to rehabilitation of the patient with osteoporosis. Osteoporos Int 2003;14(Suppl 2):S1–22.

[21] Papaioannou A, Adachi JD, Winegard K, et al. Efficacy of home based exercise for improving quality of life among elderly women with symptomatic osteoporosis-related vertebral fractures. Osteoporos Int 2003;14:677–82.

[22] Sinaki M, Brey RH, Hughes CA, et al. Significant reduction in risk of falls and back pain in osteoporotic-kyphotic women through a spinal proprioceptive extension exercise dynamic (SPEED) program. Mayo Clin Proc 2005;80(7):849–55.

[23] Kaplan RS, Sinaki M. Posture training support: preliminary report on a series of patients with diminished symptomatic complications of osteoporosis. Mayo Clin Proc 1993;68(12): 1171–6.

[24] Stillo JV, Stein AB, Ragnarsson KT. Low-back orthoses. Phys Med Rehabil Clin N Am 1992;3:57–91.

[25] Deramond H, Depriester C, Galibert P, et al. Percutaneous vertebroplasty with polymethylmethacrylate: technique, indications, and results. Radiol Clin North Am 1998;36: 533–46.

[26] Cyteval C, Sarrabere MP, Roux JO, et al. Acute osteoporotic vertebral collapse: open study on percutaneous injection of acrylic surgical cement in 20 patients. J Rheumatol 1999;173: 1685–90.

[27] Cortet B, Cotton A, Boutry R, et al. Percutaneous vertebroplasty in the treatment of osteoporotic vertebral compression fractures: an open prospective study. J Rheumatol 1999;26:2222–8.

[28] Heini PF, Walchll B, Berlemann U. Percutaneous transpedicular vertebroplasty with PMMA: operative technique and early results. A prospective study for the treatment of osteoporotic compression fractures. Eur Spine J 2000;9:445–50.

[29] Zoarski GH, Snow P, Olan WJ, et al. Percutaneous vertebroplasty for osteoporotic compression fractures: quantitative prospective evaluation of long-term outcomes. J Vasc Interv Radiol 2002;13(2 Pt 1):139–48.

[30] McGraw JK, Lippert JA, Minkus KD, et al. Prospective evaluation of pain relief in 100 patients undergoing percutaneous vertebroplasty: results and follow-up. J Vasc Interv Radiol 2002;13(9 Pt 1):883–6.

[31] Prather H, Van Dillen L, Metzler J, et al. Prospective measure of functional and pain improvements in patients with non-neoplastic compression fractures treated with vertebroplasty. J Bone Joint Surg Am 2006;88(2):334–41.

[32] McKiernan F, Faciszewski T, Jensen R. Does vertebral height restoration achieved at vertebroplasty matter? J Vasc Interv Radiol 2005;16(7):973–9.

[33] Martin JB, Jean B, Suglu K, et al. Vertebroplasty: clinical experience and follow-up results. Bone 1999;25(Suppl 2):11S–5S.

[34] Grados F, Depriester C, Cayrolle G, et al. Long-term observations of vertebral osteoporotic fractures by percutaneous vertebroplasty. Rheumatology (Oxford) 2000;39:1410–4.

[35] Barr JD, Barr MS, Lemley TJ, et al. Percutaneous vertebroplasty for pain relief and spinal stabilization. Spine 2000;25:923–8.

[36] Amar AP, Larsen DW, Esnaasharl N, et al. Percutaneous transpedicular polymethlmethacrylate vertebroplasty for the treatment of spinal compression fractures. Neurosurgery 2001;49:1105–15.

[37] Evans AJ, Jensen ME, Kip KE, et al. Vertebral compression fractures: pain reduction and improvement in functional mobility after percutaneous polymethylmethacrylate vertebroplasty retrospective report of 245 cases. Radiology 2003;226(2):366–72.

[38] Hodler J, Peck D, Gilula LA. Midterm outcome after vertebroplasty: predictive value of technical and patient-related factors. Radiology 2003;227:662–8.

[39] Peh WC, Gilula LA, Peck DD. Percutaneous vertebroplasty for severe osteoporotic vertebral body compression fractures. Radiology 2002;223:121–6.

[40] Gaitanis IN, Hadjipavlou AG, Katonis PG, et al. Balloon kyphoplasty for the treatment of pathological vertebral compression fractures. Eur Spine J 2005;14(3):250–60.

[41] Crandall D, Slaughter D, Hankins PJ, et al. Acute versus chronic vertebral compression fractures treated with kyphoplasty: early results. Spine J 2004;4:418–24.

[42] McCann H, LePine M, Glaser J. Biomechanical comparison of augmentation techniques for insuffiency fractures. Spine 2006;11(15):E499–502.

[43] Cotton A, Dewatre F, Cortet B, et al. Percutaneous vertebroplasty for osteolytic metastases and myeloma: effects of the percentage of lesions filling and the leakage of methyl methacrylate at clinical follow-up. Radiology 1996;200(2):525–30.

[44] Berlemann U, Franz T, Orler R, et al. Kyphoplasty for treatment of osteoporotic vertebral fractures: a prospective non-randomized study. Eur Spine J 2004;13(6):496–501.

[45] Fribourg D, Tang C, Sra P, et al. Incidence of subsequent vertebral fracture after kyphoplasty. Spine 2004;29:2270–6.

[46] Tomita S, Kin A, Yazu M, et al. Biomechanical evaluation of kyphoplasty and vertebroplasty with calcium phosphate cement in a simulated osteoporotic compression fracture. J Orthop Sci 2003;8(2):192–7.

[47] Mathis JM, Barr JD, Belkoff SM, et al. Percutaneous vertebroplasty: a developing standard of care for vertebral compression fractures. AJNR Am J Neuroradiol 2001;22(2):373–81.

[48] Liebermann IH, Dudeney S, Reinhardt MK, et al. Initial outcome and efficacy of "kyphoplasty" in the treatment of painful osteoporotic vertebral compression fractures. Spine 2001; 26(14):1631–8.

[49] Kallmes DF, Schweickert PA, Marx WF, et al. Vertebroplasty in the mid- and upper thoracic spine. AJNR Am J Neuorodadiol 2002;23(7):1117–20.

[50] Garfin SR, Yuan HA, Reiley MA. New technologies in spine: kyphoplasty and vertebroplasty for the treatment of painful osteoporotic compression fractures. Spine 2001;26: 1511–5.

[51] O'Brien JP, Sims JT, Evans AJ. Vertebroplasty in patients with severe vertebral compression fractures: a technical report. AJNR Am J Neuroradiol 2000;21:1555–8.

[52] Ledlie JT, Renfro M. Balloon kyphoplasty: one-year outcomes in vertebral body height restoration, chronic pain, and activity levels. J Neurosurg 2003;98(Suppl 1):36–42.

ELSEVIER
SAUNDERS

Phys Med Rehabil Clin N Am
18 (2007) 593–608

PHYSICAL MEDICINE
AND REHABILITATION
CLINICS OF
NORTH AMERICA

The Role of Physical Activity in Bone Health: A New Hypothesis to Reduce Risk of Vertebral Fracture

Mehrsheed Sinaki, MD, MSc

*Department of Physical Medicine and Rehabilitation, Mayo Clinic,
200 First Street SW, Rochester, MN 55905, USA*

Locomotion has always been a major criterion for human survival. Thus, it is no surprise that science supports the dependence of bone health on weight-bearing physical activities. "Bone, to be maintained, needs to be mechanically strained—within its biomechanical limits" [1].

Musculoskeletal challenges of aging

Bone loss and sarcopenia of aging cause an imbalance in the body's musculoskeletal ability to withstand extensive mechanical strain. A mechanical strain to the skeletal structure can be as low as gravity alone and as high as the impact of a moving, energized body part as it contacts a hard floor. The point of no return for fracture is defined by the quality of the bone and supportive soft tissues of the musculoskeletal structure.

Bone loss related to aging is more challenging for the female skeleton than the male skeleton. In one study comparing the ash weight of vertebral bodies (L3) in the cadavers of men and women aged 18 to 96 years, women had significantly lower ash weight than men of the same age [2]. Sarcopenia of aging affects women more than men because women start life with less muscle strength [3].

The process of bone remodeling affects bone loss more from metabolically hyperactive trabecular bone than cortical bone at menopause. The result is 47% bone loss from the spine during a woman's life [4]. The most significant bone loss occurs between ages 50 and 58 years, after sudden gonadal atrophy at menopause. In men, age-related axial bone loss is

E-mail address: sinaki.mehrsheed@mayo.edu

1047-9651/07/$ - see front matter © 2007 Elsevier Inc. All rights reserved.
doi:10.1016/j.pmr.2007.04.002

approximately 30% throughout life, and occurs more gradually because no sudden reduction in reproductive hormones occurs. The appendicular bone loss of aging is also less in men (15%) than in women (30%) [5]. In boys and girls, axial and appendicular muscle strength is approximately the same until age 10 years, when a discrepancy begins to develop (Fig. 1) [3].

Back extensor strength (BES) in women at different decades of life ranges from 54% to 76% of the strength in men (Fig. 2) [6]. This difference in BES between the genders decreases with age. By age 90, men have lost 64% of their maximal BES and women have lost 50% [6]. Sarcopenia of aging affects type II (fast twitch) muscle fibers more than type I fibers. This process expands the ratio of type I motor neuron units at the expense of the type II fibers [7]. The result of these changes is smaller, weaker muscles. Clinically, the consequence is a decrease in the protective role of muscles in locomotion and musculoskeletal health. The loss of muscle strength and bone mass creates more challenges for women than men, because women start life with less bone and muscle mass. In addition, other age-related spinal changes, such as facet arthropathies and reduction of resilience in intervertebral disks, decrease spinal flexibility [8] and can subsequently increase risk for vertebral fracture.

A person who has a fear of falling tends to decrease locomotion and weight-bearing physical activities. In one study, healthy community-dwelling subjects who had osteoporosis had a significantly higher perceived risk for falls than control subjects [9]. The fact that risk for falls increases with aging is well known [10,11]. Participation in a moderate level of physical activity is a significant component of physical and mental health in older adults and can decrease death rate; however, loss of bone and muscle mass may limit their choice of physical activity. Limitation of locomotion

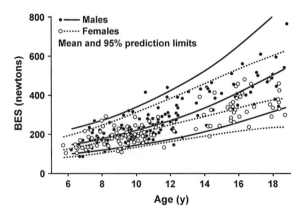

Fig. 1. Correlation of back extensor strength (BES) and age in 246 healthy children (137 boys and 109 girls). (*From* Sinaki M, Limburg PJ, Wollan PC, et al. Correlation of trunk muscle strength with age in children 5 to 18 years old. Mayo Clin Proc 1996;71(11):1047–54. Used with permission of Mayo Foundation for Medical Education and Research.)

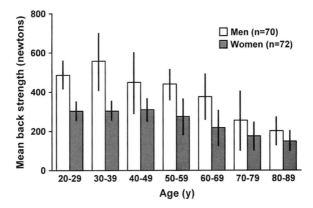

Fig. 2. Back extensor strength in men and women during the third through ninth decades. (*From* Sinaki M, Nwaogwugwu NC, Phillips BE, et al. Effect of gender, age, and anthropometry on axial and appendicular muscle strength. Am J Phys Med Rehabil 2001;80(5):330–8; with permission.)

is inevitable, whether it is caused by central nervous system disorders or the musculoskeletal changes of aging, which usually adds to premature frailty of aging. Risk for falls may increase because of extraskeletal or intraskeletal factors, which are listed in Box 1.

Maintaining biomechanical competence of bone

Proper mechanical loading can increase osteoblastic activity and the rate of bone formation, but its mechanism is not fully understood [12,13]. One study showed that job-related physical activity correlated significantly with bone mineral density of the spine (Fig. 3) [14]. This study showed that individuals working in a medical center who performed weight lifting at their jobs had greater bone mineral density than those engaged in a sedentary job. Some studies that used interventions to improve bone mass in humans did not show a significant increase in bone mass of the spine with weight-training exercises for the back extensor muscles [15,16]. This unexpected result may be attributed to the low intensity of the exercise program, the method used to expose the bone to load, the subject's compliance, or, perhaps, the genetic coding of the bone itself. However, the benefit of exercise on bone should not always be measured based on increased bone mineral density; the resulting changes in bone structure are important in increasing bone strength. One study in animals showed that mechanical loading improved bone strength by reshaping bone structure without increasing bone mineral density [17].

Preventing bone fracture, whether through increasing bone mineral density or reshaping the trabeculae, is the objective of clinical intervention.

Box 1. Factors that contribute to risk of falls

Extrinsic
Environmental
    Physical obstacles
    Slippery floor
    Uneven surfaces
    Poor illumination
    Ill-defined stairs
    Pets
    Icy sidewalks
Extraskeletal
    Inappropriate footwear
    Obstructive clothing

Intrinsic
Lower-extremity weakness (neurogenic or myopathic)
Balance disorder (eg, vestibular changes, peripheral neuropathy, hyperkyphosis)
Visual impairment, use of bifocals
Cognitive decline
Decreased coordination (eg, cerebellar degeneration)
Postural changes, imbalance, gait unsteadiness
Gait apraxia
Reduced muscle strength
Reduced flexibility
Respiratory difficulty (eg, orthopnea)
Postural hypotension
Cardiovascular deconditioning
Iatrogenically reduced alertness

Modified from Sinaki M. Prevention of hip fracture: physical activity. In: Senile osteoporosis. Ringe JD, Meunier JP, editors. Stuttgart: Georg Thieme Verlag Publications; 1996. p. 99–115; and Sinaki M. Falls, fractures, and hip pads. Curr Osteoporos Rep 2004;2(4):131–7; with permission.

Most current medical literature focuses on the role of exercise in improving bone mass. In a recent long-term follow-up of a controlled trial, however, improved back muscle strength was shown to reduce the risk for vertebral fractures several years after the exercise program was discontinued [18]. The results of this study prompted a new hypothesis that perhaps the exercises to decrease vertebral fracture should be different from loading exercises to increase bone mineral density in the upper and lower extremities.

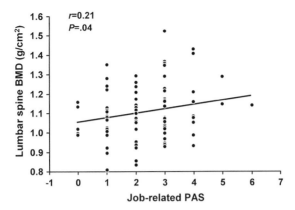

Fig. 3. Physical activity score (PAS) significantly correlated with spinal bone mineral density (BMD). (*From* Sinaki M, Fitzpatrick LA, Ritchie CK, et al. Site-specificity of bone mineral density and muscle strength in women: job-related physical activity. Am J Phys Med Rehabil 1998;77(6):470–6; with permission.)

Choosing a proper physical activity program

Determining how to perform osteogenic exercises, especially in individuals who have osteopenia or osteoporosis, without exceeding the bone's biomechanical competence always poses a dilemma and must be done under medical supervision. Not all exercises are osteogenic. Several studies support the positive effect of physical activity on the maintenance of musculoskeletal health [14,18,19]. However, the significance of the type of exercise and the exercise techniques on bone mass were investigated in recent decades, and the studies have added further information. Before 1980, spinal flexion exercises were popular for managing back pain related to vertebral fractures. The possible logic behind prescribing spinal flexion exercises was to stretch the paraspinal muscles that are in painful cocontraction while guarding the painful, fractured vertebral bodies [20]. Flexing the spine might have made scientific sense initially, but considering that these exercises flexed and compressed the osteoporotic spine, which was already biomechanically compromised, made no common sense. The clinical study, which was conducted to clarify the investigators' clinical impression, supported the fact that flexion of the osteoporotic spine would result in more vertebral compressions or fractures (Fig. 4) [20,21]. In this study, 59 women aged 49 to 60 years (mean age, 56 years) with postmenopausal spinal osteoporosis and back pain were divided into four groups. One group performed spinal extension exercises (not hyperextension), one group performed spinal flexion exercises, one group performed a combination of spinal extension and flexion exercises, and one group received only heat and massage with no prescribed exercise. All groups received instructions for proper posture principles. Follow-up time varied from 1 to 6 years (means for the groups, 1.4–2 years)

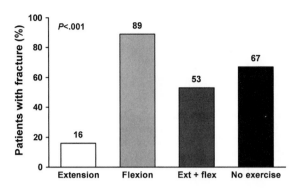

Fig. 4. Percentage of patients who experienced fracture after spinal extension exercise, spinal flexion exercise, a combination of extension and flexion (Ext + flex) exercise, and no exercise. (*Data from* Sinaki M, Mikkelsen BA. Postmenopausal spinal osteoporosis: flexion versus extension exercises. Arch Phys Med Rehabil 1984;65(10):593–6.)

dependent on the occurrence of increased back pain, which indicated a need for follow-up radiographic evaluation. The extension group had a longer period before follow-up. All subjects underwent spine radiographic studies before initiation of the treatment program and at follow-up, when any further wedging or compression fractures, or both, were recorded. Comparisons of the baseline and follow-up radiographs showed additional fractures in 16% of subjects in the extension group, 89% in the flexion group, 53% in the extension and flexion group, and 67% in the group that had no prescribed exercises for treatment and was provided only heat and massage (see Fig. 4).

The difference between the spinal extension and spinal flexion groups was most significant ($P < .001$). The P values were also significant for the extension group versus the extension and flexion group ($P < .01$) and for the extension group versus the no-exercise group ($P < .01$). The result of this study was so surprisingly supportive of the author's clinical impression that exposing the osteoporotic spine to flexion exercises in a prospective study seemed unethical. Flexion of the spine has also been shown to increase intradiskal pressure [22], which can be transmitted to osteoporotic vertebral bodies anteriorly and result in vertebral wedging and fracture.

The conclusion that physical activity affects bone has been reported repeatedly; however, not all exercises affect bone and muscle in the same way. Osteogenicity depends on the type, intensity, and duration of the exercise performed. In addition, the type of exercise must differ according to the various spinal deformities or skeletal challenges.

Reducing the risk for vertebral fractures without increasing bone mass

In one study, the author and colleagues showed that bone mineral density of vertebral bodies and back strength were correlated [23]. Later, however, they found that resistive exercises that did not load the spine vertically could not increase the vertebral bone mass, although back extensor strength increased significantly (Fig. 5) [15]. Initially, the lack of increase in bone mineral density was disappointing, but they later learned that the long-term effect of these exercises was very promising and effective in reducing the risk for vertebral fractures [18]. Exercise can affect not only bone mass and muscle strength but also vertebral structure and the horizontal trabeculae, which may individually reduce the risk for vertebral fractures [18].

Osteogenicity and site specificity

The effect of physical activity on bone is site-specific. In young and old tennis players, the bone mineral density in the dominant humerus was reportedly up to 33% greater than in the nondominant humerus [24,25]. Weight lifters have been shown to have greater bone mineral density of the spine and femur than athletes who do aerobic activity [26]. Also, swimmers have been shown to have less bone mineral density of the femoral neck than sedentary people [27]. Although swimming exercises are not osteogenic in women, their effect on improving muscle strength and general fitness should not be minimized [28]. The correlation of muscle strength at various sites of the axial and appendicular skeleton with physical activity and aerobic capacity was assessed in one study of women aged 29 to 40 years [29]. This study showed that maximal oxygen uptake is not a valid marker for the level of daily weight-bearing physical activities.

Significance of mechanical loading of physical activity in bone health

In general, physical activity increases the competence of neuromuscular structures to reduce the risk for fracture. This effect is accomplished through

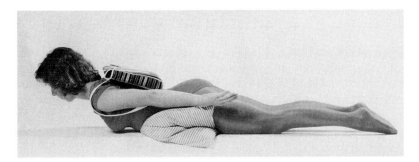

Fig. 5. Model showing the author's back-strengthening exercise with a backpack containing sandbag weights. (*From* Sinaki M, Wahner HW, Offord KP, et al. Efficacy of nonloading exercises in prevention of vertebral bone loss in postmenopausal women: a controlled trial. Mayo Clin Proc 1989;64(7):762–9. Used with permission of Mayo Foundation for Medical Education and Research.)

improvement in muscle strength, bone structure, and neuromuscular efficiency, thereby reducing the risk for falls [19]. In animal studies, the bone response to mechanical loading was proportional to the applied dose of load in cell and organ culture [30]. In human studies, the evaluation of this relationship has been hindered by a lack of proper technology. With the advancement in quantitative CT and MRI techniques, further research will help clarify these issues.

Mechanical stimulus initiates a chain of events that involves intracellular messengers. The subsequent effects on proper cellular coding can cause bone formation and increase bone mass [31]. Several studies on exercise have discovered more facts about effective exercises for managing bone health [19,27,32]. The effects of high strain from muscle contractions in non–weight-bearing exercises compared with weight-bearing exercises did not increase lumbar and femoral bone mass in eumenorrheic swimmers. In a finding of great interest, the study reported that the bone mineral density of the femoral neck and spine was significantly less in swimmers than in gymnasts but not different from that in control subjects [32,33].

Several studies report the effect of strengthening exercises on bone mass in postmenopausal women [16,20,34–36]. These reports substantiate the conclusion that bone mass is not the only factor in maintaining bone health; muscle strength is also important. Although physical exercises are needed at all stages of life, women at risk for fracture should initiate a specific exercise program rather than increase bone strain during their habitual physical activities [37]. For example, they should perform back strengthening exercises in a sitting or prone position, rather than lift heavy loads during gardening, cooking, or other strenuous homemaking activities.

Optimal physical activity for bone health

Optimal exercise programs differ according to an individual's cardiovascular health, bone density, muscle strength, and history of involvement in sports activity. The status of lower-extremity joints and neuromuscular health are also decisive factors in selecting an appropriate exercise program for patients. Considering these issues before recommending exercises increases the probability of adherence to the prescribed program. Prevention of falls also must be addressed, because frailty associated with osteoporosis increases the risk for fracture and the fear of participation in ambulatory activities. Musculoskeletal changes that increase spinal deformities, especially hyperkyphosis, may increase the risk for falls [38].

Muscular strength of the axial skeleton is important in preventing falls. The main axial support is provided by back extensors, hip muscle groups, and the quadriceps. One study showed that the risk for falls decreased when lower-extremity muscles were strengthened through resistance-training exercises [39]. Another study showed that improvement in back muscle strength increased the level of physical activity [9,40].

Prescribing optimal exercise programs is different from advising patients to stay physically active. Some physical activities may increase the risk for vertebral fracture rather than improve skeletal health. (Of these activities, the most well-documented is flexion of the osteoporotic spine with or without lifting a load with the upper extremities.) In addition, inducing flexion on an osteoporotic spine, even without loading the spine, may result in vertebral fracture (see Fig. 4) [21]. One study found that sarcopenia of aging affected the lower extremities more than the upper extremities [6]. This study in women showed that, over the decades of life, body mass index increased while muscle strength decreased significantly (Fig. 6). A gradual increase in the level of physical activity can increase muscle strength and thus improve lean body mass, which mainly consists of supportive skeletal muscles. However, extra body fat can decrease the risk for fracture in areas such as the hips by dispersing the energy of a fall-related impact.

Increasing the level of physical activity despite osteoporosis and pain

Osteoporosis-related back pain, whether chronic or acute, prevents participation in physical activities (Fig. 7) [9]. Further bone and muscle loss concomitantly occurs when immobility related to back pain persists. In addition, the pain-induced inhibition of contraction of back extensors results in overuse of spinal flexors that guard the spine, which may further contribute to hyperkyphosis. Physical therapeutic measures that facilitate the use of back extensors (eg, posture training with or without weighted kypho-orthosis) reduce back pain and immobility and increase the level of physical activity. A significant decrease in back pain and risk for falls and improvement in the level of physical activity have been achieved through the spinal proprioceptive extension exercise dynamic (SPEED) program ($P < .05$) [9]. In the

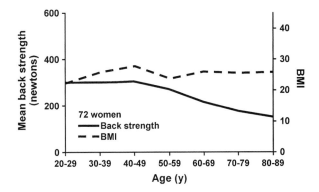

Fig. 6. Back extensor strength and body mass index (BMI) in women during the third through ninth decades. (*From* Sinaki M, Nwaogwugwu NC, Phillips BE, et al. Effect of gender, age, and anthropometry on axial and appendicular muscle strength. Am J Phys Med Rehabil 2001; 80(5):330–8; with permission.)

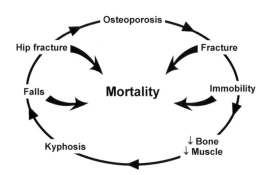

Fig. 7. "Circle of events" showing common events that can result in hip fracture and mortality.

SPEED program, joint proprioceptors are used to improve spine posture and balance disorder. Another issue is that prior fracture has been consistently associated with increased risk for subsequent fractures [41,42].

After compression fracture of vertebral bodies and its induced back pain, participation in physical activity decreases. To decrease painful contractions of the erector spinae muscles, a decrease is needed in the load over the anterior aspect of the spinal column and vertebral bodies and may be accomplished through the use of a back support. Initially, a rigid shell or brace may be considered, but most elderly patients who have spinal deformity do not tolerate them for more than a short time. If a patient has a spinal deformity, using a weighted kypho-orthosis with the weights positioned below the inferior angles of the scapulae unloads the spine in the more desired direction and thus improves the kinetics of the spine, rather than causing the spine immobilization that results from rigid bracing. This device may kinematically facilitate the use of the erector spinae muscles to protect the spine, because most compression fractures occur in the midthoracic and thoracolumbar junction and upper lumbar vertebral bodies. Kyphotic posture kinematically creates an angle for contracting the erector spinae muscles that is not advantageous.

Physical activity, whether it is in homemaking, job-related, or structured sports activities, correlates with improvement of muscle strength in the back and the upper and lower extremities according to the areas of the body involved in the activity [43,44]. Structured physical activity, such as a whole-body vibration program, has been shown to increase muscle strength, balance, and bone mineral density of the hip [45]. These exercise machines are newly available and must be evaluated further. The use of exercise machines that increase hip muscle strength (Fig. 8) contributes to improved body mechanics and body mass index [46]. A back-extension exercise program may improve posture and decrease risk for vertebral fracture and falls [9]. Back-extension strengthening exercises can be implemented with use of a progressive, resistive exercise program (see Fig. 5) [15]. In individuals who have osteoporosis, these exercises can be performed without applying weight

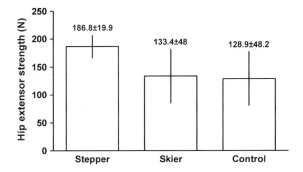

Fig. 8. Hip extensor strength was significantly higher in stepper group than in skier and control groups (stepper versus skier, $P = .03$; stepper versus control, $P = .03$; skier versus control, $P = .72$). Numbers at top of columns are mean $\pm$ SD. N, newton. (*From* Sinaki M, Canvin JC, Phillips BE, et al. Site specificity of regular health club exercise on muscle strength, fitness, and bone density in women aged 29 to 45 years. Mayo Clin Proc 2004;79(5):639–44. Used with permission of Mayo Foundation for Medical Education and Research.)

to the back (Fig. 9) [47]. Additionally, studies have shown that changes in the frequency of back-extension exercise or the repetition of weight lifting at each exercise session, or both, or changes in the exercise intensity may result in different outcomes [48].

In the postmenopausal stage, a woman's physical activity must consist of weight-bearing aerobic activities and safe weight-training exercises. Physical activity can decrease the prevalence of cardiovascular disease in postmenopausal women by 30% to 50% [49]. It is well known that physical activity contributes to the maintenance of cardiovascular fitness. Therefore, a 45- to 60-minute physical activity program must consist of cardiovascular exercise, such as walking (30 minutes); range-of-motion exercises combined with stretching; muscle strengthening (three times per week); and weight lifting (three times per week) [1]. Muscle strengthening consists of resistive exercises for the intended muscle groups, and weight

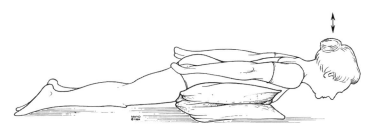

Fig. 9. Back-extension exercise performed in prone position with no added weight. (*From* Sinaki M, Grubbs NC. Back strengthening exercises: quantitative evaluation of their efficacy for women aged 40 to 65 years. Arch Phys Med Rehabil 1989;70(1):16–20. Used with permission of Mayo Foundation for Medical Education and Research.)

lifting consists of loading the spine or lower extremities with weights. Participating in a regular physical activity program consisting of weight-bearing, weight-training, and aerobic activities promotes good musculo-skeletal and cardiovascular health.

Exercise after osteoporotic fracture

Physical rehabilitative measures play a key role in preventing further fracture. To improve a patient's level of physical activity after vertebral fracture, locomotion must be facilitated and axial muscle strength improved. Improvement in BES may increase the patient's level of physical activity [9,14]. The most successful physical activity and rehabilitative programs are those that are incorporated into the patient's usual daily ambulatory activities; they must be user-friendly and site-specific to back extensors without overdoing the strain on the spine or dependence on a specific exercise machine [1].

New hypothesis on the best exercise to reduce vertebral fracture risk

A study of the late effect of back-extension strengthening exercise after 8 years showed that vertebral fracture risk can be decreased through exercise (Fig. 10) [18,36]. However, exercises to decrease the risk for fractures of the

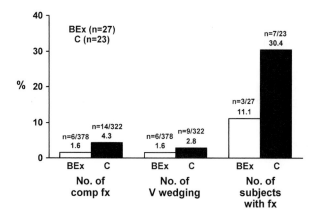

Fig. 10. At 10-year follow-up, the number of vertebral compression fractures (comp fx) was 14 (4.3%) of 322 vertebral bodies examined in the control (C) group and 6 (1.6%) of 378 vertebral bodies examined in the back exercise (BEx) group (χ^2 test, $P = .0290$). The number of subjects with vertebral fractures in the control group was three times greater than in the BEx group. The denominator represents the number of vertebral bodies that were evaluated using spinal radiographs at baseline and at 10-year follow-up; the nominator represents the number of vertebral bodies that were fractured or wedged on follow-up evaluation. V, vertebral. (*From* Sinaki M. Critical appraisal of physical rehabilitation measures after osteoporotic vertebral fracture. Osteoporos Int 2003;14(9):773–9. [erratum in: Osteoporosis Int 2006;17:1702]; with permission.)

spine are different from those to strengthen the upper extremities. The author's hypothesis is that back exercises performed in a prone position, rather than a vertical position, may have a greater effect on decreasing the risk for vertebral fractures without resulting in compression fracture. One can theorize that the risk for vertebral fractures can be reduced through improvement in the horizontal trabecular connection of vertebral bodies.

Summary

To be maintained, bone must be strained with a stimulus of specific magnitude and frequency. In postmenopausal osteopenia or osteoporosis, success depends on a combination of proper pharmacotherapy (especially adequate calcium and vitamin D supplementation) and biomechanical, bone-safe, osteogenic physical activity programs [50,51]. When the physical stimulus on bone is within a routine, daily range of physical activities, bone mass is neither lost nor increased. If the level of physical activity changes to one that is above or below the routine level, bone mass changes; if the change in activity puts more strain on bone, hypertrophy occurs. Severe repetitive loading strain that extends beyond the biomechanical competence of bone results in bone stress fracture, as observed in some soldiers, gymnasts, and long-distance runners [52,53]. If the loading physical activity is at an effective level that does not result in a stress fracture, it helps to increase bone mass. In postmenopausal women who have hormone deficiency, participation in very exertional weight-lifting exercises, such as lifting heavy objects, that applies loading beyond the biomechanical competence of bone can result in vertebral fracture. This is especially important since women with osteoporosis have lower back extensor strength [54]. Also, habitual, repetitive lifting and flexion of the spine may cause microfractures of vertebral bodies and gradual vertebral compressions that result in gradual loss of height. Therefore, flexion of the osteoporotic spine is not recommended because it strains the vertebral bodies anteriorly. If anterior loading on the vertebral bodies is beyond a woman's biomechanical competence, wedging and vertebral compression fractures can result during daily, not-so-innocent physical activities.

Successful, bone-safe physical activity for a challenged musculoskeletal status must be initiated under supervision to avoid injuries and improve adherence. The critical issue is adherence to a low to moderate level of physical activity in the postmenopausal stage.

Acknowledgment

The author thanks Sandra Fitzgerald for her secretarial assistance with the initial manuscript. Editing, proofreading, and reference verification were provided by the Section of Scientific Publications, Mayo Clinic.

References

[1] Sinaki M. Prevention and treatment of osteoporosis. In: Braddom RM, editor. Physical medicine & rehabilitation. Philadelphia: Saunders Elsevier; 2007. p. 929–50.

[2] Ebbesen EN, Thomsen JS, Beck-Nielsen H, et al. Age- and gender-related differences in vertebral bone mass, density, and strength. J Bone Miner Res 1999;14(8):1394–403.

[3] Sinaki M, Limburg PJ, Wollan PC, et al. Correlation of trunk muscle strength with age in children 5 to 18 years old. Mayo Clin Proc 1996;71(11):1047–54.

[4] Riggs BL, Melton LJ III. Involutional osteoporosis. N Engl J Med 1986;314(26): 1676–86.

[5] Riggs BL, Wahner HW, Melton LJ III, et al. Rates of bone loss in the appendicular and axial skeletons of women: evidence of substantial vertebral bone loss before menopause. J Clin Invest 1986;77(5):1487–91.

[6] Sinaki M, Nwaogwugwu NC, Phillips BE, et al. Effect of gender, age, and anthropometry on axial and appendicular muscle strength. Am J Phys Med Rehabil 2001;80(5):330–8.

[7] Lexell J, Taylor CC, Sjostrom M. What is the cause of the aging atrophy? Total number, size and proportion of different fiber types studied in whole vastus lateralis muscle from 15- to 83-year-old men. J Neurol Sci 1988;84(2–3):275–94.

[8] Adams P, Eyre DR, Muir H. Biochemical aspects of development and aging of human lumbar intervertebral discs. Rheumatol Rehabil 1977;16(1):22–9.

[9] Sinaki M, Brey RH, Hughes CA, et al. Significant reduction in risk of falls and back pain in osteoporotic-kyphotic women through a Spinal Proprioceptive Extension Exercise Dynamic (SPEED) program. Mayo Clin Proc 2005;80(7):849–55.

[10] Tinetti ME, Speechley M. Prevention of falls among the elderly. N Engl J Med 1989;320(16): 1055–9.

[11] Sinaki M. Falls, fractures, and hip pads. Curr Osteoporos Rep 2004;2(4):131–7.

[12] Lanyon LE. Functional strain as a determinant for bone remodeling. Calcif Tissue Int 1984; 36(Suppl 1):S56–61.

[13] Frost HM. A determinant of bone architecture: the minimum effective strain. Clin Orthop Relat Res 1983;(175):286–92.

[14] Sinaki M, Fitzpatrick LA, Ritchie CK, et al. Site-specificity of bone mineral density and muscle strength in women: job-related physical activity. Am J Phys Med Rehabil 1998;77(6): 470–6.

[15] Sinaki M, Wahner HW, Offord KP, et al. Efficacy of nonloading exercises in prevention of vertebral bone loss in postmenopausal women: a controlled trial. Mayo Clin Proc 1989; 64(7):762–9.

[16] Gleeson PB, Protas EJ, LeBlanc AD, et al. Effects of weight lifting on bone mineral density in premenopausal women. J Bone Miner Res 1990;5(2):153–8.

[17] Jarvinen TL, Kannus P, Sievanen H, et al. Randomized controlled study of effects of sudden impact loading on rat femur. J Bone Miner Res 1998;13(9):1475–82.

[18] Sinaki M, Itoi E, Wahner HW, et al. Stronger back muscles reduce the incidence of vertebral fractures: a prospective 10 year follow-up of postmenopausal women. Bone 2002;30(6):836–41.

[19] Smith EL, Gilligan C. Dose-response relationship between physical loading and mechanical competence of bone. Bone 1996;18(1 Suppl):455–505.

[20] Sinaki M. Postmenopausal spinal osteoporosis: physical therapy and rehabilitation principles. Mayo Clin Proc 1982;57(11):699–703.

[21] Sinaki M, Mikkelsen BA. Postmenopausal spinal osteoporosis: flexion versus extension exercises. Arch Phys Med Rehabil 1984;65(10):593–6.

[22] Nachemson A. Lumbar intradiscal pressure: experimental studies on post-mortem material. Acta Orthop Scand Suppl 1960;43:45–74.

[23] Sinaki M, McPhee MC, Hodgson SF, et al. Relationship between bone mineral density of spine and strength of back extensors in healthy postmenopausal women. Mayo Clin Proc 1986;61(2):116–22.

[24] Huddleston AL, Rockwell D, Kulund DN, et al. Bone mass in lifetime tennis athletes. JAMA 1980;244(10):1107 9.

[25] Ducher G, Courteix D, Même S, et al. Bone geometry in response to long-term tennis playing and its relationship with muscle volume: a quantitative magnetic resonance imaging study in tennis players. Bone 2005;37(4):457–66.

[26] Block JE, Genant HK, Black D. Greater vertebral bone mineral mass in exercising young men. West J Med 1986;145(1):39–42.

[27] Fehling PC, Alekel L, Clasey J, et al. A comparison of bone mineral densities among female athletes in impact loading and active loading sports. Bone 1995;17(3):205–10.

[28] Emslander HC, Sinaki M, Muhs JM, et al. Bone mass and muscle strength in female college athletes (runners and swimmers). Mayo Clin Proc 1998;73(12):1151–60.

[29] Petrie RS, Sinaki M, Squires RW, et al. Physical activity, but not aerobic capacity, correlates with back strength in healthy premenopausal women from 29 to 40 years of age. Mayo Clin Proc 1993;68(9):738–42.

[30] Snow CM. Exercise and bone mass in young and premenopausal women. Bone 1996;18 (1 Suppl):51S–5S.

[31] Rana RS, Hokin LE. Role of phosphoinositides in transmembrane signaling. Physiol Rev 1990;70(1):115–64.

[32] Taaffe DR, Snow-Harter C, Connolly DA, et al. Differential effects of swimming versus weight-bearing activity on bone mineral status of eumenorrheic athletes. J Bone Miner Res 1995;10(4):586–93.

[33] Snow-Harter C, Wegner M, Robinson T, et al. Determinants of femoral neck mineral density in pre- and postmenopausal women. Med Sci Sports Exerc 1993;25:S153.

[34] Krolner B, Toft B, Pors Nielsen S, et al. Physical exercise as prophylaxis against involutional vertebral bone loss: a controlled trial. Clin Sci (Lond) 1983;64(5):541–6.

[35] Dalsky GP, Stocke KS, Ehsani AA, et al. Weight-bearing exercise training and lumbar bone mineral content in postmenopausal women. Ann Intern Med 1988;108(6):824–8.

[36] Sinaki M. Critical appraisal of physical rehabilitation measures after osteoporotic vertebral fracture. Osteoporos Int 2003;14(9):773–9 [erratum in: Osteoporosis Int 2006;17:1702].

[37] Kemmler W, Weineck J, Kalender WA, et al. The effect of habitual physical activity, non-athletic exercise, muscle strength, and VO_{2max} on bone mineral density is rather low in early postmenopausal osteopenic women. J Musculoskelet Neuronal Interact 2004;4(3):325–34.

[38] Sinaki M, Brey RH, Hughes CA, et al. Balance disorder and increased risk of falls in osteoporosis and kyphosis: significance of kyphotic posture and muscle strength. Osteoporos Int 2005;16(8):1004–10.

[39] Nelson ME, Fiatarone MA, Morganti CM, et al. Effects of high-intensity strength training on multiple risk factors for osteoporotic fractures. A randomized controlled trial. JAMA 1994;272(24):1909–14.

[40] Sinaki M, Lynn SG. Reducing the risk of falls through proprioceptive dynamic posture training in osteoporotic women with kyphotic posturing: a randomized pilot study. Am J Phys Med Rehabil 2002;81(4):241–6.

[41] Lindsay R, Silverman SL, Cooper C, et al. Risk of new vertebral fracture in the year following a fracture. JAMA 2001;285(3):320–3.

[42] Port L, Center J, Briffa NK, et al. Osteoporotic fracture: missed opportunity for intervention. Osteoporos Int 2003;14(9):780–4.

[43] Sinaki M, Offord KP. Physical activity in postmenopausal women: effect on back muscle strength and bone mineral density of the spine. Arch Phys Med Rehabil 1988;69(4):277–80.

[44] Limburg P, Sinaki M, Bergstrahl E, et al. Correlations between physical activity, physical fitness and back extensor strength in healthy, active young women. In: Christiansen C, Overgaard K, editors. Osteoporosis, vol. 3. Denmark: Osteopress ApS; 1990. p. 1350–2.

[45] Verschueren SM, Roelants M, Delecluse C, et al. Effect of 6-month whole body vibration training on hip density, muscle strength, and postural control in postmenopausal women: a randomized controlled pilot study. J Bone Miner Res 2004;19(3):352–9.

[46] Sinaki M, Canvin JC, Phillips BE, et al. Site specificity of regular health club exercise on muscle strength, fitness, and bone density in women aged 29 to 45 years. Mayo Clin Proc 2004; 79(5):639–44.

[47] Sinaki M, Grubbs NC. Back strengthening exercises: quantitative evaluation of their efficacy for women aged 40 to 65 years. Arch Phys Med Rehabil 1989;70(1):16–20.

[48] Hongo M, Itoi E, Sinaki M, et al. Effects of reducing resistance, repetitions, and frequency of back-strengthening exercise in healthy young women: a pilot study. Arch Phys Med Rehabil 2005;86(7):1299–303.

[49] Beitz R, Doren M. Physical activity and postmenopausal health. J Br Menopause Soc 2004; 10(2):70–4.

[50] Gass M, Dawson-Hughes B. Preventing osteoporosis-related fractures: an overview. Am J Med 2006;119(4 Suppl 1):S3–11.

[51] Devine A, Dhaliwal SS, Dick IM, et al. Physical activity and calcium consumption are important determinants of lower limb bone mass in older women. J Bone Miner Res 2004; 19(10):1634–9.

[52] Lloyd T, Triantafyllou SJ, Baker ER, et al. Women athletes with menstrual irregularity have increased musculoskeletal injuries. Med Sci Sports Exerc 1986;18(4):374–9.

[53] Finestone A, Shlamkovitch N, Eldad A, et al. Risk factors for stress fractures among Israeli infantry recruits. Mil Med 1991;156(10):528–30.

[54] Sinaki M, Khosla S, Limburg PJ, et al. Muscle strength in osteoporotic versus normal women. Osteoporos Int 1993;3(1):8–12.

ELSEVIER
SAUNDERS

Phys Med Rehabil Clin N Am
18 (2007) 609–621

PHYSICAL MEDICINE
AND REHABILITATION
CLINICS OF
NORTH AMERICA

Prevention and Treatment of Frailty in the Postmenopausal Woman

Wendy S. Shore, PhD*,
Barbara J. deLateur, MD, MS

Department of Physical Medicine and Rehabilitation, The Johns Hopkins Medical Institutions, 600 North Wolfe Street, Phipps 174, Baltimore, MD 21287, USA

Frailty is a complex subject, and all aspects of frailty are intertwined. This article identifies and discusses the individual aspects of frailty. These aspects, including sarcopenia, nutrition, obesity, relative strength, inflammatory markers, osteopenia and osteoporosis, aerobic capacity, absolute strength, balance, and prevention of frailty, must be reunited, albeit in varying combinations, if the effects of frailty on women are to be understood and treated. This article does not exhaust the topic, but covers what the authors consider to be the major issues.

Definitions of frailty

Frailty can be intuitively defined as the characteristics of an individual who is thin and weak. Vulnerability, fragility, and lack of resilience are also generally considered characteristics of frail individuals. A broad definition of frailty, developed by Buchner and coworkers [1] in the Seattle arm of the Frailty and Injuries: Cooperative Studies of Intervention Techniques (FICSIT) study, states that frailty is any loss of physiologic reserves that predicts or increases the susceptibility to disability. These reserves include relative strength, bone density, and aerobic capacity, and might also include cognitive abilities, motor skills, linguistic ability, various types of memory, visual acuity, and hearing acuity. When young people become temporarily incapacitated from illness or injury, they lose some muscle mass, strength, and aerobic capacity. However, they have enough in reserve that they can recover from the illness or injury using what strength remains to return to preillness levels. If older individuals have lived sedentary lives, they will

---

* Corresponding author.
E-mail address: wshore1@jhmi.edu (W.S. Shore).

doi:10.1016/j.pmr.2007.04.004

have gradually lost so much strength that they have little or no reserves; illness or injury will weaken them and they will not have the ability to recover completely. Many families report that grandparents are never the same after the flu or a fall; their reserves, which were once abundant, are gone.

Because frailty can exist before it is obvious, and because it is such a central problem with aging, considerable effort has been expended to clearly define the concept. Using factor analysis, Speechley and Tinetti [2] identified nine variables that loaded heavily on a construct called frailty. Those variables were divided into three subgroups: (1) predictors of future loss of physiologic reserve (eg, age >80 years, depression, sedative use, sedentary lifestyle), (2) indicators of current loss (eg, decreased muscle strength in shoulder or knee, visual loss), and (3) clinical measures of disability (eg, measurements of gait, balance, and lower extremity disability). The frailty syndrome has also been elucidated by Fried, Bandeen-Roche, and co-workers [3], who characterize frailty as a medical syndrome caused by aggregate declines in multiple molecular, cellular, and physiologic systems, and is indicated by weight loss, exhaustion, low energy expenditure, weakness, and slowness. In proportional hazards models, frail women had a higher risk for losing the ability to perform activities of daily living (ADLs) or instrumental ADLs (IADLs), and a greater risk for institutionalization and death, independent of multiple potentially confounding factors.

Sarcopenia

Sarcopenia, the loss of muscle mass and strength that occurs with aging, is a term coined by Rosenberg in 1988 [4] to describe one of the most noticeable changes that occurs in older women. It has generally been considered a normal part of aging and does not seem to require the presence of disease [5]. However, because most data are cross-sectional, and the speed and degree of loss varies greatly among individuals, defining the limits of "normal" is an ongoing process. Consequently, discussion is ongoing about how much loss of muscle mass is an inevitable part of aging, and how much is caused by disuse [6,7]. Numerous studies of older athletes have found that for those who have maintained an active lifestyle, the loss of muscle mass is much less than would be predicted by age [8].

Muscle mass is also lost after illness or surgery. Each day of bed rest results in an estimated 1% loss of muscle strength [9], and an estimated 75% of hip fracture patients will lose so much muscle mass that they will never regain previous levels of function [10].

Clearly a link exists between muscle loss and disability. Janssen and colleagues [11], developed a scale of muscle loss with certain cut points below which odds for disability significantly increased. Encouragingly, even very frail nursing home residents in their 70s, 80s, and 90s can improve muscle strength by as much as 100% through resistance training, resulting in improvement in gait velocity and stair-climbing ability [12].

Because production of hormones, such as growth hormone, testosterone, and estrogen, are known to be related to strength and diminish with age, treatment of muscle loss with hormones has been investigated. Studies suggest that although some improvements can be attributed to growth hormone, the unwanted side effects are numerous and the improvements minimal [13]. Testosterone replacement therapy is considered a possible treatment of frailty for older men. Although some experts suggest that this treatment might have beneficial effects on muscle mass and strength, determining whether adverse side effects counterbalance any possible benefits is impossible. Despite the fact that testosterone levels in women are also linked to muscle mass and strength and that testosterone production diminishes with age in women, few studies have examined testosterone replacement for older women as a treatment of loss of muscle mass, and none has shown unequivocal improvement in health-related outcomes [14]. Although hormone replacement therapies have been used to try to reverse sarcopenia, strength training is the preferred treatment of age-related muscle wasting [15].

Nutrition

Aging is associated with altered sensations of thirst, hunger, sense of smell, and satiety [16,17]. When older people have no obvious reason to eat, the frequent result is diets lacking in the variety necessary to provide adequate nutrition. Older women may be at higher risk for micronutrient malnutrition because of difficulty with shopping and meal preparation and simple disinclination to prepare complex meals when the meal will be eaten alone (among women aged ≥75 years, 51% live alone [18]). Not unreasonably, older persons tend to adapt their diets to individual functional difficulties, such as chewing, self-feeding, shopping for basic necessities, carrying a shopping bag, cooking a warm meal, or using fingers to grasp or handle. These problems can lead to monotonous food consumption and, as a consequence, inadequate nutrient intake. Reporting difficulties in three or more nutrition-related activities has been shown to significantly increase the risk for inadequate intake of energy [19,20]. Bartali and colleagues [19] found evidence that low intakes of energy and selected nutrients are independently associated with frailty. Semba and colleagues [21] found that low serum micronutrient (various vitamins and minerals) concentrations are an independent risk factor for frailty among disabled older women, and that the risk for frailty increases with the number of micronutrient deficiencies.

Individuals do not need to be thin to be malnourished. In a study examining the nutritional status of rural, homebound elderly, virtually all were deficient in recommended nutrients, but only 5% of those interviewed were underweight (body mass index [BMI] <18.5). In fact, 22% were overweight (BMI 25.0–29.9) and 33% were obese (BMI >30.0) [22]. Overweight and obese older women, particularly those living alone, may be at greater nutritional risk than men who have a high BMI [23].

Experts have suggested that, although older people's caloric needs may diminish with age, their need for protein may not, and the current recommended dietary allowance of 0.8 g per kilogram of weight per day is probably insufficient to meet the needs of most older people [24,25].

Inadequate diet, and especially inadequate protein, results in low energy, which leads to reduced activity and therefore loss of muscle mass and aerobic capacity, which then diminishes appetite. This vicious circle is further exacerbated by the fact that poor diet, inadequate activity, and (often) inadequate intake of water contribute to constipation, which also diminishes appetite and discourages physical activity (Fig. 1).

Some suggest that aerobic activity can improve the absorption of nutrients in malnourished older individuals, and resistance training seems to effectively lower dietary protein needs by improving the efficiency of protein absorption [25,26]. Some studies have suggested that supplementation with essential amino acids can help offset the muscle wasting produced by prolonged bed rest [27], but no evidence exists that it is a useful way to maintain muscle mass in community-living elders. A study investigating nutritional supplementation and strength training in frail nursing home residents found that nutritional supplementation alone had no effect on muscle mass, and

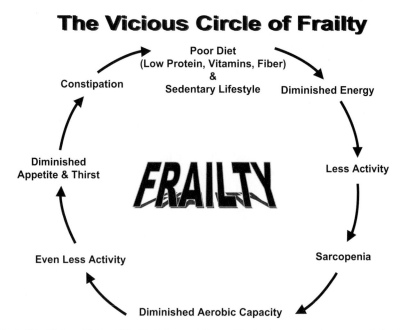

Fig. 1. The Vicious Circle of Frailty links poor diet and hydration, reduced energy and physical activity, and sarcopenia.

that the supplementation was related to diminished caloric intake in those who did not participate in resistance training. The resistance training had a significant positive effect on strength, gait speed, and overall physical activity [12]. Evans [25] stated that resistance training seems to have the greatest potential for stopping or reversing sarcopenia in malnourished older individuals. This article's authors would add that it should be combined with proper diet and aerobic exercise.

Clearly, educating older women, and the general population, about the importance of eating adequate amounts of fruits, vegetables, and protein is essential. Proper diet must be combined with enough exercise to stimulate appetite and elimination and maintain enough muscle mass to enable individuals to continue performing (at least) ADLs.

Obesity

An obese individual rarely comes to mind when thinking of a frail person, but in fact the two are not mutually exclusive, and are actually closely linked. By the time an obese woman reaches 80 years of age, she will almost certainly evince the symptoms listed by Speechley, Tinetti, Fried, and Bandeen-Roche [2,3] of sedentary lifestyle, weakness, exhaustion, low energy expenditure, slowness, difficulty with gait and balance, and lower extremity disability. Obesity as a factor is further elucidated in the following section on relative strength.

Relative strength

As Buchner and deLateur [28] pointed out, an intuitive understanding exists that strength and ability to function are closely interrelated. They were the first to understand that, in terms of function, the key is not absolute strength, but strength relative to height and weight. A woman may be able to leg press 100 lb, but if she weighs 300 lb, she will not be able to stand up. This relationship has recently been corroborated in a longitudinal study that found that *sarcopenic obesity*, or low muscle mass in relation to fat mass, predicted onset of IADL disability in community-dwelling elders who had no disability [29]. Those who did not develop subsequent disability had significantly higher activity levels than those who developed disabilities, whether obese or not.

Inflammatory markers

Indicators of frailty can be found among blood tests. Low Insulin-like growth factor-1 (IGF-1) levels have been shown to be associated with markers of frailty, especially inflammatory markers, such as interleukin 6 (IL-6) [30]. This finding might partially explain the effectiveness of low-dose aspirin in the prevention of heart attacks. That is, not only does the acetylsalicylic acid decrease the tendency of platelets to aggregate, it also has an anti-inflammatory effect. High levels of cytokines, particularly IL-6, are often observed in elderly people and can apparently accelerate sarcopenia, because IL-6 inhibits the production of IGF-1, an important anabolic stimulus for muscle growth [5].

The apparent interaction between elevated inflammatory markers and reductions in growth factor signals may be a root cause of progressive muscle wasting [31]. Cappola and colleagues [32] found that older women who had the lowest levels of IGF-1 and high levels of IL-6 showed the greatest decrements in walking performance and functional ability, and increased mortality.

Therapies directed toward inflammatory factors have been available for many years, but their efficacy in treating muscle wasting is either questionable or has not been tested [31]. Reducing the blood levels of IL-6 has not been shown to be as effective in preventing frailty as has, for example, lowering total and low-density lipoprotein cholesterol in preventing coronary artery disease. More likely, correcting frailty causes reduction in the levels of IL-6 and C-reactive protein.

Although a common assumption is that age is the underlying cause of increased inflammatory markers, evidence shows that it may be related to inactivity. McFarlin and colleagues [33] investigated the relationship among age, physical activity, and biomarkers of inflammation. The findings of that study supported previous reports, which inferred that acute exercise or a physically active lifestyle may possess anti-inflammatory properties.

Osteopenia and osteoporosis

One of the most obvious results of increased frailty is the higher incidence of fractures in older women. After menopause, bone turnover continues, but more bone is lost than is built. Because women frequently have small bones, as age increases this loss of bone density results in more porous, and therefore more fragile, bones. A fall that might result in a quickly forgotten bruise at 20 years of age may result in a fractured hip at 80 years of age. Although hip replacements have helped maintain mobility for some individuals who fracture hips, the femur must be dense enough to receive the implant, which can be a problem for older women, whose bones are often brittle and porous [34].

Discussion is ongoing about whether lipid-lowering drugs slow bone turnover, thereby improving bone mineral density. One large case-control study (498,417 cases) in Denmark suggests that among lipid-lowering drugs, statins, but not non-statins, protect bone density [35]. The Women's Health Initiative Observational Study (93,716 women) in the United States concluded that statin use did not improve fracture risk or bone density and that the cumulative evidence does not warrant use of statins to prevent or treat osteoporosis [36].

As in sarcopenia, some evidence shows that testosterone replacement therapy may slow or reverse bone loss in older women and men, but no large randomized controlled studies have adequately investigate the safety and efficacy of this treatment [14].

Aerobic capacity

Another aspect of aging and frailty is diminished aerobic capacity. It is common knowledge that maximal aerobic capacity declines with age, although the decline is much less debilitating if regular physical activity is part of the aging person's lifestyle. Although the possible peak workload diminishes with age, trained older athletes still perform better than most sedentary young individuals [37]. Older women's participation in vigorous aerobic activities is only now becoming socially acceptable, so the available data on women who have maintained a very active lifestyle are limited. Currently, studies referring to active lifestyles often consider women who report an hour of activity a week to be active. Even using that lenient criterion, active lifestyles are consistently linked to better function and overall health. Studies that measure actual aerobic fitness, such as the recent studies by Barlow and colleagues [38], Kara and colleagues [39], and Ades and colleagues [40], report an inverse relationship among aerobic fitness and hypertension, cognitive function, and overall function in women.

It is becoming much more common for older women to participate and even compete in aerobic activities such as rowing, running, tennis, cross-country and downhill skiing, swimming, water aerobics, and hiking. It will be interesting to see what will be discovered when there are more very active older women.

Absolute strength

Although seeking a concise definition of frailty and understanding its underlying causes are interesting and useful, identifying an indicator that can be quickly identified without multiple sophisticated tests is also helpful. A very simple indicator of frailty does seem to exist: absolute grip strength seems to be inversely proportional to disability. As part of the Women's Health and Aging Study, Rantanen and colleagues [41,42] found that absolute grip strength was a powerful predictor of cause-specific and total mortality. Presence of chronic diseases or the mechanisms underlying decline in muscle strength associated with chronic disease, such as poor nutritional status, disuse, and depression, all of which are independent predictors of mortality, did not explain the association. They concluded that handgrip strength may predict mortality through mechanisms other than those leading from disease to muscle impairment. In a study of 75- and 80-year-old community-dwelling individuals, Portegijs and colleagues [43] found that a high level of regular physical activity seemed to compensate for low muscle strength, resulting in lower mortality than would normally be predicted by the low muscle strength.

Balance

Another problem associated with frailty is loss of balance. As women age, many experience repeated falls, often resulting in hip fracture or other injury. Loss of balance can sometimes be attributed to conditions such as Parkinson's disease, vestibular disorders, vision problems, stroke, or side effects of drugs. Often no cause is obvious. Understandably, fear of falling increases as falls increase, usually resulting in diminished activity, even if no injury resulted from the fall [44,45]. Diminished activity leads to loss of muscle mass and bone density, which lead to more falls and more injuries. Fortunately, this downward spiral can be reversed with exercise [12,46,47].

Prevention of frailty

With the ever-increasing number of active and strong older women, the fact that frailty is not an inevitable part of aging is becoming apparent. This condition can at least be postponed, and at best prevented.

Each section that addresses aspects of frailty ends with the same refrain: exercise is the key to prevention of frailty. As other authors have shown (such as in the articles on bone health and those on prevention and management of compression fractures found elsewhere in this issue), building physiologic reserves during adolescence and young adulthood is important. Even more important, however, is developing and maintaining the habit of regular exercise to develop and maintain these physiologic reserves. This activity must be as integral to normal life as brushing the teeth.

Several important types of activity prevent frailty. One type is strength training, which wards off sarcopenia and helps maintain bone density and balance. Another type is aerobic exercise, which maintains cardiovascular health. Flexibility and balance exercises should also be included in an exercise program. The question, of course, is how, in this time of ever-diminishing need to be active, exercise can be integrated into daily life; how can sedentary patients be convinced to become more active.

The authors believe this question must first be answered at a personal level. Do physicians themselves participate in regular exercise to show that they understand its importance? And if not, can they expect patients to believe them if they do not demonstrate what they claim is so vital? Finding time in a busy day for some exercise is no less challenging for patients than for physicians.

The problem is rarely lack of general knowledge that exercise is beneficial; most people are already aware that exercise should be part of life, so physicians do not need to spend much time explaining this to patients. However, many people are not aware of the long-term effects of not exercising, nor are they aware that many of the effects are reversible. Many people think that they must join a gym or an organized exercise group to achieve the appropriate levels of physical activity. Although group support has been shown to help maintain exercise adherence [48], perceived lack of time and lack of value for exercise are major barriers to exercise [49]. Another significant barrier is the misconception that bed rest, or a lot of rest, is beneficial, when in fact it rapidly accelerates loss of muscle mass, strength, and cardiovascular decline [50].

Although some debate continues about how much information is retained after a physician visit, elderly adults who receive exercise advice from their physician have been shown to perform more moderate to heavy levels of exercise per week than those who did not [51]. Physicians must communicate the need and importance of daily exercise to all patients [52].

Explaining to patients how physicians themselves manage to fit exercise into their busy lives, to help patients understand how this can be done, can also be helpful. Box 1 provides some suggestions. The authors, who exercise regularly, have found that these guidelines work.

If patients are not exercising at all, suggesting incremental changes in behavior works best. Even considering a major lifestyle change might seem overwhelming to them. Rather than asking them to buy weights, tell them to go the pantry and get a couple cans of soup or bags of rice (something soft is preferable because it is easier to grasp and hurts less when dropped, but cans also work well) and put them on their favorite chair. This way, when the patients sit down to watch television, they can do 10 biceps curls; when a new show comes on, they can do 10 more. Voila! They have an exercise schedule! Because evidence shows that presenting patients with written material after giving exercise advice increases adherence [55], physicians should literally give them a list of things they can do with the "new toys." For example:

1. Place the cans or bag on each knee and raise them to shoulder level.
2. Take one in the left hand and touch it to the right hip, then touch the right one to the left hip.
3. Bend over and touch them to the floor several times.

Physicians should also add several blank lines to the list and provide patients with an assignment: they should add two new exercises that use the toys and must demonstrate them at the next visit. Successive approximations should be rewarded. If patients return with only one new exercise, they should still be praised and encouraged to think of another exercise for next time.

Some additional suggestions include doing a hula dance while brushing teeth, which will strengthen abdominal and leg muscles and is fun. When grocery shopping, they can walk half an aisle on the toes and the other half on the heels, and can do a few biceps curls with a milk jug. If they

Box 1. Suggestions for finding ways to fit exercise into your life

1. Think about why exercise is important to you. Do you want to maintain or regain mobility or strength, flexibility, or balance? Do you want to lose or keep off some fat? Do you want to improve or maintain aerobic capacity? Do you want to find new friends or enjoy the company of old ones? Whatever the reasons are, they are valid for you. Remember them and remind yourself of them often.

2. Set reasonable goals. Very few people have an hour a day to spend at the gym, and even fewer want to. Most people can find half an hour during the day, even if it is divided into two or three parts, when they can fit something in. It has been shown that multiple short bouts of brisk exercise reap almost the same benefits as one half-hour bout for previously sedentary individuals [53]. The most important part is doing it.

3. Keep the goals short-term. Commit to 1-week intervals rather than "the rest of my life." As Bandura [54] pointed out, *chunking*, or dividing tasks into manageable bits, makes getting the task done much easier.

4. Plan ahead and be specific. Opportunities for exercise rarely "just appear." "I'll try to get a walk in some time today" usually means that the day will be over and the walk will not have happened. Look for specific time in the day and literally put it in the schedule. Do the planning for exercise in 1-week chunks.

5. Do not think about it too much and do not allow yourself to question whether you really have time or whether you really feel like it. You have time because you already planned it, and you will certainly feel better after it is done.

have a sense of humor, physicians can suggest that the grocery aisles, or any long halls, are great places to practice "silly walks"; this is not only good exercise but is also fun, and if the activity is fun, patients are more likely to repeat the exercise.

Physicians should keep in mind that patients who do not exercise probably do not know how [56], and therefore simply telling them they should is not likely to produce a change in behavior. Physicians should discuss ways to get some movement into their lives and provide patients with written suggestions to take home, because all patients forget what doctors tell them to do, especially if it is something novel.

At no age does one no longer need to be active to maintain good health. The recommendations from the Centers for Disease Control and Prevention/American College of Sports Medicine [57–59] that every adult in the

United States should accumulate 30 minutes or more of moderate-intensity physical activity on most, preferably all, days of the week do not put an upper age limit on the guidelines. Throughout the lifespan, regular exercise is vital. No one wishes to one day discover that she has fallen and cannot get up.

References

[1] Buchner DM, Cress ME, Wagner EH, et al. The Seattle FICSIT/MoveIt study: the effect of exercise on gait and balance in older adults. J Am Geriatr Soc 1993;41:321–5.

[2] Speechley M, Tinetti M. Falls and injuries in frail and vigorous community elderly persons. J Am Geriatr Soc 1991;39:46–52.

[3] Bandeen-Roche K, Xue QL, Ferrucci L, et al. Phenotype of frailty: characterization in the women's health and aging studies. J Gerontol A Biol Sci Med Sci 2006;61:262–6.

[4] Rosenberg IH. Sarcopenia: origins and clinical relevance. J Nutr 1997;127:990S–1S.

[5] Roubenoff R, Hughes VA. Sarcopenia: current concepts. J Gerontol A Biol Sci Med Sci 2000;55:M716–24.

[6] Bortz WM 2nd. Disuse and aging. JAMA 1982;248:1203–8.

[7] Marzetti E, Leeuwenburgh C. Skeletal muscle apoptosis, sarcopenia and frailty at old age. Exp Gerontol 2006;41:1234–8.

[8] Hawkins SA, Wiswell RA, Marcell TJ. Exercise and the master athlete—a model of successful aging? J Gerontol A Biol Sci Med Sci 2003;58:1009–11.

[9] Creditor MC. Hazards of hospitalization of the elderly. Ann Intern Med 1993;118:219–23.

[10] Wilkins CH, Birge SJ. Prevention of osteoporotic fractures in the elderly. Am J Med 2005; 118:1190–5.

[11] Janssen I, Baumgartner RN, Ross R, et al. Skeletal muscle cutpoints associated with elevated physical disability risk in older men and women. Am J Epidemiol 2004;159:413–21.

[12] Fiatarone MA, O'Neill EF, Ryan ND, et al. Exercise training and nutritional supplementation for physical frailty in very elderly people. N Engl J Med 1994;330:1769–75.

[13] Liu H, Bravata DM, Olkin I, et al. Systematic review: the safety and efficacy of growth hormone in the healthy elderly. Ann Intern Med 2007;146:104–15.

[14] Padero MC, Bhasin S, Friedman TC. Androgen supplementation in older women: too much hype, not enough data. J Am Geriatr Soc 2002;50:1131–40.

[15] Borst SE. Interventions for sarcopenia and muscle weakness in older people. Age Ageing 2004;33:548–55.

[16] Morley JE. Decreased food intake with aging. J Gerontol A Biol Sci Med Sci 2001;56:Spec No 2:81–8.

[17] Hays NP, Roberts SB. The anorexia of aging in humans. Physiol Behav 2006;88:257–66.

[18] Federal interagency forum on aging related statistics. AgingStats.gov. Available at: http://www.agingstats.gov/. Accessed February 28, 2007.

[19] Bartali B, Frongillo EA, Bandinelli S, et al. Low nutrient intake is an essential component of frailty in older persons. J Gerontol A Biol Sci Med Sci 2006;61:589–93.

[20] Bartali B, Salvini S, Turrini A, et al. Age and disability affect dietary intake. J Nutr 2003;133: 2868–73.

[21] Semba RD, Bartali B, Zhou J, et al. Low serum micronutrient concentrations predict frailty among older women living in the community. J Gerontol A Biol Sci Med Sci 2006;61:594–9.

[22] Millen BE, Silliman RA, Cantey-Kiser J, et al. Nutritional risk in an urban homebound older population. The nutrition and healthy aging project. J Nutr Health Aging 2001;5: 269–77.

[23] Ledikwe JH, Smiciklas-Wright H, Mitchell DC, et al. Nutritional risk assessment and obesity in rural older adults: a sex difference. Am J Clin Nutr 2003;77:551–8.

[24] Campbell WW, Trappe TA, Wolfe RR, et al. The recommended dietary allowance for protein may not be adequate for older people to maintain skeletal muscle. J Gerontol A Biol Sci Med Sci 2001;56:M373–80.

[25] Evans WJ. Protein nutrition, exercise and aging. J Am Coll Nutr 2004;23:601S–9S.

[26] Bermon S, Hebuterne X, Peroux JL, et al. Correction of protein-energy malnutrition in older adults: effects of a short-term aerobic training program. Clin Nutr 1997;16:291–8.

[27] Paddon-Jones D. Interplay of stress and physical inactivity on muscle loss: nutritional countermeasures. J Nutr 2006;136:2123–6.

[28] Buchner DM, deLateur BJ. The importance of skeletal muscle strength to physical function in older adults. 1991;13:91–8.

[29] Baumgartner RN, Wayne SJ, Waters DL, et al. Sarcopenic obesity predicts instrumental activities of daily living disability in the elderly. Obes Res 2004;12:1995–2004.

[30] Cappola AR, Bandeen-Roche K, Wand GS, et al. Association of IGF-I levels with muscle strength and mobility in older women. J Clin Endocrinol Metab 2001;86:4139–46.

[31] Roth SM, Metter EJ, Ling S, et al. Inflammatory factors in age-related muscle wasting. Curr Opin Rheumatol 2006;18:625–30.

[32] Cappola AR, Xue QL, Ferrucci L, et al. Insulin-like growth factor I and interleukin-6 contribute synergistically to disability and mortality in older women. J Clin Endocrinol Metab 2003;88:2019–25.

[33] McFarlin BK, Flynn MG, Campbell WW, et al. Physical activity status, but not age, influences inflammatory biomarkers and toll-like receptor 4. J Gerontol A Biol Sci Med Sci 2006;61:388–93.

[34] Barrios C, Brostrom LA, Stark A, et al. Healing complications after internal fixation of trochanteric hip fractures: the prognostic value of osteoporosis. J Orthop Trauma 1993;7: 438–42.

[35] Rejnmark L, Vestergaard P, Mosekilde L. Statin but not non-statin lipid-lowering drugs decrease fracture risk: a nation-wide case-control study. Calcif Tissue Int 2006;79:27–36.

[36] LaCroix AZ, Cauley JA, Pettinger M, et al. Statin use, clinical fracture, and bone density in postmenopausal women: results from the women's health initiative observational study. Ann Intern Med 2003;139:97–104.

[37] Tanaka H, Seals DR. Invited review: dynamic exercise performance in masters athletes: insight into the effects of primary human aging on physiological functional capacity. J Appl Physiol 2003;95:2152–62.

[38] Barlow CE, LaMonte MJ, Fitzgerald SJ, et al. Cardiorespiratory fitness is an independent predictor of hypertension incidence among initially normotensive healthy women. Am J Epidemiol 2006;163:142–50.

[39] Kara B, Pinar L, Ugur F, et al. Correlations between aerobic capacity, pulmonary and cognitive functioning in the older women. Int J Sports Med 2005;26:220–4.

[40] Ades PA, Savage PD, Cress ME, et al. Resistance training on physical performance in disabled older female cardiac patients. Med Sci Sports Exerc 2003;35:1265–70.

[41] Rantanen T. Muscle strength, disability and mortality. Scand J Med Sci Sports 2003;13:3–8.

[42] Rantanen T, Volpato S, Ferrucci L, et al. Handgrip strength and cause-specific and total mortality in older disabled women: exploring the mechanism. J Am Geriatr Soc 2003;51: 636–41.

[43] Portegijs E, Rantanen T, Sipila S, et al. Physical activity compensates for increased mortality risk among older people with poor muscle strength. Scand J Med Sci Sports 2006 (OnlineEarly Articles). doi:10.1111/j.1600-0838.2006.00606.x.

[44] Fletcher PC, Hirdes JP. Restriction in activity associated with fear of falling among community-based seniors using home care services. Age Ageing 2004;33:273–9.

[45] Murphy SL, Dubin JA, Gill TM. The development of fear of falling among community-living older women: predisposing factors and subsequent fall events. J Gerontol A Biol Sci Med Sci 2003;58:M943–7.

[46] McMurdo ME, Rennie L. A controlled trial of exercise by residents of old people's homes. Age Ageing 1993;22:11–5.

[47] Madureira MM, Takayama L, Gallinaro AL, et al. Balance training program is highly effective in improving functional status and reducing the risk of falls in elderly women with osteoporosis: a randomized controlled trial. Osteoporos Int 2007;4:419–25.

[48] Estabrooks PA, Carron AV. Group cohesion in older adult exercisers: prediction and intervention effects. J Behav Med 1999;22:575–88.

[49] McAuley E, Jerome GJ, Elavsky S, et al. Predicting long-term maintenance of physical activity in older adults. Prev Med 2003;37:110–8.

[50] Convertino VA, Bloomfield SA, Greenleaf JE. An overview of the issues: physiological effects of bed rest and restricted physical activity. Med Sci Sports Exerc 1997;29:187–90.

[51] Balde J, Figueras DA, Hawking DA, et al. Physician advice to elderly about physical activity. Journal of Aging and Physical Activity 2003;11:90–7.

[52] Myers J. Physical activity: the missing prescription. Eur J Cardiovasc Prev Rehabil 2005;12: 85–6.

[53] Macfarlane DJ, Taylor LH, Cuddihy TF. Very short intermittent vs continuous bouts of activity in sedentary adults. Prev Med 2006;43:332–6.

[54] Bandura A. Self-Efficacy: the exercise of control. New York: W.H. Freeman; 1997.

[55] Kreuter MW, Chheda SG, Bull FC. How does physician advice influence patient behavior? Evidence for a priming effect. Arch Fam Med 2000;9:426–33.

[56] Schutzer KA, Graves BS. Barriers and motivations to exercise in older adults. Prev Med 2004;39:1056–61.

[57] American college of sports medicine position stand. The recommended quantity and quality of exercise for developing and maintaining cardiorespiratory and muscular fitness, and flexibility in healthy adults. Med Sci Sports Exerc 1998;30:975–91.

[58] American college of sports medicine position stand. Exercise and physical activity for older adults. Med Sci Sports Exerc 1998;30:992–1008.

[59] Pate RR, Pratt M, Blair SN, et al. Physical activity and public health. A recommendation from the Centers for Disease Control and Prevention and the American College of Sports Medicine. JAMA 1995;273:402–7.

ELSEVIER
SAUNDERS

Phys Med Rehabil Clin N Am
18 (2007) 623–629

PHYSICAL MEDICINE
AND REHABILITATION
CLINICS OF
NORTH AMERICA

Index

Note: Page numbers of article titles are in **boldface** type.

1047-9651/07/$ - see front matter © 2007 Elsevier Inc. All rights reserved.
doi:10.1016/S1047-9651(07)00072-1   *pmr.theclinics.com*